the new b[...]

east-west teachings

in the

beauty of body & soul

michelle dominique leigh

Illustrated by michelle dominique leigh

KODANSHA INTERNATIONAL
Tokyo • New York • Lodon

Distributed in the United States by Kodansha America, Inc., 114 Fifth
Avenue, New York, N.Y. 10011, and in the United Kingdom and conti-
nental Europe by Kodansha Europe Ltd., 95 Aldwych, London WC2B
4JF. Published by Kodansha International Ltd., 17-14 Otowa 1-chome,
Bunkyo-ku, Tokyo 112, and Kodansha America, Inc.

First edition, 1995.
95 96 97 10 9 8 7 6 5 4 3 2 1

ISBN 4-7700-1869-X

Library of Congress Cataloging-in-Publication Data

Leigh, Michelle D.
    The new beauty : east-west teachings in the beauty of body
and soul / by Michelle Dominique Leigh : illustrated by Michelle
Dominique Leigh.
        p.   cm.
    Includes bibliographical references
    ISBN 4-7700-1869-X
    1. Beauty, Personal. 2. Cosmetics—Japan. 3. Toilet
preparations—Japan.   4. Acupressure.   I. Title.
RA778.L533 1995
613—dc20
95-8161
 CIP

the new beauty

for my children
amber lundy and gabriel william
and for
my mother joy
my father jack and my stepmother song sun
and
for my grandmother dolly
with love

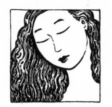

acknowledgments

I wish to thank Mr. Junichiro Suzuki, editor in chief of the *Japan Times*, for his interest in having me write the column "Beauty East & West" for his venerable newspaper. I wish to thank Ms. Yoshie Yamaguchi, the Arts & Entertainment editor at the *Japan Times*, for her ongoing support and understanding, and to extend as well a big thank you to the entire fleet of editors who have assisted in the publication of "Beauty East & West" during the nine years it has been running thus far. I wish to thank all those who have offered material or aided me in the gathering of it, most particularly Michiko Kohama and Megumi Abe, and I especially wish to thank the many faithful readers with whom I enjoy an active communication and whose input has been essential to this work. And for their help in the bringing to fruition of this book, I wish to thank William Miller, Elmer Luke, and especially Meagan Calogeras, my gracious editor at Kodansha, who is herself the embodiment of harmonious East-West beauty.

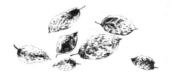

note to the reader:

This book is presented as a collection of natural remedies and as an aid in understanding the theories and practices underlying their use. The book does not represent an endorsement or guarantee as to the efficacy of any remedy or of its preparation. The remedies are not intended to replace or supersede medical consultation and treatment. Neither the author nor the publisher may be found liable for any adverse effects or consequences resulting from the use of any of the suggestions or preparations in this book.

table of contents

teachings east and west

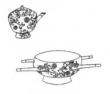

introduction

an invitation to beauty

With this book I invite you to discover whole beauty. I invite you to learn how to bring your own inner beauty to the surface and to take pleasure in the rituals that bring this about. In the discovery of whole beauty, we will draw upon both sides: East and West, the whole world. We will draw upon old and new. We will find in the ancient ways of tending body and soul those rites and plants that can have meaning for us now.

I have long been interested in women's beauty rituals and have examined these in diverse parts of the world: Africa, Asia, Europe, North America. When I began to explore the Japanese tradition, I was struck by several things:

—The orally transmitted wisdom has begun to die out. (My previous book *The Japanese way of Beauty* [in paperback, *Inner Peace, Outer Beauty*], published in 1993 by Carol Publishing under the Birch Lane Press imprint, is a documentation of that tradition in an attempt to preserve it.)

—Japanese beauty rituals draw on the rich Chinese medicine tradition yet have evolved in ways distinctly Japanese. Many of the techniques, such as *shiatsu*, render the Chinese traditional practices accessible, more adaptable to self-care.

—Zen Buddhism, an eminently practical spiritual tradition that continues to cross cultural boundaries and influence Western thought, has informed Japanese aesthetics with interesting applications to the human image. Mind/body unity and inside/outside beauty are natural elements in this influence.

—The Japanese feminine beauty tradition is imbued with the same purity and design sophistication found in that culture's art, architecture, cuisine, crafts traditions, and fashion. Just as the West has found abundant inspiration in these Japanese forms, the ways of beauty can also offer a rich resource, a truly comprehensive botanically based system that is both practical and elegant. In the Japanese culture the beauty of woman has been raised to a high art.

I attempt in this book to offer a practical blend of Eastern and Western traditions. As in "world music" and "nouvelle cuisine," the principles and practices offer endless room for experimentation. Along with the Japanese and Chinese ways, we draw upon the European and the American; there is a sprinkling too of Indian, Russian, Polynesian, and others. My hope is that readers will be inspired to create from this their personal forms of "world beauty."

One might also call this approach to beauty "Zen beauty," not only because it is in large part inspired by Asia and especially the Japanese tradition but also because it starts with the inner being. First in this approach to beauty is the peaceful spirit, the mind in balance, the imperturbable serenity that glows from within. This inner beauty is the only true beauty, and from it can blossom the outward forms. When we encounter in others beauty of this depth, we know it, don't we? When we begin to nurture it within ourselves, we understand the meaning of beauty as harmony, as truth.

The simplification of the rituals of beauty makes it possible to bring clarity to daily life. A reorientation must take place for the rituals to be understood, to be reduced to what is necessary and no more, but also to understand the rituals themselves as enactments of love for the body, enactments of women's traditional gestures. We must begin to understand the inside/outside nature of the being, the interrelatedness of what goes into the body, what surrounds the body, and the condition the body is in. We must learn to pay attention. We must learn respect.

The rituals: rather than adding to, we wish to take away. We do not want greater complexity, more to do, more to think about. We wish to purify, to simplify, to allow ourselves to exist outwardly as the embodiment of health, as the reflection of balanced self. We wish to create the conditions by which the body may function with ease and efficiency. To this end, and for the sake of our ancient bond with the earth and the plants that grow upon the earth, we seek the essential, natural ways to beauty. We plant seeds in the earth, we harvest the young leaves, we infuse them for tea, and we drink the tea and bathe in it for its ability to bring health and balance to the being. Whole beauty is not only the connection of body and soul but the connection of human being to earth.

Like the practice of everyday Zen, this approach to beauty is practical. The teachings of East and West presented here are those that have endured the centuries. The teachings are simple. They have been preserved for their efficacy and streamlined by time and use so that they now are very pure. Because of their simplicity and purity, these teachings seem to me very modern.

Beauty is a convergence of things. One might think it is no more than the external image. This is not enough. Why? Not only is the external image relatively unstable—we change from day to day: we grow older; we finally disappear entirely—but to approach beauty from the outside in is backwards. That is the way of make-up as disguise, last-resort wrinkle creams after 20 years of baking in the sun, liposuction instead of eating a healthy diet over the years, plastic surgery; it is the way of the desperate beauty-cultist, the woman who can't bear the thought of aging. The end result of this approach carried to its extreme can be a kind of assembly-line, artificial-doll appearance. At the center is often someone who is frightened and unhappy and frantically concerned with others' judgments. This viewpoint sees the fleeting surface beauty of youth as the only true beauty and seeks to recreate it when it is gone. (I am not saying that artifice has no place in whole beauty! But do not mistake it for the real thing....)

Another component of beauty, of what appears to be beauty, is indeed illusion. But it is illusion created by a palpable sense of self, of entitlement, confidence, an air of pride and *je ne sais quoi* that comes across in the carriage, the air, the presence. It is so powerful an effect that one need not possess the ideal physical features—in fact, this quality of presence is what gives the so-called *belle-laide* her unique allure. When a woman finds herself attractive, this thinking, this knowing makes her so! It is wise to learn this way of finding beauty's confirmation within and not without.

Then there is that more ephemeral aspect of beauty—all that is expressed through the body as vehicle, not the plastic arrangement of features and forms, but everything that is life and style, grace and charm: the voice, the manner of expression, the gestures, the posture, the way one relates to others and to the physical world. This is an art, the art of being, and to master it requires awareness.

All that supports physical health and well-being is fundamental to beauty: diet, exercise, cleanliness. Inner balance, peace of mind, and emotional health, as we've said, are there at the very heart of it. How one thinks about beauty, how one defines it, will be the key too to whether or not the aging process will be graceful.

The rituals of bathing, of applying lotions to the skin, of caring for complexion and hair—the rituals of attention and care for the body—are integral to a presence that speaks of self-love and self-respect. The artistry of make-up, grooming, adornment, and fashion, all these come last, and they are a wonderful way to play. As in theatre, these things can bring the image to life.

The core of this book is woven from a collection of newspaper columns taken from those I have written for the *Japan Times* over a period of about nine years. "Beauty East & West," as the continuing column is called, began as a forum for the presentation of the Asian beauty practices I was uncovering in my research on Japanese folk medicine, a project I undertook over a period of six years.

The column is written for a sophisticated urban readership made up of a truly international mix, Western and Eastern women and, as I gradually learned, a good number of men as well. With the immediacy of the communication offered by newspaper writing, and with the development of my column into an arena inviting the participation, comments, questions, and suggestions of readers, I gradually adapted the approach to the expressed needs and interests of my readers. While retaining the fundamentally natural, botanical orientation, I enlarged the field to include access to Western as well as Eastern ways of beauty. My readers have increasingly sought practical information that will broaden their horizons, that will reflect the even more global, East-West community of which many of us are now a part. This multicultural approach to beauty informs the book you are about to read.

how to use this book

The "rituals" section of the book is devoted to the process of stripping down, simplifying one's beauty routine. In this section, you will learn the principles and the priorities of beauty.

In working with the "botanicals" section, where you begin to concoct treatments using leaves, flowers, nuts, seeds, and oils, I advise you to play. There are many ways, for example, to achieve a smoother complexion, and the choice is often simply a matter of what appeals. Choose a particular botanical and experiment with it, then try another and compare the results. Have fun, and feel free to create your own variations of the recipes!

Throughout the book, you will find listings in the margins with the headings *inside* and *outside;* these tell you what internal and external recipes or techniques are found on each page of the text. In the "botanicals" section, these refer to techniques described for each botanical selection.

the

way

to

inner

beauty

True beauty is the outward embodiment of inner harmony and grace of spirit. The challenge lies in achieving this delicate state of balance in a high-stress world.

Traditional Asian medicine tells us that an excess of any of the seven emotions—joy, anger, anxiety, concentration, grief, fear, and fright—can be damaging to the body, causing illness or disease if not kept in check. If we allow the emotions to pass through us with lightness, the body is able to maintain the vital flow of *ki*, the essential energy of the being. It is not repression that is required, but a relaxed poise that prevents stress from settling into the body. By remaining neutral and softly detached, one maintains vitality, health, and beauty. The spirit orchestrates the harmony of heart, mind, and body. We feel good about ourselves on every level, and it shows.

exercises for inner beauty

The exercises presented here are simple. Approach them like games. They are designed to define and develop inner balance through precisely focused practice. I have tried here to approximate elements of what in Japan is called "polishing the heart," a spiritual task that is understood in that culture as the inner work of each individual. Without a polished heart there can be no harmony, no compassion, no faith, no generosity, no loving kindness, no peace, and certainly no beauty.

This approach to inside/outside beauty is a most practical one. By working with the body, with the mundane activities of life, and with everyday tools, we engage the spirit in right relationship to these outward things. We constantly test ourselves in this regard; we nourish the soul from the outside in. With true inner beauty achieved thus, the woman ages gracefully; the nobility of her inner nature is gradually revealed on her face. Without such inner loveliness, what we see with age is but the loss of the external beauty of youth. For aging is the true test of beauty: what has been easy, the surface prettiness of youth, must evolve into a visible inside beauty that has become richer over the years.

The exercises here have harmony as their goal: harmony within the self, harmony between the self and others, harmony between the self and the physical world. These exercises were inspired by my observations of daily life in Japan, by my experiences pursuing the Zen-imbued study of crafts in Japan, by certain Zen disciplines and training practices, and by the Japanese therapeutic system known as Morita. By playing these simple games, which are easily integrated into any lifestyle, it may be possible to enrich and deepen one's inner beauty, to polish one's heart, and to create the kind of loveliness that deepens with time.

the stretching cat

Lying in bed in the morning, flex the feet and stretch the arms far above the head. Lengthen the neck, tuck the chin, flatten the spine toward the mattress, and stretch. Stretch luxuriously, deeply, lengthening every muscle, and breathe. The cat, fully present in its body, is the best teacher in the art of awakened relaxation.

the essence of air

There are breathing techniques in many mind/body traditions. One can benefit from deep breathing without any complicated technique, however, as long as one follows two rules: breathe as deeply and fully as possible, taking air into the abdominal area and not just the upper chest, and control the exhalation and inhalation by breathing through the nostrils. One may further control the passage of air by slightly tightening the throat, which will create a very soft hissing sound there. For conscious breathing practice, recline or sit comfortably, eyes closed and body relaxed. Air fills the lowest part of the abdomen first, then gradually moves upward until the whole chest expands. The exhalation too proceeds from the lowest part of the abdomen. Breathing continues at an even, slow pace. Only a couple of minutes daily will improve the general condition. To breathe properly returns us to ourselves. Breathing, we are in constant relationship to the earth.

the moveable retreat

For a few hours or a whole day, don't speak. Don't utilize words in any way. Don't watch television, don't look at a newspaper or a book or a magazine, don't listen to a radio. Try not to notice clocks and watches. Communicate when necessary by writing notes.

The elimination of noise, stimulation, mass media chatter,

and countless distractions occurs naturally during a wilderness retreat, but it is also possible to re-create this sense of deep quiet within one's everyday life. Being quiet for sustained periods will nurture in you a quality of spiritual density, self-containment, and detachment. An amusing side-effect: your quiet air of poise and secret knowing will draw others to you like a magnet. And they will all want to talk.

thanking the tools

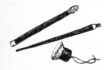

Choose some tools or utensils that frequently serve you in daily life. Spend 30 minutes or more cleaning, arranging, repairing, sorting, and caring for the tools. Offer focused attention to each object and renew it in whatever way is necessary. Silently thank each tool for its help and good work, and employ a careful loving touch as you clean and polish it. Appreciate the tools consciously.

For this exercise, one may attend to kitchen utensils; calligraphy brushes and inkstone; paintbrushes and palette; pottery tools; computer, typewriter, pencils and pens; carpentry tools; home or car repair tools; beauty-ritual tools like brushes, combs, cosmetics, and powder puffs. To invest the mundane objects of existence with love is to bring one's world to life, and to love oneself within it. To practice this ritual of thanking the tools will bring a new grace to your use of them, and a relationship of respect that will give greater success in the tasks the tools are used for.

looking for teachers

Set aside a few hours or a whole day for this exercise. Regarding every object, living thing, or situation as your teacher, try to discover what it is you are being taught. Learn it!

The most useful lessons are often presented in the form of challenges. The object that breaks or is misplaced, the individual who is irritating, the situation in which everything seems to go wrong. Fear, of course, is a supreme teacher. But one may also learn interesting lessons simply by observing the very nature of things: holding a lump of wet clay, one may find much there to be realized. Approach each moment as an opportunity for discovery.

baby steps

Choose a goal that you have always wanted to achieve. (Why not? Choose your secret dream!) Each day, devote 15 minutes to that goal. Set aside a regular time for attention to the goal and take even the tiniest silliest steps toward achieving it. Never spend less than 15 minutes on it, although you may decide to spend more. Don't set a date for completion, just work on it a little every day. Sometimes our dreams are so big that we are intimidated by them; as you weave a vision little by little into a reality, you will watch the dream become ever more accessible. When you are actively making it real, in however small a way, the dream will begin to gather an inner momentum in its passage from fantasy to reality.

freedom

Experiment with a very different identity. For one day, dress in a very different way than you usually do; break all your customs, rituals, and habits. Surprise yourself! If you always drink coffee in the morning, drink tea instead. If you always walk down a partic- ular street, take a different route. Change your look, your way of walking, the timbre of your voice. Invent a new you. Your old identity was no more the real you than is the new one.

purification

Set simple endurance tasks for yourself occasionally, small every- day disciplines. Eat small, austere meals. Rise before dawn. Take cold showers. Push yourself further in your exercise routine. If you are in good health, take brisk walks in cold weather or ice-cold plunges into mountain streams. Walk across town instead of tak- ing a bus; take the stairs instead of the elevator; temper yourself with small difficulties. Make some of these practices part of your lifestyle. In this way, the spirit becomes taut, toned, tuned into the essential.

focus

Choose a solitary activity that is part of your daily routine, some- thing you must do or something you do for pleasure. Washing the floor … throwing pots … weeding the garden … walking in the forest … soaking in the bath … exercising … some activity that you are so accustomed to doing that you hardly think about it. 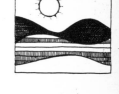 Give your full and focused attention to the activity for 30 minutes. Execute it as consciously as possible, observing each action and attempting to fill it with mindfulness, perfecting it, completing it. Don't hurry or think of other things; just do what you are doing fully in the here and now. Imagine that this is the last time you will do this thing. Rediscover the richness in doing something that you do well, something whose gestures seem to be a part of your being, and give it the freshness of attention that you applied to it the first time. Train your attention; teach yourself to give such focus, such presence, to everything.

the gift of tea

The tea ceremony is an exercise in full presence. To prepare tea with the highest degree of attention and consciousness as an

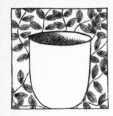

offering to another person is a way to approximate the experience. Using tea leaves instead of bags is important. Assemble leaves, teapot, and cup and set them out so that the arrangement is beautiful. The cup and teapot and leaves are chosen with the other person, as well as the season and the surroundings, in mind. Clean the preparation area and the implements and utensils carefully. Prepare the area where the tea will be enjoyed, perhaps with a flower arrangement and a special cloth. Make the tea in the presence of the person to whom you will offer it. With each gesture, pay deep attention to what you are doing. Offer admiration to the cup for its beauty, love to the teapot for its warm shape and its work, appreciation to the leaves for their fragrance. Remember the great tradition of tea, going back thousands of years. Slowly and quietly, when the tea is ready, offer it to your friend. Enjoy the ancient gesture of presentation of the tea. Drink tea together. Discover the fullness of the moment.

soft face

Look at your face in the mirror, not to see how beautiful or unbeautiful you are, but to locate signs of negative feelings, worries, anxieties, anger, fear. These will be areas of tightness or hardness, perhaps around the eyes, the mouth, or on the forehead. The jaw and the chin may hold such tensions as well. Relax and soften those places. Picture the soft, relaxed face of a baby. Put a happy, light, open feeling into your eyes; relax your lips without trying to smile. Nothing is forced. After learning to do this as you watch your face in the mirror, remind yourself to make a soft face at other times, too.

compassion practice

For a few hours or a whole day, don't judge, but sympathize. Regard objects, living things, people, and situations with compassion, understanding, and love. Try to think of the sadness that may underly an individual's rude behavior. Even if only internally, find a way to feel empathy toward a difficult person or situation.

It can sometimes be useful to apologize to a person who is angry at you, even if you feel they have an inaccurate perception of what is going on. This can be a very effective way to make the person feel better, bringing quick harmony, peace, and balance rather than prolonging the conflict by engaging in it. This is not giving in out of weakness; it is a way of intelligently controlling the situation. This practice requires distancing oneself a bit from the ego! Sometimes ego gets in the way, so it's good to learn how to work around it.

detachment practice

For a period of a few hours or a whole day, practice the path of least resistance. When an irritating incident takes place, observe your feelings, recognize them, but don't act in emotional response to them. Let the feelings flow through you. Let them go. Forget about them. Just accept the situation, saying, It is, and my feelings are, but I choose not to be moved by either. The state of mind is soft, imperturbable, and free.

Many irritating situations or people will not be positively influenced by our actions, though we may we feel compelled to react with expressions of outrage, indignation, or frustration. What often occurs is that the initial situation not only does not improve, but another layer of stress and conflict is added. In the cases where an action appears to offer a solution, that action should be carried out in a detached, ego-free way, merely in an attempt to soften or heal a situation. Humility may be required.

service practice

For a few hours or a whole day, practice being of service to others. Notice what might need doing and do it. Think of what might make a person happier or more comfortable, and offer it. Do helpful and kind things anonymously. Don't seek recognition. Go out of your way to help, expecting nothing in return. Practice kindness not only toward people but toward animals, insects, plants, and your home and surroundings.

serenity *shiatsu*

It can be useful to have at one's disposal a knowledge of certain pressure points—these spots, when pressed firmly with two fingertips, will help immeasurably in righting both short- and long-term imbalances. While *shiatsu* is an art requiring years of study for true mastery, everyone should know some pressure points for use in self-treatment.

For calming the mind and improving the quality of sleep, increasing general stamina, eliminating pimples, and remedying weight problems, a point called CHŪ-KAN may be pressed. CHŪ-KAN is 12 cm/4 1/2 inches up from the navel in a direct line. TAI-KEI is another good pressure point, located just behind the protruding ankle bone on the inner side of the leg. Pressing TAI-KEI is said to calm the mind, improve circulation, and muscle tone and increase vitality. It is also pressed to get rid of pimples, alleviate menstrual problems, tone the reproductive organs, and to make the legs more shapely. Finally, to relieve stress, firmly press the thumb-pad and middle fingerpad together. Both hands may be used.

foods for the spirit

In the pursuit of inner beauty, the diet should be examined for overstimulating foods that may contribute to mental or emotional disequilibrium. Substances that may be sources of nervousness or even anxiety in some are white sugar, chocolate, alcohol, coffee, and tea. Some food additives may have adverse chemical effects on the brain, while heavy metals like lead, mercury, cadmium, and copper pose problems to both mind and body. Food allergies to such substances as wheat, milk, and sugar may produce symptoms of nervousness or hyperactivity. In the Japanese diet soybean products, whole grains, shiitake mushrooms, burdock root, and other foods are considered to encourage calm and equilibrium. Avoid heavy, rich, spicy, sugary, and oily foods; instead eat small amounts of plain, simple food. Prepare dishes that harmonize, so that nourishment makes no huge demands upon the organism. A favorite medicinal tea for calming the mind and purifying the system is made from powdered pearls: 1 teaspoon of pearl powder is stirred into $1/2$ cup of hot green tea and sipped slowly.

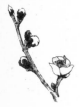

true beauty

To polish one's heart may be likened to the process of polishing a gemstone; one makes use of the grit, the roughness, the hard edges of existence to bring out an initially hidden beauty. In the lessons for inner beauty, one learns to keep a tranquil mind in the midst of the disturbances of life by training one's responses. This is freedom from reaction, or detachment. One develops the ability to direct attention outward in a spirit of compassion and service, and this in turn nourishes the true beauty that is found in those who think not only of themselves. Endurance training enables us to direct ourselves rather than be directed. In this training we also exercise the capacity to maintain inner peace in the face of difficulty. The training in focused attention nurtures a centered, calm consciousness, along with a deeper sense of relationship to the world in which we live. What is developed over time in the process of heart-polishing is a constantly increasing ease in achieving a state of harmony. Relaxation, renewal, and a refreshed body/mind become a way of life.

in the beginning, woman was the sun

The image of feminine beauty in Japan has ancient origins. The mysterious pale-skinned woman with the secret rosebud smile and the downcast eyes, wrapped in silks and moving with the quiet grace of a breeze fluttering through green bamboo—this woman may be traced far, far back to the time of early Shinto, to a time when shamans were women.

In the Japanese as in all cultures, the beautiful woman serves as a kind of sacred being, a reminder and representative of the good and of goddesses. While the outward forms and ideals of beauty vary from place to place, there is at the deepest level a universal unity. The woman's body contains the secret of life, and while this truth arouses a primitive fear and awe, it is ultimately regarded as the embodiment of a divine good. The beauty evokes by her presence both the fear and the worship of woman; in her physical form we are confronted with mystery. The beauty guards her secrets carefully; she veils her strength with softness and a flower's silence. She offers us this truth: in the silence of pure being, the spiritual mystery of beauty is most resonant.

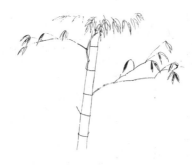

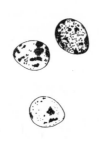

rituals

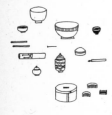

To simplify is good. To become conscious of what one does, and why, is good. In the area of beauty, we need to know what is essential and what is not, how to prevent undesirable conditions and how to treat them if they arise. The concrete things one does for beauty—the beauty rituals—are straightforward and direct and have to do with basic care and maintenance. There are other factors at work in beauty, but these ways of caring for the body should help to keep the skin, hair, and body in proper working order.

In this section of the book we'll take a fresh look at the core rites of beauty. Most of what is presented here has to do with encouraging the development of habits or practices that protect one's natural beauty or provide uncomplicated natural means for its illumination. These rituals are derived from the traditional wisdom of East and West; they are based on common-sense knowledge of physical existence and the way the skin and hair function in relation to both the organism as a whole and the environment. These simple ways instill a respect for the body, allowing an enduring beauty to blossom.

a note on *shiatsu*

The holistic approach to beauty and health, the inside/outside connection, is a basic premise of Asian herbal medicine. The ancient art of *shiatsu*, in which the pressure points, or *tsubo*, are manipulated or stimulated, plays an important role in the Japanese rites of beauty. *Shiatsu* is widely practiced by the layman in Japan, even if only in a rudimentary way. This simple, direct method for affecting the conditions of body and mind is integral to Japanese folk medicine and self-treatment of minor ailments. Most people know a few of the more important *tsubo*, and while for serious or chronic problems they will consult a specialist, in less dire circumstances or purely as part of an ongoing health-maintenance program they will press or massage these spots.

Tsubo are vital points on the surface of the body by which internal organs and areas of the body may be affected or their conditions diagnosed. Together with meridians, the pathways of vital energy flow or *ki* that connect groups of *tsubo* with specific areas of the body, they form the basis for the systems of acupuncture, *shiatsu* massage, reflexology, and moxabustion.

In self-treatment, *tsubo* manipulation is most simply accomplished by the application of finger pressure, though in Japan another common method involves the application of heat, with the aid of a hand-held hairdryer, a heating pad, or even a lit cigarette held close to the *tsubo*. Portable handwarmers are also employed for this purpose, wrapped in gauze and laid over a spot for a brief or extended period of time.

Sitting in front of a small heater will also supply heat stimulation to the *tsubo*, as will the application of a hot ginger, garlic, or mustard compress or a "heating" cream. Small "hot plasters" are sold in Japan for the sole purpose of heating the *tsubo*. The technique of moxabustion consists of burning a small cone of dried and powdered mugwort that has been placed directly on the skin over the *tsubo*; a piece of garlic or ginger may be inserted between the moxa and skin as an alternative method. Although nowadays it is possible to buy boxes of cones over the counter, those who wish to embark on an exploration of self-treatment by moxabustion should initially consult a specialist.

Also available in Japan for use in self-treatment through *tsubo* manipulation are specially designed tools of various kinds: a variety of brushes of different shapes and sizes, wooden sticks to effectively stimulate a *tsubo* anywhere on the body, even small wands with which a weak electric current may be applied to the pressure points. Magnet bands and plasters containing metal grains are other devices used on the *tsubo*.

Because the hands and feet are particularly abundant in *tsubo*, with correspondences to every body part and internal organ, there are devices designed specifically for the stimulation of these areas. One that is widely used for the feet is a length of split bamboo, upon which one may tread, bounce, and rock to relax and stimulate not only the soles of the feet but the entire body. For the hands an enormous range of small exercise-toys and *tsubo* stimulators are available: sets of steel balls to roll in the hand, rubber porcupine-shaped balls that press the vital points when squeezed, tiny rings connected by heavy rubber with which to strengthen the fingers isometrically, rings with protuberances for squeezing and rotating, tension-spring flexers—all arcane-looking gadgets that resemble nothing so much as futuristic teething toys. Two unhulled walnuts rolled simultaneously in the hand will achieve the same effect.

By diligently practicing the thorough daily facial massage either with an emollient or with bag, sponge, brush, or fingers in the process of cleansing; by doing the same for the scalp during washing or as a separate treatment; and by scrubbing the body with scrupulous enthusiasm at bathtime, one automatically stimulates the *tsubo*. By incorporating into one's daily routine a short stint on the split bamboo for the feet or a workout with a finger tool for the hands, one may benefit from *tsubo* stimulation without ever learning the precise points.

From here the beginner may wish to proceed further, but to confront an entire body of knowledge so intricate and complex is a daunting prospect. It is perfectly possible, however, to learn to locate some important *tsubo* and experiment with their manipulation as the need arises. Presented with each of the "simple beauty" chapters that follow are directions for locating and stimulating a few *tsubo*, specifically those that may benefit the face, the hair, body tone and vitality, and state of mind. The reader is reminded, in this as in all things, to exercise the ancient Asian principle of moderation—press the *tsubo* for the duration advised, and never to the point of severe pain. Further, those with serious health problems are advised to seek treatment from a specialist.

simple skin beauty

I propose that you rethink your face-care routine. Start over from scratch. If you are like most of us, whatever you are now doing for your skin is a combination of habit, negligence, and occasional bursts of zeal (with one outward result being a small fortune invested in high-tech creams). Let's think about this. Has the Western woman forgotten what the Asian woman has not? There are two simple things that should be the backbone of your skin-care ritual. What are they? Protection and purification.

Protection means first and foremost protection from the sun, and further it means protection from all the forms of internal or external aggression: bad diet, toxins, dry air, chemicals, stress. Purification means keeping your skin scrupulously clean through external cleansing and through a diet that emphasizes cleansing medicine foods and teas.

Ninety percent of your skin-care routine should consist of protection/purification. The rest—all the packs and creams and elixirs and lotions—are fun and can offer real benefits, but only when added to a sound fundamental skin program.

The modern woman works her skin to death. Give your skin a vacation! Less is more. Find just one or two products—do get the best you can afford rather than a lot of lower-quality ones—and follow a simplified routine. Keep your skin clean. Protect it from the sun, wind, and pollution. Watch your diet. Exercise regularly, and practice an antistress discipline. Unless you have really serious skin problems your energy is better spent elsewhere. And think loving thoughts! It's the best beauty treatment in the world.

In this section we'll go through the steps of the ideal skin-care routine. We'll talk about sun protection, and skin lightening, and damage control when the sun has already gotten to you. We'll see how to shield the skin from the cold dry air of winter. We'll look at skin that's very young and at skin that's aging, at the special needs of each. We'll have a play session with face packs, in which you will raid your refrigerator and cupboard for do-it-yourself beautifiers. And in all of this, we'll take it from the East-West angle, which offers a wider world of possibilities.

the simplest of face-care rituals

Let's get down to basics. Is the typical face-washing routine of cleanser-tonic-moisturizer really necessary? What is and what isn't important for the skin? Is there any simple, easy regime for the skin that will allow it to be healthy and to function at its best? Is there any connection between the growing incidence of sensitive skin and the overuse of commercial products on the skin?

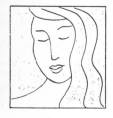

Faced with high-powered advertising featuring the retouched, impossibly creamy complexions of supermodels, the promise from every company to delay wrinkles and deliver to Everywoman that elusive state of ultimate beauty, the overstocked cosmetics counters and their predatory salesclerks, and then, *chez soi,* the dressing-table mirror that reveals actual—horrors!—pores, many women feel a sense of confusion.

These days, dermatologists are seeing sensitive skin on nearly everyone and calling it normal. It was not always thus. What this means, one conjectures, is that the combined effects of a modern diet, a polluted environment, stress, and the overuse of complicated chemical substances on the face have resulted in complexions that are in an aggravated condition.

My advice to anyone who is experiencing skin trouble of any kind, including skin sensitivity, is to start with the diet. Get rid of all the junk! Try living without refined carbohydrates, sugar, alcohol, and chemicals for a couple of weeks and see what happens. If you're really serious, cut down on pork, beef, and milk products (except, perhaps, for yogurt). Borrow from other cultures to find dishes based on healthy, natural foods. A traditional Japanese diet, for example, offers plenty of foods for skin beauty, with fish, soybeans, vegetables, and seaweed. Substitute brown rice for the usual white, of course. Shop organic to avoid pesticides.

Next, examine what is coming your way from the outside. Are you exposed to pollutants? Are you getting too much sun? What can you do to shield yourself? For the sun, the best protection in any season is a hat. In the winter, wrapping the face and neck in scarves will protect against the drying winds. If you're getting a blast of chlorine—damaging to skin and hair—every time you step under the shower, invest in a water-purifier. If you think there are other forms of pollution in your daily life, take any steps you can to rectify the situation. If you hail a taxi and it's full of cigarette smoke, tell the driver you want a smoke-free taxi: get out and hail another one.

Stress. It shows up on the skin, too. Solutions are individual, but increased exercise often works. And, of course, the improvement in circulation, metabolism, and skin and muscle tone will give you a better-functioning, better-looking complexion.

Now you've set the scene for your skin to start functioning properly. And function it does; the skin is not only a convenient protective cover for the rest of the organism but it also acts as an organ of elimination. This is where the idea of letting the skin "breathe" comes in. If you cover the face up with heavy creams and don't give it proper cleansing, it will react by behaving badly in the elimination department.

It is important to cleanse the skin thoroughly, and this may be done by whatever means seems to work! For some, it's soap. For others, an elegant French *lait demaquillant*. For some, an oil; for others, a gel. Only experimentation will tell you what's right for you. For the record, however, here's the old-fashioned, simple, natural Japanese method:

First apply camellia oil to the face with the fingers. Remove with a gauze pad or a patch of silk. Next, massage the face with a *nukabukuro*—a small cotton or silk drawstring bag containing pure rice bran—that has been soaked for a few minutes in warm water. Rinse, then pat dry with silk. Follow with an application of *hechimasui*, or loofah-vine water (diluted brown rice vinegar or soybean vinegar could be used instead). This last step both lightly moisturizes and protects against the elements.

outside

camellia oil demaquillant

rice bran face wash

loofah-vine facial water

vinegar facial water

One can't discuss skin care without a mention of make-up. Again, less is more. The important thing is to look as good as possible using as little as possible. Consider using oil-free products and those that contain few additives. Hypersensitive skins may react well to a make-up-free period every now and then.

in the sun

If you observe only one skin-beauty rule, let it be "protect your skin from the sun."

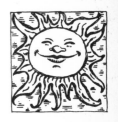

Even in these enlightened times of 48-SPF sunscreens, total blocks, skin cancer alarms, and premature-aging propaganda, people are baking on beaches everywhere, toasting to brown under ozone-depleted skies. And even those of us who want the beach without the tan will occasionally find ourselves burned. For the glory of a day at the ocean is that we meld with nature; we give ourselves up to sun, sand, and sea, discarding all routines and responsibilities. Under such conditions, what an effort to remember the sunscreen every two hours, what an intrusion into the sweet floating-away of it all.

So here, some sage advice for sun-worshippers.

To fortify your body and skin, take vitamins A and C. Both are depleted by exposure to the sun. Zinc may also protect against sunburn when taken internally.

Do remember your sunscreen; apply it before you go into the sun and reapply obsessively. Start with high-SPF sunscreen and

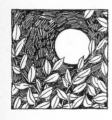

work to a lower number gradually if you want a bit of color. A special sunscreen for the lips is an excellent idea.

Use an umbrella or wear a hat. Sit under a palm tree. The sun will still reach you, but less brutally.

Wear the best sunglasses you can find. Poor-quality glasses will allow the harmful high-intensity rays to enter, and the eyes could be damaged.

Build up resistance by spending a short time in the sun the first few days, then gradually increasing sun sessions. This way you will avoid painful, harmful burns on vulnerable skin.

Drink a lot of water!

Carefully protect your hair from the sun. My hair stylist has always recommended applying any sunscreen used on the body to the hair as well. There are also specific sunscreen products for the hair. Sunlight and salt can combine to give you a head of lifeless straw.

A good beauty treatment for the hair is to apply a nourishing oil (camellia, olive, sesame or, coconut) mixed with a sunscreen and leave it on while you are in the sun. You will have to shampoo several times to remove the oil, but results are worth it. Your hair will be luxurious—shiny and strengthened.

Walking in sand will give you beautiful legs and feet. Muscles are used that usually aren't; calluses and rough skin soften and disappear.

Run, play, swim: your body will exult as it grows stronger and more agile. Appreciate the sea; the salty, mineral-rich water will beautify and tone the skin, rev up the circulation, nourish the soul.

To heal a burn, use tea bags, rice bran, or peach leaves in the bath. Rub fresh aloe or cucumber juice on the skin.

When your tan is fading and you want to be rid of it, take a sulphur bath. The results are astonishingly quick! A lemon-juice-and-yogurt face or body pack will serve the same purpose.

Has the sun already gotten to your skin? From "Delightes for Ladies," written by Sir Hugh Plath in London, 1602, the following remedy:

> To take Away the Freckles in the Face Wash your face, in the wane of the Moone with a sponge, morning and evening, with the distilled water of Elderleaves, letting the same dry into your skin. Your water must be distilled in May. This from a Traveller, who hath cured himself thereby.

CUCUMBER JUICE TONIC: Cleansing, healing, cooling, smoothing, lightening, wrinkle softening, freckle bleaching. Grate a cucumber and squeeze through cheesecloth to extract juice. Apply daily to a clean face and pat dry.

outside

oil treatment for hair

tea bath for sunburn

rice bran bath for sunburn

peach-leaf bath for sunburn

aloe skin-soother

cucumber skin-soother

lemon & yogurt pack for skin lightening

sulphur bath for skin lightening

cucumber skin-lightener

The traditional Japanese methods for skin lightening include the following:

LOOFAH-VINE WATER (*hechimasui*): Cooling, soothing, smoothing, moisture balancing, and lightening, this lovely "water" will also erase wrinkles and freckles. Use pure *hechimasui* (store in the refrigerator) and apply as a tonic after washing; do not rinse. Daily use recommended.

AZUKI BEAN POWDER (*azuki no kona*): A face wash that tightens, smoothes, exfoliates, cleanses, and whitens the complexion. See under "bean" in the botanicals section for the bean powder recipe. Add to the powder a few drops of warm water to make a creamy paste; use instead of soap and massage softly into the skin before rinsing.

BUSH WARBLER OR NIGHTINGALE DROPPINGS (*uguisu no fun*): A most venerable beauty tradition, this face wash smoothes and lightens the skin, giving it a pale glow. In Japan, buy *uguisu no fun* as a commercially prepared powder. Soap your hands with a mild face soap, then add some *uguisu no fun* powder and enough water to make a paste. Massage into the skin and rinse well. This one should not be used daily—once a week is about right.

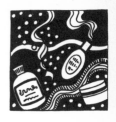

outside

loofah-vine skin-lightener

azuki *bean powder skin-lightener*

bush warbler droppings skin-lightener

Fact: In 1991, the United Nations Environment Program projected a sustained 100 percent decrease in ozone, linking this to an annual increase of more than 300,000 cases of non-melanoma skin cancers worldwide.

Fact: In areas of susceptible fair-skinned population, like Australia, the United States, and Scandinavia, skin cancer figures have doubled during the past 10 years.

Fact: Not only is more UVB sunlight reaching us due to the reduction in ozone, but sunscreens designed to guard against UVB in some cases do not provide adequate protection against UVA, until recently thought to be harmless but now recognized as a catalyst in skin damage.

The traditional Japanese insistence upon maximal sun protection and white skin has meant that the Japanese cosmetics companies were paying serious attention to the sun problem long before the rest of the world caught on. Many companies have allocated substantial portions of their research budgets to the development of products that afford protection from the sun.

There is a significant difference between Japanese and standard Western approaches to the problem of sun. For many European and American companies, the underlying paradigm has been "women want a safer tan"—thus the dizzying proliferation of complex sun systems.

One starts with SPF 2000 and moves slowly but surely toward the SPF 2 or 4 level, the idea being that in this way the skin's natural sun-defense, melanin, gently turns the skin a safe, biscuity brown. Of course there are exceptions—products that aim for total protection rather than the "safe" slow bake do exist. But take a stroll upon any Mediterranean beach in August—the pearly pale complexion is not present. Why are Western women still tanning?

One of the dangers of the tan is that it appears to benefit the skin: by acquiring a golden glow, skin problems, a pasty, dull complexion, wrinkles, lines, and even sun damage all may seem suddenly erased. It is only a temporary illusion, but it is certainly one of the reasons that those who know better continue on the suntan course. The cultural switch to "pale is beautiful" has yet to be made, though there are signs that the tide is turning.

In Japan, of course, there has never been any widespread attempt to satisfy a tanning urge. Thus the Japanese sun-protection products are designed to shield the skin as thoroughly as possible with no thought of a compromise.

To guard the skin from the sun is the number one rule in skin beauty. Need convincing? Compare the complexion of an eighty-year-old woman who has avoided the sun religiously with that of her sixty-year-old daughter raised on a lifestyle of sun worship. The sixty-year-old's skin almost certainly looks older.

in the cold

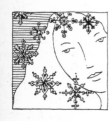

When winter is upon us, with its cold air (drying) and winds (drying) and artificial heat (drying) and lack of sunshine (depressing) and short, dark days spent indoors under—too frequently—fluorescent lights, we must take measures!

Use a humidifier to moisten indoor air; wear moisturizer on the skin; wrap up well to shield skin and hair from chilly breezes. Get exercise to bring a healthy glow to your complexion, speed up your metabolism, and increase your resistance to colds and the cold. Drink lots of mineral water.

outside

rice bran moisturizing bath

camellia oil moisturizer for skin & hair

The bath, or Japanese *ofuro*, is wonderful for warming up in wintertime, but the hot water is also very drying. Try a Japanese-style *nuka* bath: Wrap a few handfuls of pure, fresh *nuka* (rice bran) in a large square of cheesecloth; add this to the bath. The *nuka* bath will not only cleanse your skin and give it a silky texture but will impart the natural, vitamin-rich oils of whole rice. A great beauty treatment to be repeated often! Use a small *nukabukuro* bag instead of soap to further guard against dryness.

Camellia oil is a lovely all-purpose moisturizer. The oil, which is light and odorless, may be used on skin, hair, and nails in small amounts to reduce dryness. Apply the oil to lips to prevent chapping; add a few drops to a basin of warm water for soaking chapped hands.

Fluorescent lights are really dreadful for both health and beauty. The lower cost does not make up for the drawbacks. If you must be exposed to fluorescent lights, be aware that studies have shown that prolonged exposure causes adverse effects in some people (problems with eyesight, headaches, lowered resistance to illness). Not to mention the bleached-out look these lights give your complexion!

To combat winter pallor and bleak lighting you can liven up your complexion with a tea tan! An old European remedy for giving a sunny glow to the skin is to bathe in tea—not Japanese green but basic English black. An easier and less costly method is to rub a freshly soaked and drained tea bag over your face after washing. If you do this daily, eventually you will acquire a subtle tan. An alternative approach is to eat lots of orange things like carrots and tangerines.

outside

tea bath for skin darkening

And of course, since winter is dark and dim, dress yourself up in bright shining colors. Create your own light!

skin that's young

There is an old Japanese saying that goes, "A lovely complexion will conceal seven flaws." The look of the skin has a profound impact upon not only others' impressions of us but also upon our self-image. It seems unfair that just when children are going through the awkward and unsettling process of becoming adults—that stage when the appearance can constitute one of life's major dramas—skin trouble arrives on the scene.

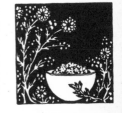

The first thing to do when a pimple appears is to say to the child: "Don't panic. This is normal. It will pass." It is important to take a calm and unflustered approach, since any anxiety will be picked up by the child. Undue concern about his or her attractiveness and worry about the skin often leads to an unconscious habit of picking.

Now this situation clearly is moving in the wrong direction. Picking at the skin is going to worsen it. And then there will be more picking, and more shame, and more worrying. Finally there will be an ongoing skin problem and an ongoing state of panic. Worst of all, the child will feel ugly. (And this unfortunate self-image can be one that will endure for years, long after puberty has ended.)

In adolescence the skin often enters a state of imbalance, visible in the form of bumps and oiliness. The skin's appearance is the reflection of many factors: diet, sleep habits, mental and emotional states, general physical health, hormone activity, climate, pollution, cleansing habits, and so forth. Breakouts are a relatively normal phenomenon and should not be cause for undue alarm. However, it is important to attend to any controllable factors in order to ameliorate the skin condition and to prevent it from worsening.

The daily routine should include plenty of sleep, preferably not in a stuffy environment, and lots of exercise and fresh air. A sedentary existence indoors will result in sluggish circulation and an unhealthy, dull-looking complexion. The young person should have some kind of active exercise or sports program; this will help not only in improving all body functions and circulation but in reducing stress.

Stress can be further alleviated through establishing a harmonious and open family relationship (talk about problems and worries) and setting aside sacred time reserved for pure play. School pressures can be intense for many young people, and play that is not goal-oriented is often devalued, so that there is no time or energy for fun.

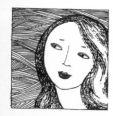

Follow these general guidelines, and overall health should improve, the complexion along with it.

The mother of a child entering puberty should by this time have already taught the child the simple rules of skin care. A basic cleansing routine should be established. Washing should be carried out with a high-quality cleanser rather than the standard bar of soap. The use of a washcloth or other fabric is good, provided it is laundered after each use. When the child begins to show signs of spots, an antiseptic or astringent facial tonic may be applied after the face is washed.

Three fundamental truths should be taught: first, the food one eats will show up on the skin; second, one need *never* touch the skin except to wash it; and third, the oily, easily blemished adolescent skin condition is normal, and it will pass.

Regarding diet, many dermatologists and nutritionists generally believe that an imbalanced diet—especially one high in sweets and processed foods—can have an adverse effect on the skin. The adolescent who is experiencing hormonally caused skin changes will not help matters by surviving on junk food. The child should eat the healthiest diet possible—with lots of whole grains, fruits, vegetables, and protein sources that are low in saturated fat—and drink plenty of pure water. If the basic diet is excellent, occasional indulgence in "bad foods" won't do as much damage as it might. The vitamins A, B, C, and E are particularly important for the skin. Cleansing foods and teas should be taken regularly.

inside

pearl barley for skin clearing

As a supplement to a balanced diet, an internal treatment for any kind of skin trouble is *hatomugi* (pearl barley), taken in tablet form as *hatomugi ekisu* (pearl barley extract), as a tea, or as a cooked grain dish. Ingested daily over a long period, this traditional Asian remedy should clear up the skin. Western dietary supplements include brewer's yeast, wheat germ, vitamin C, vitamin A, and zinc.

When administering any diet supplement to a young child, first check with your doctor regarding appropriate dosages. When supplements are taken in their food form—cooked pearl barley, wheat germ flakes—there is less danger of overdosage, so this would be the advisable method.

Many products on the market are designed to reduce oil, kill germs, or exfoliate the skin (which helps to unblock pores and release sebum). The problem is that often such products are overused, which leads to a very irritated skin condition, manifested by excessive drying, flaking, and blotchy redness. Use something gentle, and don't overdo it.

As long as a child has only mild skin problems, it may be best just to wait for them to go away. If there are persistent blackheads or comedos, go to a dermatologist for treatment. Don't treat the problem yourself. A monthly salon facial with steaming and deep cleansing can help maintain a good skin condition.

For the routine cleansing of sensitive or troubled skin, I cannot recommend anything more highly than the traditional Japanese *nukabukuro* (rice bran bag). The rice-bran-bag wash will calm and cleanse, effectively restoring skin health without abrasion or the removal of natural oils.

The Western alternative is the oatmeal scrub. Fine-ground oats may be wrapped in cheesecloth or a *nuka* bag, or applied as is with a little water. No soap is needed in either case. Change the cloth or bag daily to avoid the proliferation of bacteria.

An occasional at-home face pack can be effective, and most kids love them. The oatmeal-honey pack and the rice bran pack with grated *daikon* and tofu are both known for their antipimple benefits. First cleanse and steam the face, then apply the pack and leave on for 20 minutes before rinsing.

More treatments to try:

THE JAPANESE BLACK SUGAR RINSE: Dilute *kurozato* (the darkest, least-refined form of sugar) in warm water and splash on the face as a final rinse.

THE EUROPEAN HONEY PACK: Apply honey to a well-cleansed face. Let sit until it becomes sticky and "tacky," then tap face all over with fingers for a pleasant boost to the circulation. Rinse with cool water.

THE TOFU PACK: Mix tofu with a little rice bran or ground oats, honey optional. Apply to a well-cleansed face and let it remain for 15 minutes before rinsing.

All external treatments outlined here may be used safely by even the smallest children.

outside

rice-bran-bag wash for troubled skin

oatmeal scrub for troubled skin

oatmeal & honey pack for troubled skin

daikon & tofu & rice bran pack for troubled skin

black sugar rinse for troubled skin

honey pack for troubled skin

tofu pack for troubled skin

skin that's aging

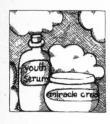

There are now many wonderful creams, emulsions, gels, and serums that can do more than was ever possible before to improve the look of aging skin.

But still, modern science, as sophisticated as it is, cannot perform miracles. Understand the various factors that contribute to the visible signs of aging, know the process involved, and you will learn that there must be limits to your expectations But there is also much that *you* can do to help improve your appearance as you age.

Everyone's skin ages, but the process takes place at different rates and with varying manifestations from individual to individual. Factors involved include biological age, genetic inheritance, internal physical condition (the result of nutrition and exercise), level of stress, external care (or neglect) of the body, and environmental realities (sun exposure, pollution). While there is little you can do about the first two factors, it is possible to influence the rest to one degree or another. Proper attention or the lack of it to these areas will help determine how fast and how gracefully your skin ages.

Whatever the factors, skin aging follows a definite pattern. It is usually in the 30s that the first visible signs of aging are seen: fine wrinkles and expression lines. As the process continues in the 40s and 50s and beyond, there may be dryness, loss of tone, uneven pigmentation, and sagging areas. Between the ages of 35 and 80, the rate of cell division and replacement decreases by half. With diminished cell activity, cells on the surface of the skin—the old dead ones that give your complexion a dull appearance—stay there longer. Cell metabolism slows down; cells receive less nourishment and eliminate wastes less efficiently.

On the level of the dermis, elastin molecules lose their elasticity, and collagen and elastin fibers fuse into an inflexible substance termed elastone. The epidermis thins. With the decrease in estrogen at menopause, the skin is likely to suffer from increasing dryness, which contributes to dullness and roughness and the accentuation of wrinkles and lines.

Most modern aging-skin treatments attempt to "revive" cellular activity, supply potent nutrients, and moisturize, basically encouraging aging skin to behave as if it were younger. Before examining the various external treatment options, what changes can you make in your lifestyle to safeguard your beauty as you age?

Relative to biological age, some menopausal women undertake hormone replacement therapy, which is said to drastically improve skin tone and suppleness. Those who wish to consider this therapy must discuss it with a doctor. The estrogen-rich soybean, so prevalent in the Japanese diet, has attracted scientific attention for its potentially beneficial role in menopause.

Regarding the body's internal condition, of fundamental importance is a nutritious diet high in vitamins A, B, C, D, and E (that's easy to remember!). Because the skin of smokers wrinkles up to 20 years sooner than that of nonsmokers, the habit of smoking must be given up. Alcohol, too, when it is consumed without moderation, can contribute to more rapid aging by depleting the body of vitamins B and C, causing cellular damage, and by harming metabolism and blood circulation—both functions fundamental to beauty. (Wine, on the other hand, is viewed as life-prolonging when taken in moderation. Recent French studies indicate that wine, when accompanying high-fat, high-protein foods, actually helps to clear the bloodstream of some cholesterol and aids in the digestion of the meal. *Sake* in small amounts is used in a similar way as a purifying tonic by the Japanese.)

Scientific studies have shown that exercise, performed regularly, helps the skin retain a youthful appearance longer. Exercise of the whole body, especially of the cardiovascular variety, brings visible benefits within a very short period of time. Facial exercises and facial massages can improve circulation and tone in specific areas of the face.

Because sun exposure does enormous damage to the skin, with results being cumulative and largely irreversible, as said earlier it is wise to forgo tanning completely. Adopt the regular use of a high-SPF sunscreen, or take a lesson from Japanese women and use a parasol under the summer sun.

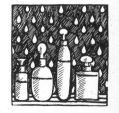

Retin-A, the vitamin A derivative that has been found to greatly ameliorate sun-caused wrinkles and skin damage, has various side-effects and is available by prescription for use under a doctor's supervision. The jury is still out on the long-term effects of alpha hydroxy acid and the acid peels that remove the outer layers of skin cells, often leaving the skin looking smoother and younger. New versions of these substances and others are emerging rapidly, as scientists work to find solutions to visible aging.

Pollution of air, food, and water is difficult to avoid—but it is possible to make an effort to lessen exposure. Eat organically grown natural foods, avoid processed foods with additives, and drink pure water, whether bottled or filtered. Supplements that encourage the elimination of toxins may be useful— the Japanese *chlorella* supplement has been shown to be particularly effective in this regard. Vitamin C is also very useful.

Finally, learn to control the amount of stress you undergo through exercise and conscious relaxation. Your face (and the rest of you) will benefit.

Now let's have a look at the range of external skin-care options—all those expensive, sophisticated, high-tech creams and serums that tantalize the customer with promises of a more youthful beauty.

Women face a familiar dilemma in shopping for such products; there is a huge choice available, and each product on the market vaunts its own unique, state-of-the-art, scientifically revolutionary, active deep-penetrating ingredient. And how many of us understand the vocabulary?

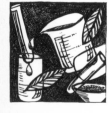

We know vaguely that free radicals are evil (but what do they look like?) and certainly we know to despise cross-linking, loss of collagen, and UV rays of all kinds, but what do we fight back with? What is a liposome? We know alpha hydroxy acid must be wonderful, because every cream ad around seems to tout its benefits ... and what about microspheres, sphingolipids, mucopolysaccharides, myopeptides, dynamized fibroblasts? It seems the only way to make an informed choice is by first going for an advanced degree in chemistry.

These products are never cheap; free samples are hard to come by. Word of mouth doesn't help; every woman's skin is different, reacting differently to the same product. How does one determine which product to invest in? A good basic rule: be faithful to the brands whose other products have worked well for you. Also, choose a product that is right for your skin type, age, and particular preferences and needs. Sample the testers at cosmetics counters—by seeing how a product sits on your skin, you can learn about its texture, penetrability, and other characteristics.

There are three basic categories of daily-use anti-aging skincare products: A) rejuvenating creams or emulsions, B) rejuvenating gels or fluids, and C) "active" moisturizers.

The first category includes oil-containing products that may be used morning and night for hydrating and smoothing the skin—at the same time they supply nourishment and stimulate cell activity. Some of these products incorporate sunscreens and skin-lighteners (to improve the appearance of liver spots or uneven pigmentation).

These products contain very high-powered active ingredients and can improve the appearance of the skin with regular use, but they may be too rich for oily skins.

The gels and fluids are lighter in texture and are non-oily. They generally offer the same benefits as the creams but without the rich moisture. Instead, these products tighten the skin somewhat, toning and firming the complexion. The gels and fluids may be used alone or under a simple moisturizer, morning and night.

Hydrating lotions and creams range from simple moisturizers to more complex "active" treatments. In any case, the goal is to help skin retain its own moisture while offering a good external supply as well. The texture of the skin is visibly improved: smoothed, softened, and brightened.

Also available to combat aging are the "cure" products designed to be used during limited periods, usually several weeks. These are good for fast results when one's skin is in desperate need of a lift.

Other products in the anti-aging panoply: eye-area treatments, exfoliators, moisturizing or regenerating facial packs, nourishing massage creams. All can be useful supplements to your basic anti-aging regimen, but must be chosen with your individual needs in mind.

The Japanese take a long-term holistic approach to the pursuit of beauty and health. It is perhaps most visible in the area of aging. Everything that is done to prevent undue signs of aging begins when one is young. State of mind, diet, and discipline in the external practices of beauty combine to bring grace to the process.

An important defense against wrinkles is the traditional Japanese facial massage. When performed properly, massage (always done with an emollient) will stimulate circulation, relax lines and tension, and encourage a softer, glowing, relaxed look. See "the *shiatsu* facial" at the end of this chapter.

outside

face massage for aging skin

As for diet, many Japanese foods are like medicine for the skin: fish, seaweed, *nattō, miso, daikon, shiitake, hatomugi,* tofu, ginger, black soybeans … the list is long.

Green tea is of particular interest for its ability to encourage a strong and balanced organism; in this respect green tea can be considered useful as a beauty tonic. When the body is functioning optimally, without the impediment of toxin buildup caused by an improper diet, stress, or any number of other factors, the skin is likely to be beautifully alive-looking.

inside

green tea tonic

Green tea purifies the system and helps combat health-destructive influences. By stimulating body functions as well as acting as a calming agent, green tea can be useful in helping the skin to maintain vibrant freshness.

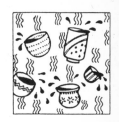

It is not wrinkles so much as the tone of the skin that is the determining factor in older skin beauty: we have all seen exquisite, radiant women in their 80s with plenty of wrinkles. What makes them beautiful is the healthy tone of their complexion—there is no dullness or grayness caused by poor circulation. This is truly beauty generated from inner health, a state well worth aspiring to.

playing with packs

First, a definition. The pack is basically a substance applied to a freshly cleansed (better yet, steamed) face and left on the skin for a length of time, anywhere from 5 to 30 minutes, then carefully rinsed off.

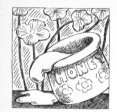

Depending on the ingredients, a pack will stimulate circulation, refine texture, deep-cleanse, soothe and calm, heal, exfoliate, tighten and tone, soften lines temporarily, hydrate, or lighten the skin. Almost any pack will bring an immediate glow to the skin along with a temporary improvement in texture.

Packs or masks exist as several basic types: clay-based, which are cleansing and often drying and thus best for oily or blemished skins: peel-off packs, which usually stimulate, soften, and exfoliate; nondrying packs, which are usually designed to moisturize and enrich; and packs that contain exfoliating substances or small particles, designed to be massaged gently over the skin to remove dead skin cells.

While the face pack is not a Japanese tradition, many of the traditional beauty-care ingredients make wonderful packs.

Any of the following may be used in a pack: bush warbler (also known as nightingale droppings), rice bran, *azuki* bean powder, camellia oil, soybean flour, rice flour, buckwheat flour, black sugar, grated *daikon*, tofu, *okara, sake*, seaweed, ground white or black sesame, and *yuzu* juice.

To experiment, choose a binding ingredient (one of the flours or powders) and add to it a treatment ingredient based on the following properties:

Nightingale droppings—exfoliating, lightening, softening; not recommended for sensitive skin

Rice bran—nourishing, cleansing, healing, moisturizing

Azuki bean powder—cleansing, lightening, refining

Camellia oil—moisturizing, softening

Soybean, rice, or buckwheat flour—soothing, nourishing, calming

Black sugar—healing, nourishing, stimulating

Grated *daikon*—purifying, beneficial to acne

Tofu—nourishing, soothing

Okara—nourishing, moisturizing

Sake—exfoliating, smoothing

Seaweed—revitalizing, nourishing, toning, refreshing

Sesame—nourishing, moisturizing, healing

Yuzu—purifying, lightening, drying

Some pack recipes to try:

For dry skin: 2 tsp each rice flour and sesame paste, 2–3 drops of camellia oil, and enough warm water to form a paste

For oily skin: 2 tsp each rice bran and buckwheat flour, 2–3 drops of lemon or *yuzu* juice, and warm water to form a paste

For sensitive skin: 2 tsp each rice flour and drained tofu, 1 tsp black sugar, and warm water to form a paste

For acne: 2 tsp each rice bran and buckwheat flour and enough juice from grated *daikon* to form a paste

For any skin, to relax, nourish, and improve texture: 2 tsp

outside

sesame & rice pack for dry skin

buckwheat & rice bran pack for oily skin

tofu & black sugar pack for sensitive skin

daikon & buckwheat & rice bran pack for acne

each soybean, rice, and buckwheat flour, 1 tsp black sugar, and warm water to form a paste

Wakame seaweed, rinsed of salt and softened, can be applied to the face in strips just the way it comes. This seaweed pack is great for reviving a dull complexion and stimulating, toning, and tightening the skin.

Any of these packs should be applied to a freshly cleansed, preferably steamed, face and left on for 15–20 minutes, then rinsed off gently with tepid water.

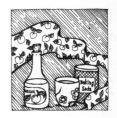

The classic face packs of both the European Old World and the New often make use of cookie-baking ingredients like honey, eggs, oatmeal, almonds, and milk. Herb teas, powdered herbs, fresh mashed fruits or vegetables, wheat germ, nut and grain flours, pure clays, seaweeds, volcanic muds, algaes, and essential oils are all used as well in the Western natural face-pack tradition. Most things that are nourishing when eaten (and unprocessed, chemical- and pesticide-free, of course) can be nourishing to the skin when applied externally, and this dictum can serve as a guideline for experimentation at home. Following, some old-fashioned recipes that generations of women have sworn by:

outside

soybean & rice & buckwheat pack for any skin

wakame seaweed pack for toning

honey & almond & egg yolk pack for aging skin

oatmeal & egg white & aloe pack for any skin

meringue pack for any skin

brewer's yeast & yogurt pack for normal skin

milk & honey pack for dry and normal skin

clay face pack for any skin

HONEY & ALMOND & EGG YOLK PACK: Grind a handful of almonds to a meal in a coffee or grain mill, then add the yolk of an egg and enough honey to make a spreadable mixture. Massage the mixture onto the face, then leave on for 20 minutes before rinsing. Recommended for any skin, but especially for aging, tired, or dry skin.

OATMEAL & EGG WHITE & ALOE GEL PACK: Mix either cooked oatmeal or oat flour (grind oats in a mill) with egg white and the fresh gel from the inside of an aloe leaf, then spread onto the face evenly. Leave on for 20 minutes before rinsing. This pack will tighten the skin and heal blemishes, so it's useful for both young troubled skin and aging wrinkled skin.

MERINGUE PACK: Whipped-stiff egg whites can be applied to the face for 10–15 minutes for a quick pore-refining pack, good for all skin types.

BREWER'S YEAST & YOGURT PACK: Leave this mixture on until it dries for a very stimulating complexion treatment. Those with sensitive or irritated skin should avoid this pack, however, as it is quite potent and may cause inflammation to skin that is delicate. Oily skin and tired, stressed skin will appreciate it greatly.

MILK & HONEY: Warm a little milk—fresh cream is even better—and add an equal amount of honey. Spread the mixture as is on the face or add a bit of almond meal to thicken it. This is the ultimate moisturizing pack for dry or winter wind-beaten skin.

REFINING PACK: Prepare some agar-agar gel (*kanten* in Japanese). Add gel to a small quantity of French clay or Fuller's earth, then mix in some egg white.

Apply to damp skin, allow to harden, then remove by rinsing with first warm, then cool water. (If enough agar-agar has been used, the mask will peel off in one piece.) This pack is good for any skin type and will refine pores, remove impurities, and stimulate the complexion. If your face is quite dry, you might add a drop or two of camellia oil or olive oil.

outside

almond & lemon face pack for oily skin

parsley & honey pack for dry skin

PACK FOR OILY SKIN: Grind almonds until fine; mash a cucumber in a mortar. Mix these ingredients together and add some lemon juice to make a thick paste. Leave on the skin for 15 minutes, then rinse well with cool water. This pack is gently astringent and soothing.

PACK FOR DRY SKIN: Blend fresh parsley until it is pulp; add some honey, and if the concoction is too wet, some ground oatmeal or whole wheat flour. Massage gently into the skin and allow to sit for 20 minutes. Steam face briefly before removing pack with first warm, then cool, water. Very nourishing, moisturizing, and tightening. If you are interested in experimenting with the Western pack ingredients, here are some basics:

Avocado—very nourishing
Egg White—stimulates, tightens, refines pores
Egg Yolk—nourishes, moisturizes
Clay—absorbs oil, refines pores
Aloe—heals and soothes irritated, burned, or blemished skin
Honey—tightens, nourishes, hydrates, stimulates
Vegetable or Nut Oil—moisturizes, nourishes, smoothes
Yogurt/Milk/Buttermilk—nourishing and calming
Flours (Oat, Corn, Wheat, Buckwheat)—nourishing, stimulating

the simple *shiatsu* facial

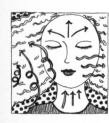

While skillfully applied make-up can simulate the natural inner glow of healthy beauty, isn't it preferable to achieve this radiance without artifice? Because *shiatsu* encourages well-being of mind, body, and spirit, the kind of beauty borne of it is truly more than skin-deep.

The very best way to put a glow in the cheeks is by getting the circulation going. A brisk walk in the mountain air, a session of cardiovascular exercise, a hot bath—any of these will do it. If you exercise with regularity, preferably out-of-doors, your skin will look better all the time. Combine this with local stimulation of the pressure points and you may be able to give up make-up!

I describe here a few key *tsubo*, or pressure points, that are among those that affect the beauty of the face. They are the most commonly known *tsubo* for the purpose and are easily found and manipulated. A complete *shiatsu* massage for facial beauty would involve the stimulation of interrelated sets of many *tsubo*—not only on the face and head but on areas far distant from the face.

While the aim is to apply firm pressure to the vital point, at the start pressure should be light, increasing gradually and intuitively until the appropriate degree of force is reached. The hands should be warm; some practitioners advise generating *ki*—vital energy—by first shaking the hands 25 times, then rubbing the palms together briskly 50 times, before applying pressure to the *tsubo*. The body should be comfortable and relaxed, and when stimulating face *tsubo* the eyes are best kept closed.

While there are many specialized pushing techniques designed for treatment of the various body areas, in applying pressure to points on the face there are basically five options, based on common sense.

Pressure may be applied with the fingerpad of the thumb; the joined fingerpads of forefinger and middle finger pressed together; the fingerpads of those fingers plus the ring finger, held together so as to form a triangular point; or the palm. In the area around the eyes, the middle fingerpad alone may be found to work most effectively.

When a pair of symmetrical points is pushed simultaneously, the same fingers and pressure should be applied to each. Each point or set of points may be pushed for a period of 3–5 seconds —with the 3–5-second push repeated 3 times at each location —and the set of 3 pushes may be executed 2–3 times per day.

It is possible to use not only a static pressure technique but also a rubbing or kneading massage technique. When sitting in bath or sauna, apply an emollient to the cleansed face, then massage for 5 minutes. Basic principles: Always move fingertips upward or outward, never downward or inward; move fingers across the skin, don't move the skin itself; apply gentle but firm pressure. Facial *shiatsu* may be practiced daily for good results. Remember never to pull or stretch the skin if an active massage technique is used. Those wishing to delve further into the possibilities of *tsubo* manipulation should consult a practitioner trained in *shiatsu*, moxabustion, and acupuncture.

KEN-RYŌ

Near the center of the cheek, below the eyes, feel along the lower edge of the cheekbone. At the place where the bone protudes, at its lowest point, place your finger, moving it slightly downward so that it is below the bone, then just slightly outward (in the direction of the ears). This point, just slightly past the lower protuberance of the cheekbone, is KEN-RYŌ, which when stimulated—on both sides of the face simultaneously—is said to beautify the face by improving circulation and muscle tone, relaxing and nourishing the drawn or fatigued areas of the face around

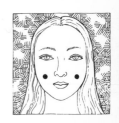

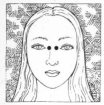

SEI-MEI

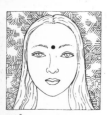

DO-SHI-RYO

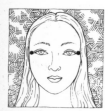

IN-DŌ

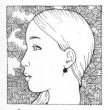

EI-FŪ

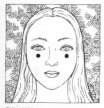

SHI-HAKU

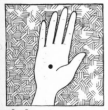

RŌ-KYŪ

the mouth and eyes, remedying eye fatigue and wrinkles and pouches in that area, and helping the body to heal and eliminate pimples and blemishes.

SEI-MEI

Located on either side of the bridge of the nose at a level with the eyes is the *tsubo* known as SEI-MEI, which when pressed is responsible for beautifying the eyes, making them clear and bright and relieving signs of fatigue. This *tsubo* is also said to have a calming effect, when pressed, on those who are over-wrought.

DŌ-SHI-RYŌ

This *tsubo* is found at the outer corner of the eye, just past the bone of the eye socket. It is used to soften wrinkles in the eye area.

IN-DŌ

The spot at the "third eye"—just above the bridge of the nose and the inner corners of the eyebrows, at the bottom center of the forehead. This *tsubo*, pressed firmly toward the center of the head, is used to improve the look of the face, bringing color by stimulating circulation, and eliminating wrinkles, sags, and roughness.

EI-FŪ

In the hollow area just underneath the earlobe, between the bones, is the *tsubo* EI-FŪ, stimulated to improve the complexion, remedy a dry, rough, or colorless skin, and relax and enliven drawn features.

SHI-HAKU

Below the center of the eyes, place your finger to locate the bony edge of the eye socket. Just below the edge by about 1 cm or $1/2$ inch, is SHI-HAKU, pressed to help lighten freckles and age spots, eliminate shadows under the eyes, and relax a drawn face.

RŌ-KYŪ

Pressing the *tsubo* just at the center of the palm of the hand will improve circulation and color in the face.

simple hair beauty

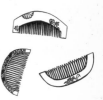

air is really a rather straightforward matter. Most of the problems one might encounter with hair are self-inflicted, and pretty often the self-inflicted damage is the result of attempting to bring beauty to the hair. The irony! Chemicals used in perming, coloring, and straightening the hair and heat applied in styling can wreak serious damage. Overuse of conditioners, gels, and mousses can burden the hair with residues and dull it into a lackluster existence. The hurry-up tempo of a busy modern life can take a toll as well, bringing stress into the equation. Hair loss among women has grown distressingly common, with stress pinpointed as the primary culprit. Inadequate sleep shows up in droopy, tired hair, and an improper diet can starve hair of the nutrients needed for healthy shine and vigor. Add environmental pollution and chemicals in the water to this picture, and you've got the average contemporary woman, unhappy with her head of hair and despairing at the situation.

The solution? Respect the nature of your hair. Refrain from torturing it into forms to which it does not take kindly. Play with color, but do it by gentle botanical means. Learn to relieve hair of heavy residues by rinsing it in vinegars and teas. Rescue your hair by improving your quality of life and reducing your stress level. The hair reflects your overall health like a barometer—while make-up can to some extent belie the true state of one's condition as shown in the skin, and clothes can conceal one's contours, the hair reveals all. In this section, the emphasis is on reducing what you do to your hair from without while enriching it from within. Respect your tresses!

the simplest of hair-care rituals

Without beautiful hair, the most exquisite face is improperly framed. The hair is the physical attribute most amenable to transformation; its color, cut, style, texture, and condition can be considerably altered, and all of these can have an enormous impact on the overall appearance.

Every woman knows the importance of the Right Haircut.

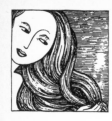

Without it you are bereft, for the right haircut is the perfect complement to your face, body, personality, and style.

With a trusted stylist taking care of your cut and color needs, all you need attend to is the condition of your hair, and in this undertaking there are two components: internal nourishment and external treatment.

Hair condition depends heavily on diet. Beautiful, healthy, luxuriant hair requires a lot of nourishment. The B vitamins, iron, sulfur, and zinc must all be included in your diet. A daily brewer's yeast supplement, whole grains, eggs, beans, legumes, fish, nuts, meat, seafood, and seaweed will all give good hair results.

Seaweed and *goma*, or black sesame seeds, are two traditional Japanese foods thought to improve the condition of hair, even to the point of restoring its natural color. Since these foods are rich in nutrients beneficial to hair, it is likely that, if one consumes them regularly, one's hair will look more vibrant, healthy, and glossy, and the dullness and faded color that characterize poorly nourished hair will be eradicated.

In the realm of beauty, it can be hard to separate what works from what doesn't. A shampoo meant to make hair silky leaves it dismally droopy; a cream against wrinkles produces red bumps instead. Sometimes the worst that happens is that a treatment does nothing—nothing discernible to the naked eye, at any rate.

Yet our spirits remain hopeful, optimistic—we want to have faith. Among the recently developed sophisticated beauty products, there are quite a few that are very good, though it is an expensive process of trial and error to discover those that suit us.

Even in the natural beauty domain, one may be disappointed. There are many treatments that are so subtle the benefits are semi-invisible. Others, however, have survived centuries—passed orally from mother to daughter—because they really offer results.

Here, some natural hair treatments that work, a very subjective list that comes from personal experience.

THE CHAMPAGNE HAIR RINSE: I'm reminded of this one after every New Year's Eve, when there's always some leftover champagne. This rinse is an old French secret for making hair shiny, silky, and healthy, and if one is fair-haired, bringing out the golden lights in it. In my experience, champagne is better than lemon or chamomile for lightening and brightening the hair—it gives results quickly, without drying or damaging the tresses.

Mix $1/2$ cup old champagne with $1/2$ cup hot water; after shampooing and rinsing well, pour the mixture through the hair. Do not rinse again. (A conditioner may precede the champagne, if desired.) The hair is left looking vital and lustrous, with pale champagne highlights.

THE RUSSIAN EGG YOLK AND OIL HAIR TREATMENT PACK: Two egg yolks, slightly beaten, about 1 tablespoon of oil (saf-

inside

seaweed for hair

black sesame for hair

outside

champagne hair rinse

egg yolk & oil hair pack

flower, almond, coconut, or walnut), and a drop of one's preferred essential oil (lemon, tangerine, jasmine, rose, sandalwood, rosemary—all good choices) are the ingredients in this recipe.

outside

camellia oil hair dressing

olive/sesame oil hair pack

incense hair fragrance

Variations of this treatment are found all over the world, East and West. Better than a simple hot-oil treatment, this pack leaves the hair looking stunning—thick, luxuriant, and shiny. The effects last a long time—even the light scent of the essential oil will linger through several shampoos.

Before applying, moisten hair very slightly by running wet fingers through it, then massage the egg mixture into hair and scalp. Wrap head in a towel (and plastic if desired) and have a sauna, take a long hot bath, or simply relax in a warm place. (The heat of a sauna is the best environment of all for this treatment.) Leave the pack on for one hour if possible, even two or three!

To cleanse, first rinse hair in warm water, then apply a lot of shampoo directly to the hair, wash well, and rinse. If you've used enough shampoo, only one wash is needed. Most commercial hair treatments don't come close to this international folk recipe.

Japanese tradition also offers some wonderful external treatments. As a hair dressing and conditioner, a few drops of *tsubaki abura*, or camellia oil, can be applied daily to dry hair. An olive-oil or sesame oil treatment pack can perform wonders: Apply warmed oil to scalp and hair, wrap head in a towel, then relax in a hot bath or sauna for 20 minutes or so. Shampoo twice and air-dry.

The following is one of my all-time favorites:
INCENSE HAIR SCENT: To perfume the hair, borrow an idea from Japanese tradition: incense. Somehow the slightly smoky fragrance seems poetically suited to the hair; it gives a mysterious, earthy suggestion of scent.

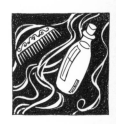

You can employ one of the incense baskets used for this purpose by Heian women of centuries past, or you can simply incline your head over sweetly burning incense (hair should be damp, so after washing is a good time) and let the smoke penetrate. Scents to choose from: sandalwood, plum blossom, pine, or whatever strikes your fancy.

The hair must be handled with care. Overprocessing through coloring, perming, and heat-styling is the source of most hair damage—but even brushing hair carelessly or when wet will hurt it severely. Comb hair gently with a wide-tooth comb when wet; brush it with a natural-bristle brush only when completely dry. A daily scalp massage will stimulate circulation and hair growth, and to top it off, it feels great.

chemicals and things

Shampooing with heavily chlorinated tap water can cause the hair to become frizzy and visibly damaged. One solution? Wash and condition hair as usual and rinse. Then apply a final rinse of warm filtered tap water mixed with apple cider vinegar, soybean vinegar, or brown rice vinegar to eliminate chlorine and tame frizziness. Even bottled mineral water alone as the final rinse will help to lessen the nefarious effect of chlorine.

Hair-beautifying tea rinses provide another interesting solution, with cherry bark or buckwheat being the teas of choice. Brew as for ordinary tea, then use as the last rinse after shampooing. And do keep a bottle of vinegar where you bathe—a vinegar rinse is a good habit to develop, whether your tap water is chlorinated or not. Vinegar is a great acid-balancer and purifier, and as such will be beneficial to skin as well.

For a more basic solution to the problem of chemical-laden water, have your water tested or do it yourself with a water-testing kit. If you feel it's warranted, invest in a water-purifying device for your shower and bath as well as for the kitchen faucet. This step should substantially reduce the drying, debilitating effects of chemicals on skin and hair.

But what about the chemicals you yourself are daily subjecting your hair to?

Hair that is overconditioned, overmoussed, gelled, and sprayed ends up coated with residues and grows sad, dull, and all but lifeless. Judging from the plethora of miracle-promising hair products on the market, many heads are being doused, slicked, sculpted, formed, misted, and molded with such modern conveniences. Ordinary washing does not remove the residues; on the contrary, shampoo, especially the conditioning type, often adds to the problem.

There are two easy and natural methods for relieving hair of its burden of chemical leftovers: baking soda rinse and vinegar rinse. Of the two, baking soda is probably the more effective in removing long-term buildup.

A half-cup of baking soda dissolved in a cup or so of warm water and poured over the hair after shampooing will efficiently clean and shine the tresses. It should be massaged into the hair and scalp for several minutes, then rinsed. If you use a lot of commercial stuff on your hair, try the baking soda rinse every week or two. Your hair will look and feel healthier.

The vinegar rinse is a very old European method for finishing a shampoo. Hair *vinaigres* are produced commercially in France and have a devoted following. A few tablespoons of some pleasant vinegar (raspberry? plum?) added to your rinse water will remove the last traces of shampoo and give the hair extra shine and a soft, smooth texture. Vinegar restores the proper acidic PH balance to hair. The technique may be used after every shampoo.

Finally, a special sybaritic beauty secret for hair. Following a shampoo/rinse, dry the hair with a piece of clean silk, a Hermés

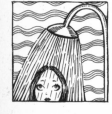

square for example. Gently rubbing the hair with silk section by section will leave you with incredibly silken locks, resplendent with body and shine.

keeping your hair in place

Hair loss in women is becoming more common. What is to be done?

While genetically caused hair loss (the type suffered by some men) has no known permanent remedy, the type of hair loss seen in women is almost always reversible. Women's loss of hair may be caused by a variety of factors: stress, overprocessing (coloring, bleaching, perming, straightening), hormonal fluctuations (such as those that occur post-pregnancy and during menopause), shock, and even brushing too vigorously or pulling hair back too tightly in styling.

A diet low in iron and vitamin B may contribute to a generally weak and 'breakable" hair strand. (Research suggests that regular consumption of soybeans may contribute to the maintenance of a healthy head of hair. Seaweed is another hair benefactor.) The aging process may result in a slowed-down process of hair regrowth, thus leading to a thinning effect as one grows older.

A certain amount of hair loss is normal: the average person can send 150 strands per day to the wind without worry. Each hair has a 3–5-year growth cycle, and an average head may have between 100,000 and 150,000 hairs.

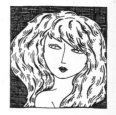

In the process of investigating Japanese folk techniques for beauty, I have come across a number of treatments for stimulating hair growth and preventing hair loss. Though traditional wisdom supports their use by both men and women, I would assume them to be most effective in the treatment of non-hereditary hair loss. When combined with proper diet, adequate rest, exercise—improvement in circulation benefits hair, too—and gentle handling of the hair, the traditional treatments may provide effective stimulation and nourishment to the scalp.

Camellia oil, the classic Japanese hairdressing oil, is recommended for use on wet hair, after shampooing. Two to three drops are applied to the scalp and massaged in well, then the hair is carefully combed with a wide-tooth comb. Never brush wet hair—it has diminished elasticity then and breaks very easily. For a variation of the camellia oil massage, combine a bit of fresh lemon juice with the oil.

Sesame oil is another traditional treatment, either the pure oil alone or in combination with grated ginger. Mix equal amounts of the juice from grated ginger with sesame oil and massage gently into the scalp. Ginger is well known in the Asian medical traditions as a stimulant and tonic; it is thought to activate

outside

silk rub for hair

camellia oil treatment for falling hair

sesame & ginger treatment for falling hair

sluggish hair cells. Always use ginger sparingly, though, as those with sensitive skin will experience a burning, stinging sensation if too much is applied.

The scalp massage in these treatments is at least as important as the materials applied. But remember that any hair loss, especially where patches of hair are missing, will take several months to reverse. And if stress is a primary factor, external treatment alone will not help. Relax! Don't worry! Be happy!

playing with hair color teas

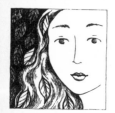

Flower-red, nut-brown, spice-yellow. Hair colored by the tints of nature can be as resplendent as a garden: a blonde dandelion-bright, a red of wild roses, a brown of chestnut, a blue or purple the color of sky in a painting by Chagall. Hair may be colored dream colors! This wild color spirit does not arise from the neon-pink punk urge that wishes to shock and cause recoil, but rather from pure playfulness. Color? Think of hair as an artist might: it can be any color you like.

The alternative to coloring the hair permanently by a method that chemically penetrates the inner cortex of the hair shaft is to apply a natural botanical substance to the hair. There are botanical hair colorings on the market now that can give you any color under the sun, but first, maybe try some gentler, subtler rinses that you make yourself as flower teas. Let's explore some of these.

all colors from gold to purple: The most well known of the natural hair coloring substances is of course henna, which in its unmodified state produces a rich deep-red color that brings volume to the hair into the bargain. While specially mixed henna is available in every color (golden yellow, copper, all the reds, browns, eggplant, and ebony), the gamut of reds generally offer the most favorable results. Henna's disadvantage is in its tendency to dry the hair.

Here's a traditional henna recipe I learned in East Africa from Indian women: using a ceramic bowl and a wooden spoon—never anything metal—mix a handful of henna with warm water and the juice from half a lemon (the lemon brightens the color). Allow the mixture to sit for 30 minutes, then apply to the hair, ends first and finally the roots. The skin will take the tint as well, so apply vaseline to the skin near the hairline or be careful around the edges. Wrap head in plastic and a towel, and let the henna work for 30 minutes. *Don't* sit in a sauna with henna on the head; the final color will be adversely affected. Shampoo and rinse well. Henna should not be used on hair that has previously been treated chemically, either by a permanent or by chemical coloring compounds. Henna works best on very thick, slightly coarse-textured hair that is not susceptible to damage. Be warned that the effects of henna are difficult to control at home. Best to have a henna treatment professionally done. Even so-called neutral henna can be unpredictable—I once turned my blonde hair a distinct shade of green with it!

reds & browns: Nothing compares with henna in this category. (It should be noted that blondes will have a hard time getting a realistic red, brown, or black at home—it is simpler by far to add highlights than it is to darken the hair.)

HENNA FOR CHESTNUT LIGHTS IN DARK HAIR: For a subtle chestnut effect, brunettes can use only a small amount of red henna mixed with neutral henna, and proceed as above. For a deeper tone, mix with strong espresso coffee rather than water. Some colorists add spices like cinnamon, nutmeg, or turmeric to vary the effects slightly. Don't try red pepper!

BLACK TEA & CHERRY BARK FOR AUBURN LIGHTS IN DARK HAIR: Prepare a strong tea from black tea leaves and cherry bark. Use as a rinse after shampooing, finishing with a water rinse.

MARIGOLD FOR RED LIGHTS IN FAIR HAIR: Blonde or brown-haired women who want to try putting reddish lights in their hair can try marigold, also known as *Calendula officinalis*. (Note: effects may be unpredictable on chemically treated hair.) Marigold will not only impart a red-gold tone to the hair, but will condition it, giving it shine and body.

The rinse technique is the gentlest way to color the hair with herbs: simmer 75 g/ $^1/_3$ C of crushed marigold flowers with 600 ml/ $2^1/_2$ C of water in a nonmetal pot for 20 minutes. Remove from the heat, then strain when cool, saving the liquid.

After washing your hair, apply the marigold decoction as a final rinse, pouring it over the hair and catching it in a basin to reapply several times. (Red wine may be added to the liquid to intensify the effect.) Allow hair to dry naturally in the sun, if possible. Repeat the rinsing process with subsequent shampoos until you achieve the desired shade.

yellows/lighteners: Rhubarb, chamomile, marigold—these are the European standbys.

RHUBARB FOR BRIGHT LIGHTS IN FAIR HAIR: Rhubarb will appreciably lighten hair of all shades. Simmer 50 g/ $^3/_4$ oz of the root in 1 liter/4 C of pure water in a covered nonmetal pot for one hour. After cooling and filtering out solids, apply to the hair as a final rinse, pouring the liquid through again and again. Effects are permanent warm/bright overtones. Red wine may be used instead of water for a warmer tone.

Lemon juice may sometimes be added to any of the lighten-

outside

espresso & henna for chestnut lights

black tea & cherry bark for auburn lights

marigold for red lights

rhubarb for golden lights

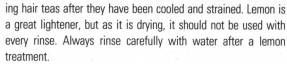

ing hair teas after they have been cooled and strained. Lemon is a great lightener, but as it is drying, it should not be used with every rinse. Always rinse carefully with water after a lemon treatment.

CHAMOMILE FOR GOLDEN LIGHTS IN BROWN, BLONDE, OR RED HAIR: A chamomile rinse after every shampoo is the classic herbal method. This is the traditional French *recette de bonne femme* used by mothers on their fair-haired children—chamomile prolongs the blondness of youth.

If you wish to try chamomile to brighten your hair, use yellow, or Hungarian, chamomile, *Matricaria chamomilla* or *Matricaria recutita* in Latin, *manzanilla* in Spanish.

The other type of chamomile, which should *not* be used for cosmetic purposes, is Roman or English chamomile, *Anthemus nobilis* in Latin.

The preparation method for a hair rinse is the decoction, as outlined for the marigold rinse. Simmer 75 g/$^1/_3$ C of chamomile blossoms or powdered chamomile in 600 ml/2$^1/_2$ C of water in a nonmetal pot for 20 minutes. Remove from the heat; when cool enough to use, strain, saving the liquid.

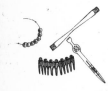

After shampooing the hair, apply the chamomile liquid as a final rinse, pouring it over the hair and catching it in a basin to reapply several times. Try to allow hair to dry naturally in the sun. Repeat this rinsing process with subsequent shampoos until you achieve the desired effect.

If you wish to pursue subtle gradations of golden tone, various herbs and spices may be added to the basic chamomile recipe. The color of the herb is the tint that will be imparted to the hair—though usually the effect on hair is less intense.

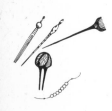

Other plants to try: turmeric, saffron, golden seal, gold thread, marigold, quassia (chips), rhubarb (root), yellow mullein (flowers), and broom. Lemon peel may also be used. Remember that your own hair color will determine the final effect. These herbs will have particularly nice results on mousy darkening blonde hair, bringing vivid lights, and they will also give brightness to brown shades.

It is not really possible to *substantially* lighten hair herbally, though on already fair hair chamomile may do this slightly. Brightening, not bleaching, is what you may expect from the golden herbal hair rinses.

dark browns/blacks: The classics for darkening hair are walnut shells, black tea, cherry tree bark, and cloves. All of these act as temporary stains when infused as described above, first grinding the bark or nutshells. The infusion of any one of these ingredients, or two in combination, may be applied to the hair as a final rinse. Following is a lovely recipe from the European tradition:

BLACK TEA & SAGE FOR DARKENING GRAY HAIR: In a teapot, steep 3 T/1 ½ oz each of black tea and sage in freshly boiled water. Allow to cool and use as a hair rinse, pouring the tea repeatedly over the hair. (Doing this over a basin, using a cup, is the easiest way.) Rinse with tepid water.

Because the results of any of these color applications will vary—the original hair color being the most obvious determining factor—it is advisable to experiment cautiously at first.

All of the above rinses may be used after every shampoo; over a period of a few weeks you will begin to see new highlights and color tones in your hair. If you stop applying the herbs, their effects will gradually disappear, except in the case of chamomile. Exposure to sun or chlorine may alter your hair's hue.

Every herbal rinse described here has the happy side-effect of conditioning and strengthening the hair as well as giving it color. You may find you can do away with your commercial rinse/conditioner altogether.

the beauty that is simple and pure

Wabi: the beauty of the simple, the commonplace, the beauty of that which is restrained. The beauty of the ordinary, the lowly, the poor, the modest, the humble. *Wabi* is quiet and pure and rich in spirit. *Wabi* beauty requires a reciprocal quietness of regard on the part of the observer.

In *sabi* is the beauty bestowed by time, the beauty of that which has faded, which possesses just a faint suggestion of a former brilliance, the soft glow of a tarnished surface; the feeling aroused in the viewer is one of lonely, detached sadness mingled with a sense of comfort and contentment.

Shibui is noble simplicity, unassuming and profound, spare and understated, the quietest possible, most spare, most pared-down kind of beauty.

Wabi, *sabi*, and *shibui* come together in a loveliness that is quiet, sober, and pure, less rather than more, always humble, never proud of itself.

simple *shiatsu* for beautiful hair

The head possesses many useful *tsubo* that may be pressed to affect the appearance of the hair, among other things, but many of these are extremely difficult to locate with accuracy. As in the section on *shiatsu* for facial beauty, described here are only a select few *tsubo* that are easy for the beginner to find and stimulate.

For simple finger-pressure *tsubo* therapy, the same basic guidelines discussed earlier hold true: the hands should be warm, the body should be relaxed, and pressure should increase gradually until the appropriate degree of force is reached.

The pushing techniques for the head are the following: forefinger, middle finger, and ring finger gathered to a point, to push with the three fingerpads at once; for the sides of the head, the palms of the hands; and for the spot at the very back of the head known as NŌ-KO, the left middle finger is placed atop the nail of the right middle finger, for pushing together. It is also possible to apply all the fingers of both hands to several points on the head at once, but this method supplies less pressure to the specific points.

Points may be pushed for 3–5-second periods, repeated in sets of 3 for each location, with each session of 3 sets of pushes being carried out 2–3 times per day.

It should be noted that if your usual shampoo massage is comprehensive and attentive, you will be stimulating pressure points on the head automatically. Also, anything you do for your feet in the way of massage or other pressure-point stimulation methods will benefit the head and hair by improving circulation.

TOKU-MYAKU MERIDIAN

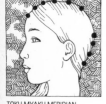

TOKU-MYAKU MERIDIAN

On the center line of the head (imagine a line that runs between the spinal cord at the back of the neck to the front of the head between the eyes)—the TOKU-MYAKU MERIDIAN—lie many *tsubo*. To remedy hair that is graying, falling, or merely lacking in shine and vitality, the points on this line may be stimulated. Using the 3-finger push, start at the forehead and push firmly toward the center of the head at that point, then move a finger's width further back and push there, repeating the process until the point HYAKU-E is reached. There should be six separate points pushed altogether, and the 6-point process should be repeated 3–5 times to make one set.

HYAKU-E

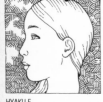

HYAKU-E

This topmost point along the TOKU-MYAKU MERIDIAN, straight up from the midpoint of the ears at the center of the head, which should feel slightly tender when pressed, may be stimulated to improve circulation in the scalp. It should be pressed strongly toward the center of the head.

ZEN-CHŌ

Just two fingers-width forward of HYAKU-E is ZEN-CHŌ, which may be pressed in the same manner and with similar benefits.

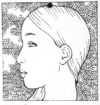

ZEN-CHŌ

NŌ-KO

This *tsubo* is located along the same meridian at the back of the head, in the middle of the bony protuberance at the center of which is a slight dent. The *tsubo* is pressed with both middle fingers, one atop the other, and is said to remedy hair loss and graying.

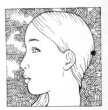

NŌ-KO

TEN-CHŪ

Located on another meridian, this pair of *tsubo* is at the back of the head at the neck hairline, just at the outside of the ridge of muscle that runs up along either side of the spine. Pressed firmly upward and toward the center of the head, these points are said to improve circulation in the scalp and relieve tension and fatigue as well.

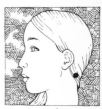

TEN-CHŪ

FŪ-CHI

One finger-width forward of TEN-CHŪ, this point is located at the bottom edge of the hairline closest to the ears. Pressed upward and toward the center of the head, these points will improve circulation and tone in the scalp area and beautify the hair.

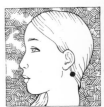

FŪ-CHI

YŌ-CHI

At the back of the wrist, at the joint, just slightly past center toward the outside, is a *tsubo* that may be pressed to increase general vitality and improve one's overall condition, hair included.

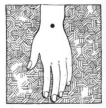

YŌ-CHI

simple body beauty

the simplest of body-care rituals

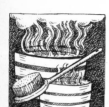

In body beauty it is skin texture and tone, muscle tone, and the silhouette that receive our attention. Beyond these, and no less important, is the quality of the body in motion. The total presence. To make your body beautiful as an object is not enough; it is essential to move through life with harmony, grace, and an understanding of the beauty of movement.

The simplest body-care ritual would consist of a devotional approach to bathing, where the bath provides not only stimulation of the circulatory system and relaxation, but moves body and soul into a state of timeless well-being ... the Zen of bathing. The bath offers too the opportunity for the full-body scrub, which I place high on the list of beauty essentials. Healthy circulation, baby-soft skin, and glowing skin tone are the rewards of the scrub. Purifying, stimulating mineral salts or botanicals set adrift from time to time in the bath add their own special powers to the cleansing soak.

Exercise should be a matter of course. Body awareness gained through a regular program of stretching, strengthening, and cardiovascular training will help you know how to move. You've got to inhabit your body with consciousness to move it well, and it must be a finely tuned instrument for you to be at your best.

How you eat is important. Combine good eating with bathing, bath-scrubbing, and exercise, and you will be in fine shape. Start now, and you'll never have to wonder if there is such a thing as cellulite. For you, there won't be. Preventive maintenance is so much easier than the cure.

It is in winter—especially in the season of *Daikan*, the time of the Greater Cold by the old solar calendar—that the pleasures of the Japanese hot spring are best appreciated. With more than 2,000 hot-spring areas gracing the archipelago, it is a short trip from almost anywhere to a spirit-warming soak. To relax in a steaming outdoor pool surrounded by snowdrifts and tall pines in an atmosphere of serenity is one of life's great luxuries. Europe too maintains a long tradition of the hot-spring cure, and America has recently come into her own in this area as well.

It is possible also to approximate the hot-spring soak at home, if only in small degree— it's hard to duplicate the ambience—by adding mineral-rich bath salts to the hottest tub one can stand. The powdered hot-spring salts marketed by many Japanese companies give one a choice of all the famous *onsen* in Japan, claiming to offer exactly the same cocktail of minerals found, for instance, in the hot springs of Beppu, or Shirahama, or Atami. These packets are unfortunately lacking in the authentic hot-spring aroma, which is a disappointment to the purist bather. However, for those who prefer gardenia- or citron-scented baths, and vividly green, orange, or pink waters, the packets are fine.

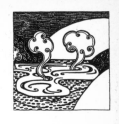

The bath tablets manufactured by many Japanese companies are another bathing option. These tablets are often alkaline, which means they offer the benefits of sodium hydrogen carbonate and fizz effervescently when plopped into the tub. They are often scented and colored, like the powder packets.

outside

alkaline bath

sea salt bath

sea salt & seaweed bath

sulphur bath

Alkaline water is softening to the skin and beautifying to the complexion; it also deeply warms the body, relieves aches, pains, and tension, and encourages the elimination of lactic acid after exercise. An alkaline bath is easy to make from scratch: just add 60 ml/^{1}/$_4$ C or more of baking soda to the hot water, then soak. A purifying bath.

Another simple *onsen*-type soak may be created by adding lots of sea salt to the bath. 500 g/17 ^{3}/$_4$ oz in your hot bath will cleanse and tone the skin, encouraging the departure of minor skin problems and the healing of blemishes. Add seaweed powder and you have the kind of toxin-eliminating, cell-rejuvenating, metabolism-activating bath featured by luxury spas in France. (For the total experience, after the seaweed-salt bath bundle up in a robe and quilt and recline for 20 minutes, then take a shower and scrub yourself. This is the real thing, if it's maximum regeneration and gorgeousness you're after.)

The sulphur bath is another high-powered beauty treatment. I once took a sulphur bath in the wilds of Honduras, and an hour in the natural jungle spring removed every trace of the suntan two weeks of ocean swimming had given me! For those who want whiter skin, the sulphur bath is a miracle-worker. It's also detoxifying, softening, and encouraging to the circulation (leading to rosy cheeks and healthier skin), but sulphur can irritate sensitive skin, so bathe with care. Don't wear jewelry in a sulphur bath unless you like your ornaments midnight black.

You can buy sulphur for the bath in well-stocked Japanese

drugstores (usually in liquid "flowers-of-sulphur" form), or you can bring *yunohana* home with you from a Japanese sulphur spring. Chemistry-supply stores also sell sulphur powder. Add the little pebbles of sulphur powder to the bath sparingly—suddenly your bathroom is a volcanic primeval paradise! (Some tubs are discolored by sulphur; package instructions advise emptying the tub immediately after bathing and washing the sulphur water away.)

For the Westerner who is unused to the intensely hot Japanese-style bath, some guidelines:

Health experts usually advise taking baths in water that is just a little above normal body temperature—around 38° C/100° F. While water that is very hot, say over 42° C/107° F, may not be dangerous to a normally healthy person, for those who suffer from high blood pressure, heart disease, or hypertension, a very hot bath is not advised. The average temperature for a Japanese-style bath is 45° C/112° F. It takes some getting used to.

Even in the healthy, dehydration and dizziness can occur as the result of a long hot bath. Babies, whose bodies are not yet finely tuned enough to adapt well to sudden and extreme temperature changes, may suffer in water that is too hot. Thus, for the very young or for those with health problems, even a bath of 42° C/107° F may be too hot. For adults and older children who want to enjoy a long hot soak, there are several basic rules to follow:

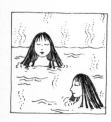

—Prior to getting into the tub, always bathe the body repeatedly with water of the same temperature. The head should also be doused well; this process helps to avoid the shock of a sudden rise in temperature. Health experts recommend about 10 minutes of this preparation.

—Drink water before and after bathing to avoid dehydration.

—Do not stand up suddenly when emerging from a very hot bath; this helps prevent dizziness or fainting.

—If you are not accustomed to high temperatures in the bath, build up your tolerance gradually over a period of time, going from warm to hot and increasing soaking periods, starting with very short soaks of 2 or 3 minutes and building up to the standard 15 or 20.

Experts say that a tepid bath provides the same advantages as a hotter one: deep relaxation, improvement of circulation, elimination of toxins through sweating, and invigoration of the metabolism. But who doesn't love a really hot bath, Japanese-style? Experiment to find the right bath for you. Enjoy your soaks by bathing wisely.

The tradition of scrubbing the skin with an abrasive device spans many cultures. In the Middle Eastern *hammam*, or communal steam bath, a small abrasive cloth mitt is used to remove the top layers of skin cells. In northern Europe and Russia, bundled birch leaves are applied vigorously to the skin to stimulate it, and strong-bristled brushes are used for exfoliation. The Japanese woman describes her skin-scrubbing ritual as one of the primary elements in beauty and health.

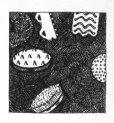

The benefits include stimulation of the local circulation; exfoliation, with the elimination of dry dull skin cells and debris; stimulation of the pressure points; and stimulation of underactive tissues, to bring blood and nutrients to the skin. The result is smoother, softer, more glowing skin, as well as improved resistance.

Tools of every description are available for scrubbing in both East and West. Choose these with a thought to the surfaces to which they will be applied. Soft materials for the face, harder ones for the body, hardest of all for the feet and elbows.

Begin gently with skin scrubbing; don't induce pain, but aim to stimulate. You must treat the face, breasts, and inner arms and thighs with delicacy, while callused areas will need a vigorous rub with a pumice stone. Over time, you will be able to apply greater pressure to the brush or mitt when you execute your body scrub. The traditional tool in Japanese is the *tawashi* brush, also used for vegetable scrubbing.

To scrub properly, the skin should be softened by heat and moisture. For a wet scrub, add soap or another cleanser to your scrubber. (A dry scrub takes place prebath, without added cleansing materials.)

outside

the skin scrub

Scrub in a circular motion, working toward the heart from the extremities. Avoid moles, blemishes, warts, and varicose veins. Rinse well afterward, first warm and then cold. Any treatment cream or pack applied post-scrub will penetrate much more easily.

To make the most of your bath, have a soak, get out and scrub, then get back in for another soak. Rinse cold! You will feel brand new....

The Japanese bath-soak is one bathing tradition in a world rich in them. There are natural hot springs to be enjoyed in many places on the globe; a favorite memory of mine is the impromptu bath I took one hot day in the mountains of Taiwan, in a sulphur-spring rapids, birds high overhead in the trees. Meg, one of the editors for this book, remembers fondly the simple hot springs in Baños, in the Ecuadorian Andes—the waters were clay-laden and opaque, and many Andean Indians had come to soak. In Western Europe there are venerable spas for taking the waters, with coastal locations offering heated seawater baths as well as freshwater mineral ones. In the Middle and Near East and in North Africa, there are the wonderful *hammam*. In Eastern Europe and Russia, soaking, steam, and mud baths. In Scandinavia, the sauna, one of life's simple luxuries.

While you may have occasion to bathe in a variety of interesting fashions during your travels, the Scandinavian sauna is, along with the Japanese-style soak, a bathing tradition you may be likely to indulge in close to home, no matter where you live.

The sauna: a wooden room in which one relaxes, bathed in dry heat, until ready to emerge and take the icy plunge into a cold pool, or even better, snow. The basic ritual, repeated as often as desired, leaves one glowing, clearheaded, relaxed to the bones, regenerated.

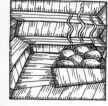

I am often dismayed to see that many sauna-takers lack a basic understanding of what the sauna is for and how it should be used. Erroneous information is passed on to first-timers, with potentially dangerous consequences.

I recently encountered a couple of women in their 70s, in the sauna for the first time, agonizingly awaiting the first drops of perspiration—having been instructed that they could not leave until they began to sweat. Some habitual "sauna-dwellers" spend three or four hours in the sauna encased in plastic weight-loss suits, now and then running out to the scales to check their kilos. To gain real benefits from the sauna without endangering one's health, it is wise to know the rules and understand the ritual.

The basic function of the sauna is to raise the body temperature and encourage the elimination of toxins through sweating. Other benefits include the stimulation of circulation, the speeding up of the metabolism, muscle relaxation, heightened immune response, greater resistance to illness, and the calming of the mind. For long-term benefits, of course, the sauna must be taken periodically, as a regular part of one's health-and-beauty regimen.

To take a proper sauna, one must first shower and scrub. Removing all surface dirt and dead skin cells will enable the skin to eliminate deeper-lying toxins more efficiently. There are two schools of thought on first entry into the sauna—some say you must be dry, some say wet. This is not a crucial detail.

The one point upon which there should be no uncertainty: it is best to sit in a sauna unclothed. Preferably, no plastic suits, no swimsuits, no towels. No jewelry should be worn, as it will heat up and burn your skin. You should have a good hour set aside for your sauna, even longer if possible.

You should not be ill when you take a sauna, say doctors. I find, however, that if I feel the very beginnings of a cold coming on, some time spent in the sauna is likely to send it on its way. Use your own judgment; certainly, if you have a serious respiratory condition, a fever, or anything more than the simplest malaise, call your medical practitioner for advice. Don't ever take a sauna on a full stomach—wait for a couple of hours after eating.

So you are entering the sauna, clean and naked. Since the heat in the sauna is dry, your hair should be protected—wet, wrapped in a towel, or slathered with a treatment pack or oil. I find the sauna a perfect place to do a hot-oil treatment for hair; apply sesame oil, camellia oil, or coconut oil and let it penetrate, to be well shampooed when you're finished.

In the sauna, some people like to apply face packs and body moisturizers. Because the skin will perspire, such substances will usually slide right off, but a light pure oil, like high-grade sesame oil or an aromatherapy oil, can be nice. African karite butter, from the nut of the shea tree, may be applied to skin and hair for potent nourishment. Sweating will not remove the oil. It's a good idea to sweat unoiled for 20 or 30 minutes, then apply oil.

The time spent in the heat should be relaxing. Lie down or sit quietly. Five or ten minutes is fine, then get out and take a cold shower or sit in the cold pool. Return to the heat when your temperature seems lower. The hot-cold routine should be repeated many times; by the end of many such repetitions, you will feel deliciously regenerated—stimulated but deeply relaxed.

Another careful full-body scrub at the end of the sauna routine will provide the final cleansing touch. Afterwards, sauna purists recommend up to one hour of resting—Scandinavian saunas always have cots for post-sauna relaxation.

If you are pregnant, elderly, in ill health, or very young, do not embark on a sauna program without a doctor's consent. The sauna is off-limits to those with heart disease. However, if you are not in those categories, a regular sauna can be a perfect addition to a regimen of healthy eating, exercise, and external beauty treatments. Those who suffer from stress, a polluted environment, or such toxin-related ailments as cellulite or troubled skin will find the sauna a magnificent oasis of purification.

the graceful silhouette

What does it mean to have a beautiful body? In its simplest definition, one will find this beauty expressed in the silhouette: the lines of the body harmonious, balanced, neither obscured by fat nor reduced to a skeletal appearance. The muscles will have presence, seem functional and vital; their curving forms will display the natural beauty of their development. The body in stillness will possess a quality of relaxed aliveness, an erect posture without distortion, without tension. The body in movement will display grace and fluidity, and its gestures will express a vital presence and awareness. And seen over time, a body that has this complete beauty will easily maintain these qualities through old age, for such beauty is derived from a conscious way of life, a life lived physically.

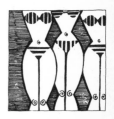

Although all aspects of one's lifestyle contribute to the outward physical presence, and certainly the food one eats is an essential element in this, the body's health and beauty and longevity depend greatly on activity. It is important to *move*. To be truly present in the body requires an exploration and cultivation of all its aspects, and a working and training of the innate potential of the physical being.

Disciplines of the body are integral to the great philosophical traditions of the East. To undertake physical training is to undertake spiritual training as well; it is via the body that the mind and soul may be engaged and illuminated. While any physical training system properly pursued can provide a means for such an evolution, those that belong to the Eastern traditions have been shaped by centuries of spiritual focus.

"Movement is nonmovement; nonmovement is movement." To grasp the meaning of this Buddhist saying, one applies not linear thinking but whole-being knowing. To be alive is to be in body, and thus to approach the mystery and adventure of human existence with the body as conscious vehicle is both convenient and direct. To learn from one's body in the process of perfecting it is one goal of most Eastern disciplines. One learns to harness and focus the vital energy, what is known as *ki* in Japanese, *chi* in Chinese, and *prana* in the tradition of yoga. In the West, we might refer to this flow of energy as the "subtle body" or the life force.

To "train one's stomach" (*hara* in Japanese, *tan tien* in Chinese) is to develop mastery over the center of the body, the origin of movement, the seat of emotion, of power, and of breath. To locate one's center of strength in the belly enables controlled being, whether in action or stillness. In martial arts training this is the starting point. The stance too is important; the foot meets the earth with aliveness and power, and with this comes a palpable energetic "grounding," a placement on the earth that serves to maximize the body's force.

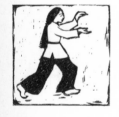

The *-dō* of the word *budō* (martial arts), *kendō* (the art of the sword), and *kyūdō* (the art of the bow), is a Japanese word meaning path or way. A *-dō* of any kind is a system of training by which one polishes oneself, and as such it is a noble path in which body and mind are one. In the strengthening of mind and body, two Buddhist sutras are employed as teachings: *Ekikin* (literally, "change/muscle"), which leads one to discipline and toughen the body, and *Senzui*, which refers to the polishing of the mind and the training of the will to achieve illumination from within.

The study of one of the many Eastern forms of physical training—yoga, *tai chi chuan*, *zazen*, *qigong*, aikidō, karatedō, among many others—can provide a path whereon a range of achievements is possible, with a beautiful, vital body being one outcome. A further benefit of most of these systems is their far-reaching health benefits. Emerging from a foundation of traditional medicine—with an underlying respect for the body's inner workings and the links among breath, energy meridians and points, the inner organs, the bones, and the muscles—a simple posture or movement can affect far more than just the parts of the body mechanically involved.

One may also devise one's own very individual physical system of training. Remember to attend to the following elements in your work: power, flexibility, and flow. Work to understand and increase your power, the strength of your muscles; work to keep your muscles and joints flexible and supple, with full range of movement; work to give your body the gift of flowing, sustained movement, the kind of action that activates breath, circulation, and heart. Train yourself in endurance as you work at these things. In everyday states of either stillness or action, train yourself to stand upon the earth with strength and harmony, with respect for the proper alignment of your body.

In the most practical terms, you should find a form of physical discipline that appeals strongly enough that perseverance will come naturally, because such a program is by its nature challenging. You must enjoy its difficulties. If existing disciplines don't seem attractive, design an individual program of movement that suits you. Read books, talk to experts, take movement classes of all kinds, and then create from such sources a way of your own. You should plan a minimum of four sessions per week, an hour each time. (If you can, devote 20 minutes on the remaining three days to a simple routine of basic exercises.)

For strength, 20 minutes should be devoted to some form of muscle-building exercise; for flexibility, there should be 20 minutes of stretches and isolation exercises; for cardiovascular training, there should be 20 minutes of some type of sustained activity like running, dancing, or swimming.

As you embark on your program, take time to examine your posture. Look in the mirror at your side view; study the way you habitually stand. Now correct it: lower the shoulders, lengthen the spine, tuck buttocks under. Lengthen the back of your neck toward the ceiling. Watch the results of this adjustment: your abdomen will appear flatter and your waist smaller; you will look taller; your chest will acquire new dimensions; even the line of your chin will appear more elegant. (Relax the muscles of your face, too!) At the beginning of each exercise session, reestablish this alignment.

Place your feet on the ground with solidity. Draw your breath in through your nostrils to fill your abdomen completely; exhale just as fully. Remind yourself that the body is a whole system, not disconnected parts. Try doing your movements with the stomach as origin. Enjoy what you are doing, but keep making your program more difficult as you progress. Allow your body to teach you, and you will be rewarded with a beautiful presence in both body and soul.

goodby cellulite

What, if anything, can be done to eliminate the scourge known as cellulite? Let's take a look at what happens when East and West join forces to battle it.

First, it is essential to understand that there is a difference between "normal" fat and cellulite. The former develops when more calories than necessary are consumed, and especially when the diet is unbalanced, containing large quantities of refined carbohydrates and fats. Unless there is some causal health factor (in which case medical treatment must be sought), the normal type of fat may be eliminated simply by eating less of the wrong foods and more of the right ones—those of a nutritious and health-giving nature—and exercising.

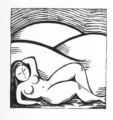

Cellulite looks different from regular fat, and it often exists in local deposits only on parts of the body, causing unsightly bulges even on bodies that are basically slim. Cellulite looks grainy and dimply, and areas where it has settled look "dead," lacking in suppleness. Women appear to be more prone than men to the development of cellulite.

While eliminating regular fat is largely a matter of diet, cellulite is different. Cellulite may diminish somewhat in response to a slimming regime, but in many cases the stuff will not budge. To understand what might be done in a cellulite situation, it is necessary to know the factors in its development.

During the 4–8 years it takes for cellulite to form, several things are happening. First, local blood circulation is poor, causing an accumulation of wastes and toxins and fluids as well as inefficient nourishment of the cells. The tissues swell and thicken as fluids build up, impeding circulation still further. The lymphatic system operates inefficiently.

To this condition is added an excess of fat in the fat cells, with nodules of collagen forming around the engorged cells, gradually causing hardened areas of lumpy, saggy tissue. An overweight condition exacerbates the situation by stimulating the further production of fat in the cells.

Once cellulite has formed in earnest, it is difficult to eliminate, but not impossible. The battle must be fought on all fronts: diet; surface exfoliation to facilitate penetration by active ingredients; surface application of substances that stimulate circulation, firm the tissues, or eliminate excess fluids; massage and scrubbing to stimulate circulation and break up the hard nodules of collagen peculiar to cellulite; exercise; and the encouragement of fluid- and toxin-elimination and the stimulation of the general circulation through specially chosen dietary supplements, beverages, and foods. Because the program that is recommended for cellulite elimination may also be followed for prevention, even the cellulite-free body will benefit.

The traditional Japanese body scrub, carried out with a *tawashi* or a wooden-backed body-scrubbing brush, is thought to be one of the best ways to prevent the formation of cellulite, and it can also contribute to its elimination. Whether one chooses a stiff-bristled brush, a gentle loofah sponge, or even an old-fashioned *tenugui*, the scrubbing process should be both vigorous and thorough, while care is taken to avoid bruising tissues. Tender areas require a softer touch; moles and blemishes must be avoided. Brush strokes begin at the extremities and move toward the heart.

While the Japanese body scrub is practiced as part of the prebath washing ritual and generally calls for soap or a cleansing powder—rice bran or bean powder—other traditional treatment recipes may be used in scrubbing.

For cellulite, one of the best is the ginger juice rubdown, prepared by grating one large ginger root, then squeezing the gratings through cheesecloth to obtain juice, into which one dips one's warm, moist *tenugui* for scrubbing. Ginger is a stimulant to the circulation and a potent purifier as well. A word of warning to those with sensitive skins: ginger may cause burning or irritation to those susceptible, in which case it must be diluted or avoided altogether.

The Japanese scrub, when carried out as outlined earlier, is said to stimulate the *tsubo* (pressure points) as well as exfoliate the skin and stimulate circulation. Because the *tsubo* are manipulated in order to balance and revitalize all functions of the body, it is likely that all body malfunctions, of which cellulite is one, will diminish. A soak in a hot bath further purifies and tones the tissues.

Certainly, a good professional massage or a vigorous self-massage, with the hands and fingertips on trouble spots, can be of enormous benefit to a body with stubborn cellulite. Whatever method is chosen, the program should be practiced once daily—twice, even, for the zealous—with unerring faithfulness. When such a regime is coupled with the application of special creams, gels, oils, or serums, results should begin to be seen within a month or so.

Cosmetic store shelves are overflowing these days with a fascinating genre of beauty product: the body-shapers, toners, slimmers, and fat-melters.

outside

anticellulite body scrub

ginger rub for cellulite

It seems an exciting, futuristic approach to refining the silhouette—just massage in some cream, gel, or oil, and watch the plump spots vanish! Is this possible? Coffee, tea, ivy, seaweed, horse chestnut, sandalwood, ginkgo, and lavender … the list of active ingredients being used in the most advanced external slimming products reads like a rather offbeat menu of nouvelle cuisine.

Although the products themselves are formulated with the latest scientific technology and often employ extremely sophisticated processes for tissue penetration or time-sustained effects, the ingredients that actually do the work of fat-fighting are nearly all botanicals.

Many of the cheaper products are very simple: they bring heat to the tissues or are diuretic, antiswelling agents that one applies to areas of bloating. A hot bath with added seaweed, salt, or even tea leaves can supply similar effects.

The more expensive products offer a more comprehensive approach. Basically, most of these products stimulate blood circulation and encourage fat cells to release excess fat. Other actions include the elimination of fluids and toxins, the reduction of inflammation, the oxygenation and nourishment of the cells, tissue repair, and the restoration of suppleness and tone to tissues and veins.

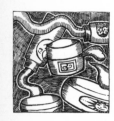

How do these products work? Read the list of ingredients and you are likely to find caffeine. Caffeine, like theophylline (tea extract), is used for its stimulating properties; it acts as a trigger, setting off the fat-burning process within the cells. The fact that both caffeine and theophylline are diuretics means they are useful in drawing out excess fluids as well.

Another of the popular botanical extracts used in slimming products is ivy. Ivy tones and firms the skin, soothes and relaxes tissues, draws out fluids, and is said to help eliminate stretch marks.

Other ingredients include: seaweed extracts, employed for their draining action on wastes and toxins, their high iodine content (important in fat-burning), and their toning, diuretic properties; *Centella asiatica*, or Gotu Kola, which stimulates tissue repair, acts as a tonic to the veins, reduces swelling, and stimulates the circulation; and ginkgo leaves, said to be instrumental in increasing blood flow and in combating the free radicals that hasten the aging process.

Also included in the antifat cocktail may be oligo-elements, synthetic amino acids such as *L. carnitine*, butcher's broom, sage, rosemary, horse chestnut, horsetail, lavender, geranium, sandalwood, and patchouli, each with its own unique properties.

When applied religiously once or twice daily, with the appropriate massage tool or scrubber, these sophisticated slimming products based on ancient herbal ingredients can be useful in the battle against cellulite. The person with ordinary fat might just as well ignore them, although some may be useful in helping to eliminate fluids where water retention is a problem.

Traditional Japanese techniques for fighting fat externally use seaweed, ginger, chrysanthemum greens, and *daikon* radish. The fact that cellulite is an uncommon problem in Japan does not mean that there are no treatments for it. In fact, built into the Japanese diet and the Japanese beauty tradition is an extraordinary panoply of cellulite-preventers. And where this sort of "abnormal fat" is concerned, prevention is all. Cellulite takes years to develop, and once it has settled in comfortably it is very stubborn about giving up its conquered territory. Best not to get it in the first place.

The traditional Japanese diet places an emphasis on purification; translated into down-to-earth terms this means foods and beverages that encourage the elimination of fats, wastes, toxins, and excess fluids—all important components in the cellulite-making process.

Foods like *daikon,* burdock, ginger, *umeboshi* (pickled plums), *shiitake* mushrooms, and soybean products all act to improve circulation and elimination functions. *Mugi-cha* (roasted barley tea), oolong tea, *polei* or *puerh* tea, and *hatomugi-cha* (pearl barley tea) are cleansing diuretic teas that encourage slenderness by washing away fats and excess water. Even ordinary green tea possesses stimulating, diuretic properties.

The Japanese bath and body-scrubbing ritual provides external stimulation to both general and local circulation. The bath, which warms the body and induces sweating, may be preceded by a tea that will further encourage elimination: mashed *umeboshi* in a cup of *ban-cha* (a coarse, basic tea), or ginger juice (obtained by grating ginger and squeezing through cheesecloth) in *ban-cha.*

The body scrub, practiced with a stiff-bristled brush such as a *tawashi* or a wooden-backed scrub brush, has the same effect upon the body as expensive modern anticellulite massagers. The scrub, as described earlier, is always carried out with respect for delicate areas, and proceeds from the extremities in long strokes moving toward the heart.

The purifying diet, the daily bath soak, and the daily bath scrub are an effective combination in the prevention of cellulite. If cellulite already exists, to these practices may be added some potent baths: the ginger bath, the chrysanthemum bath, and the *sake* bath. Each of these stimulates the circulation, raises body temperature (scientists have found that areas of cellulite are colder than adjacent areas, an indication of poor circulation), and strongly activates elimination processes. These baths should be taken at most once or twice a week.

inside

cleansing umeboshi-ban-cha *tea*

cleansing ginger-ban-cha *tea*

outside

anticellulite body scrub

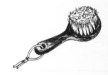

Prepare the ginger bath by grating a larger ginger root, then squeezing the gratings through cheesecloth to obtain juice. The juice is added to a hot bath, in which one should soak for 20 minutes. For the chrysanthemum bath, use edible chrysanthemum greens. Wrap generous bunches of the greens in a large muslin square and tie it closed with an elastic. Tie the bundle to the bath faucet when filling the tub; for the first 10 or 15 minutes run only hot water into the tub and through the leaves, infusing them. Later, adjust the temperature of the water, then soak for 20 minutes or so.

The *sake* bath is prepared by filling the tub with hot water and adding 2 liters/2 quarts of *sake*. Soak for as long as possible. This bath will not only deep-cleanse the pores and stimulate the circulation but will leave the skin as soft and smooth as a *mochi* rice dumpling.

In the prevention and treatment of cellulite, then, one need not invest a small fortune in sophisticated creams and scientific massage tools. It is enough to follow the simple Japanese system: purifying diet, bath soak, and bath scrub.

The way of eating that is recommended for one who is burdened with cellulite follows the simple principles of healthy nourishment, and thus may be undertaken as well by anyone wishing to maintain a slender body and youthful-looking skin. It is not necessary to follow a strict daily menu-plan (such ambitious regimes rarely endure in real life) but just to eliminate certain foods from one's diet.

Remove all full-fat dairy products, red meats, refined carbohydrates, and sweets. Restrict alcohol and spicy, salty, and fried foods. Cut down on caffeine; don't smoke. Eliminate processed foods and those containing preservatives, artificial color, and flavoring agents. Foods which are cleansing should be included in the diet: *daikon* radish, *umeboshi* (pickled plums), ginger, *shiso* (perilla leaves), parsley. Natural diuretic teas like *hatomugi-cha* (pearl barley tea), oolong tea, and *mugi-cha* (roasted barley tea) may be taken, along with plenty of good water and lots of fresh, high-fiber, high-water produce.

By removing the chemicals, dairy products, heavy meats, white flour, white sugar, and alcohol from one's diet—or substantially reducing the intake of these substances—one not only becomes naturally slender, but the system is cleansed of the toxins and fats that contribute to cellulite formation, rapid aging, and a multitude of health and beauty problems. The body is allowed to function as it is designed to, with efficient toxin-elimination, and smoothly running circulatory, metabolic, and lymph systems. Whether one has cellulite or not, the diet should be carefully examined, and all foods that threaten the body's delicate balance are then best banished or restricted.

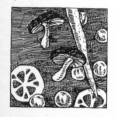

With diet, the other essential element in creating and maintaining a healthy body is of course exercise. Cellulite may be battled by any comprehensive exercise program—one that includes stretching, muscle-strengthening, and cardiovascular training. Although the particular area affected by cellulite should be focused on specifically with spot exercises, without all three forms of full-body exercise the circulation and elimination systems will suffer, as will the silhouette.

changes

With menstrual cycles, pregnancy, birth, and menopause all enacting their transformations upon us, the one constant of feminine physical existence is change. Pregnancy and weight loss can result in stretched-out skin that lacks elasticity and tone. Women's bodies bear the transformations of pregnancy and birth with varying degrees of ease; as women wait until their late 30s, and longer, to have babies, when the skin is often naturally less elastic due to aging, postpartum complaints of severe loss of tone, especially in the abdominal region, have become more common. What can be done to remedy the problem?

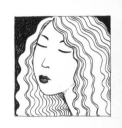

First, it is important to prepare for the physical stresses of pregnancy and birth by taking precautionary measures. During pregnancy, weight gain should be moderate. Regular exercise should be a priority, with attention given to strengthening the muscles of abdomen, back, and hips. Don't shun external devices—there is a lot to be said for the traditional Japanese belly-band, which effectively holds and supports the growing belly as its weight begins to exert a gravitational pull on skin and muscles. The Western equivalent is the pregnancy girdle.

Massage the skin with tonic oils such as lavender, lemongrass, or frankincense. Ingest herbal teas that promote skin and muscle tone: buckwheat, burdock, seaweed, raspberry leaf. Devise a diet rich in tonic foods and minerals, poor in empty calories, sweets, and hard-to-digest ingredients. Among the nutrients that may contribute to the maintenance of skin tone are zinc, vitamins B_6, B_2, and B_{12}, iron, folic acid, and vitamins E and C.

Note: if you choose to embark on a new dietary regime when pregnant, always consult a physician or qualified nutritionist. Not only is it important to determine the balance of foods appropriate for pregnancy, but each individual has her own special needs as well as potential allergies or sensitivities. Always check herbal teas and supplements for possible contraindications and to make sure you are not allergic to any of the ingredients.

If you find that six weeks after giving birth your body skin seems to have lost tone, it's time to begin taking whatever steps you can to ameliorate the situation. There are three important ways you can make a difference: diet, exercise, and external treatment. Dietary measures continue as for prebirth; one takes the same herbal teas and supplements and cuts down on all that is unnecessary for health. Exercise should be appropriately rigorous, preferably daily sessions of stretching, strengthening, and cardiovascular training. External applications of oils and toning products should be supplemented by full-body abrasive scrubs with loofah, brush, or friction sloughing towel. Sauna and steambath can help the body to function more efficiently, as can hot-spring soaks or the *ofuro.*

Women "bounce back" at different rates, so don't despair if your body does not return to normal as quickly as you'd like. The idea is to create the ideal conditions for the physiological system to repair itself and regenerate. It can take time, depending on factors such as amount of weight gain, basic metabolism, original muscle and skin tone, and age.

Professional toning treatments and specialized massage can provide good adjuncts to your personal three-part program. *Shiatsu* can also help the body to function properly. I would say that a good year should be devoted to this kind of serious regimen—though certainly in some cases results will be seen in a matter of weeks or months. If a severe problem with tone persists beyond this time, you can consider the final option, the last-resort surgical solution of a tummy-tuck. In some countries, such an operation is covered by insurance plans, often for cases where the abdominal muscles have ruptured and are causing a subsequent condition of weakness and pain.

As we become better informed about beauty and health, we can make a difference in what happens to our bodies. Judging by the way women look these days, I'd say the chances are good we can all actually improve with age!

simple *shiatsu* for a beautiful body

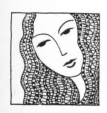

Most of the *tsubo* connected to body vitality and overall condition are located upon the body's larger expanses: the back, the chest, and the rest of the torso. For the beginner, locating such points with accuracy can be problematic. To find them exactly often requires a knowledge of the location of the underlying bones, tendons, muscles, or internal organs. In this section, therefore, I present only one easily located foot *tsubo* and a description of two important general areas of *tsubo*, one on the back of the body and one on the front.

The *tsubo* in these areas are of particular importance in maintaining the vitality and general health of the body. Stimulation of them will help to restore the proper flow of energy, or *ki*, promote self-healing of imbalances, and open areas of mental, physical, or emotional energy-blockage. The improvement of the circulation, the relief of stress and mental or physical fatigue, the toning and strengthening of internal organs, the elimination of toxins, the improvement in nervous-system functioning, weight regulation, and the toning of muscles and skin are further effects.

The application of heat to these areas, with the aid of a hairdryer, heating pad, hot poultice, or pocket handwarmer, is a good way to stimulate the various *tsubo* concerned. Brush stimulation during prebath scrubbing is also useful, and a general massage can be extraordinarily effective, particularly for the *tsubo* in the back area.

For finger pressure, the recommended techniques for the area of the chest and torso are the open palm push, the three-finger push (forefinger, middle finger, and ring finger pads together in a point) using either one hand alone or two hands together, and the two-finger push (forefinger and middle finger pads together). For the back, both thumbs may be used to apply pressure simultaneously to pairs of *tsubo*. For the sole of the foot, one thumb may be placed atop the other for pushing, or the two-finger push with forefinger and middle finger pressed together may be used. The 3–5-second, 3-set push to each point may be executed 2–3 times daily, as described earlier in the book.

Massage devices like the split bamboo for the feet or a wooden back-massage bar upon which one lies, rolling back and forth slightly, are useful for some of the *tsubo* described here.

As stated earlier, an expert practitioner should be consulted for further exploration of *shiatsu*, acupuncture, or moxabustion. As well, there are many movement systems based on the flow of *ki*; *tai chi chuan*, the ancient Chinese system of breathing and exercise, is one of the most well known in the West. In Japan, along with *tai chi* are practiced *dō-in* breathing, a simple system of coordinated breathing and movements, and *taikyoku-ken* stick breathing, which is similar but makes use of a pole that is held and moved in harmony with the body. The taking in of *ki* through regulated breathing is considered to be of fundamental importance in achieving and maintaining a state of vitality and balance.

YŪ-SEN

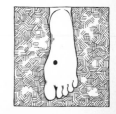

This point is located on the sole of the foot directly behind the ball of the big toe. To press there in the direction of the center of the sole is said to have a profound effect on the energy welling up from within, the name for this *tsubo* meaning "welling spring." One's vitality, stamina, and basic life force are stimulated by this point, which is also said to improve functions of the female reproductive system.

BACK *tsubo*

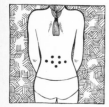

There are several important *tsubo* located in the waist area at the back, on the spine and at either side of the spine. MEI-MON is located in the center of the spine, just slightly below the waistline. Just above and to either side of the spine, $4\,1/2$ cm/$1\,5/8$ inches from the center line, is JIN-YU, on the waistline and at the same level as the bottom edge of the lowest rib. Above JIN-YU is SAN-SHŌ-YU, one vertebrae higher along the same vertical line. About 9 cm/$3\,1/2$ inches from the center of the spine, slightly higher than the waistline, level with the top edge of the lowest rib, is SHI-SHITSU. The beginner can best stimulate these *tsubo* by applying pressure, heat, or massage to the whole general area of the waist, concentrating on the areas to either side of the spine. One may place one's clenched fists under one's back while reclining, then move the body slightly to create a massaging effect. Rubbing the palms together 36 times, then placing the hands on the area is another technique. Attaching a handwarmer or a heating pad to the area will supply heat stimulation. Using a stiff brush to stimulate the area of the *tsubo*, keeping the area flexible through waist-bending and -turning exercises, and protecting the area from chills by dressing the waist warmly (during wintertime or in times of fatigue or illness) are all commonly practiced methods in Japan for maintaining vitality by attending to these *tsubo*. Simply applying strong thumb pressure to the area will also be of benefit. The *tsubo* here are important for the body's overall condition, release of tension, digestion, sexual functions, the maintenance of clear facial skin and firm body tone, relaxation and restful sleep, and vitality.

FRONT *tsubo*

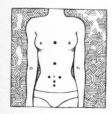

Along the central front line of the body, running from below the navel to exactly between the nipples on the breastbone, there are several important *tsubo* for energy and vitality. KAN-GEN, located 9 cm/$3\,1/2$ inches below the navel, is a point that can be helpful in clearing the skin of pimples, regulating the weight, improving circulation, toning the reproductive system, and making the legs more beautiful, as well as increasing general vitality. 3 cm/$1\,1/8$ inches above KAN-GEN is SEKI-MON. Above that point, just $1\,1/2$ cm/$1/2$ inch to either side of the navel and slightly below it, is KŌ-YU. CHŪ-KAN is located 12 cm/$4\,1/2$ inches above the navel, and DAN-CHŪ is at the midpoint between the two nipples. All of these points are useful for improving the overall condition, vitality, and circulation. To stimulate them, simple finger pressure may be applied, along with brush stimulation or the application of heat. Except for the point located around the navel (KŌ-YU), all of these *tsubo* are single points along one central line.

simple beauty for men

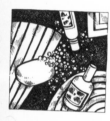

When it comes to beauty, there is a subtle but pervasive cultural bias in East as well as West that tends to tip the balance in the female direction. Men are not supposed to be concerned with appearance. The same skewed bias is applied to the woman of intelligence, of course: the implication is that to be attentive to beauty is to be superficial. As a result, there is a kind of embarassed subterfuge about the whole thing. The fact is, men are well acquainted with their mirrors but often at a bit of a loss about what to do with themselves in this regard. Thus, for he (or she) who would embark on a beauty exploration but is lacking in the most basic information, what follows is a lighthearted primer. These are emergency tips and instant tricks for rapid transformation. When you see what's possible, you may be inspired to go further.

THE SMILE: This is simple but effective, the very fastest illuminator of your appearance. To smile is also physiologically relaxing, with a proven chemical effect on the brain, as well as being highly alluring to others.

THE WHITE SHIRT: There is no man alive whose appearance is not measurably improved by the wearing of a white shirt. If it is a very good white shirt and it fits well (roomy is far better than tight), then it need not even be ironed. A pure white well-designed rumpled white shirt projects a rare combination of fascinating qualities: you will look nonchalant, modern, clean, and classy. But the primary virtue of the white shirt is that it makes your face look fantastic. This goes for women too.

THE GOOD HAIRCUT: Far less important than the actual style of your hair is that the haircut be superb. Short hair needs a trim about once a month; if the hair is worn long then every two months or so. One must shampoo the hair regularly. If you are going to go to the trouble of wearing a discernible style (ponytail, slicked-back, partially shaved, whatever), then, of course, you must keep your hair even more scrupulously clean and conditioned, for everybody will always be looking closely at your head. But men's hair must look great in an accidental way, so never let anyone see you applying mousse.

THE GLOW: The easiest safe way to suddenly glow with healthy, vital color is to use tanning gel or a bronze-tinted face cream. It's not make-up, really, just a hint of color and some nourishing moisture to give your skin a nice luster. If you're reluctant to go into a store and buy the stuff, you can try eating lots of carrots and tangerines, but then you'll have orange hands and feet as well. Another pretend-tanning method is to soak your face daily in strong tea.

OTHER POINTS: You're off to a good start if you've got the smile, the shirt, the haircut, and the glow. To be a beautiful man is not so complicated. But there are some small matters of style that you might also consider:

SHOES: Avoid bad shoes. Shoes should not be cheap or strange-looking, and they should possess no giant buckles, tassels, or high heels unless that's the kind of person you are. POSTURE: Only Marlon Brando was ever allowed to slouch, and then only when wearing an old white T-shirt. Slouching is forbidden for everybody else. NAIL POLISH: Many people are suspicious of men wearing nail polish, even the transparent kind. Just buffing is fine.

Actually, the basics of masculine beauty and feminine beauty are not so different—there are only a few areas of divergence. Men have facial hair to consider, men usually can't conceal their faces behind lots of make-up, men don't easily get cellulite, and—the essential difference—men have got to look beautiful by accident.

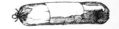

The most important thing in masculine beauty, as in the feminine version, is to start out with good raw materials. You need good skin, good hair, good muscle tone, and plenty of energy. A lot of people try to get these things by taking vitamin supplements, but this won't work. You have to eat well, exercise, and get enough sleep.

Let's look at the easier factor first: sleep. It's incredible how refreshing, rejuvenating, and relaxing sleep can be. If one has trouble getting to sleep or staying asleep, it's probably due to stress, which is a condition that is largely improved by another factor:

Exercise. That exercise will not only relax the mind and body but produce good health, firm muscles, and great skin tone, makes it a beauty-factor of major importance. Exercise should attend to three areas: strength, flexibility, and endurance. A program should include stretching, vigorous use of the muscles, and something like running, cycling, or racquetball that gets your heart pumping faster for at least 20 minutes straight. The Japanese tradition offers the option of serious martial arts study, which will give a complete workout in each of the three important categories. Any sports or exercise program should be practiced as frequently as possible—every other day or more often, depending on the sport. A cross-training program of several different activities is best. And to fuel all this activity, your primary source of energy:

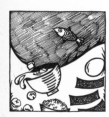

Food. Where diet is concerned, the most important thing to know is that you've got to eat real food. Eliminate all the refined and processed items and concentrate on whole grains, vegetables, fruits, the great Japanese soybean foods (tofu, *nattō*, *miso*, *okara*), nuts and seeds, seaweed, eggs, grilled fish and chicken, and you'll be pretty well nourished. In fact, if you start the day with a standard Japanese breakfast of rice, *miso* soup, grilled fish, *nori* seaweed, pickles, and maybe a raw egg, replacing the white rice with brown, you'll be taking in an amazing abundance of skin- and hair- and energy-nourishing vitamins and minerals, plenty of B vitamins, lots of iron, sulphur, and calcium, high-quality low-fat protein, and not too many calories. By comparison, the standard Western breakfast seems quite begrudging of nutrients.

What about all those Japanese and Chinese energy-drinks for men that are on the market in Asia? Some of them offer potent doses of vitamins and, depending on the brand, quite a bit of *kampō*—Oriental herbs—which can have a beneficial tonic effect on the system. Some, however, deliver their kick with a huge amount of caffeine, so unless that's what you want, check the label carefully. And by the way, most of the concoctions may also be drunk by women—though certain *kampō* (reindeer horn, snake extract, sea horse, praying mantis chrysalis, and so forth.) are traditionally meant for men only. Ingredients like garlic, ginseng, *shiitake* mushrooms, and ginkgo are for both sexes.

Along with the quick tricks for looking better fast—white shirt, tanning gel—and the fundamentals of long-term handsome healthiness—sleeping, eating, exercise—it's necessary to develop expertise in daily maintenance. This is perhaps the most mysterious aspect for many men, dealing as it does with the realm of bottles, jars, creams, lotions, soaps, serums, and cosmetics counter salespeople, always exhilarated by the sight of a male shopper. Many men avoid the whole problem by opting out entirely. But if you want to take things into your own hands, this guide's for you: what you need and why you need it, in the simplest terms.

face care

The essential steps in face care are these: cleansing, shaving, toning, and moisturizing, with an occasional special treatment applied as needed.

CLEANSING: The most important aspect of this step is thoroughness. Try rice bran or a good cleansing bar.

SHAVING: A few drops of camellia or almond oil rubbed onto the skin can give a smoother shave.

TONING: This is the step that refreshes and tones the skin, removes any cleansing-product residues, and restores acid balance. The simplest natural method is to rub a well-steeped tea bag over the skin, which will tone it and gradually give it a subtle tanned look. Loofah-vine water is also wonderful for toning and acts as an oil-free moisturizer as well.

MOISTURIZING: This comes after toning, and is important not only for skin comfort and suppleness but for prevention of dryness, roughness, and early wrinkles and lines. Again, camellia oil is good, or aloe gel if you don't like oil.

TREATMENTS: Men tend to like clay packs, but any of the face packs mentioned in this book will work wonders for skin.

outside

rice bran face wash

camellia oil preshave

tea bag facial tonic

*loofah-vine water
    facial tonic*

camellia oil moisturizer

aloe gel moisturizer

hair care

This is simple: shampoo, condition, and occasionally apply a treatment pack. Try any recipe given in this book. For dandruff, be attentive to diet (see section on "simple hair beauty" for details on hair-beautifying foods); after shampooing, tone with vinegar; practice scalp massage.

body care

For the body, the steps are cleansing, moisturizing, and an occasional treatment bath.

CLEANSING: Any good soap will do, but try using a scrub brush or loofah for maximum exfoliation, cleansing, and stimulation of the circulation and *tsubo*.

MOISTURIZING: Camellia oil.

TREATMENT BATH: Try any recipe given in this book.

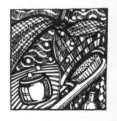

🌿

There you have it: eight steps a day, with three extra occasional ones—just eleven steps to follow in the art of basic masculine beauty. Simple.

For women, wrinkles; for men, hair loss—these two greatly

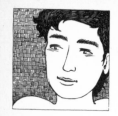

feared conditions inspire the expenditure of masses of money on the part of cosmetics companies and individuals in search of the magical cure. In both cases, men and women who feel strongly enough opt for surgical refurbishment, and even that drastic measure does not always give entirely satisfactory results.

It is a well-known fact that perceptions of beauty are cultural and subject to change and so one may hope that people will someday acquire the wisdom to see a different kind of appeal in their laugh lines and their wider, higher foreheads.

Already, changes in the concept of beauty are visible in our younger-looking and longer-lived population: professional beauties like Lauren Hutton who pronounce their wrinkles to be well loved and not subject to renovation by the knife, gray- and silver-haired models in the pages of fashion magazines. These are the vanguard, the first signs of a shift in perceptions of what is beautiful—and most importantly, in the long-held idea that beauty is youth (smooth skin, thick hair), which has caused frustration and despair to many.

It is curious, though, that men still find it difficult to accept gracefully the fact of hair loss. Male-pattern baldness occurs as the result of high levels of male hormones—usually androgen—in the system. Androgen is associated with virility, and thus it is that many women find bald men sexy, in spite of the general assumption among men that the opposite is true. Those who are connoisseurs of such things say that bald men are good lovers, and the balder the better. No small compensation for a bit of hair loss!

For those who are not compelled by this information to rush out for a complete head-shave, and who still want to know what might be done to hold onto any remaining hair or to make what they have thicker, following are some natural remedies that may be worth a try.

outside

oil scalp-massage for falling hair

sesame & ginger scalp-massage for falling hair

loquat & ash & fruit juice treatment for falling hair

One aromatherapy approach consists of daily scalp massage with a specially prepared oil. Here is the recipe: 60 ml/2 oz of carrier oil (grapeseed or avocado), 1 tsp wheat germ oil, 15 drops essential oil of rosemary, 15 drops essential oil of cedar wood. This treatment followed for six to eight months is said to allay thinning and even to revive shutdown follicles.

The traditional Japanese remedy is sesame oil and a dash of ginger juice massaged regularly into the scalp, while the Chinese might recommend the juice of loquat leaf (*biwa* in Japanese) mixed with wood ashes and fresh fruit juice, applied to the scalp and dried in the sun.

inside

alfalfa & nettle for hair vigor

The internal approach relies upon the nourishment of a good diet especially rich in B vitamins and all the important minerals. Further, a twice daily dose of the herbs alfalfa and nettle is said to restore vigor to the hair growth process.

Best is to choose one external regimen, follow it faithfully for six months at least, all the while consuming vast quantities of whole grains, brewer's yeast, wheat germ, and extravagant raw-vegetable salads dressed with extra-virgin olive oil or cold-pressed safflower oil. Certainly, try as well to cultivate an appreciation for the high-visibility message conveyed by the head that is bald. Be grateful that you have an entirely uncontrived way to flaunt your masculinity!

words found on a japanese teacup

1. Eat less meat and eat more vegetables.
2. Eat less salt and have more vinegar.
3. Eat less sugar and eat more fruit.
4. Eat a small amount of food slowly and chew it thoroughly.
5. Dress lightly and bathe often.
6. Control your chatting, and practice something regularly.
7. Control your desires, and often give alms to others.
8. Don't be anxious, and sleep soundly.
9. Don't use a car, use your feet.
10. Don't be angry, but always smiling.

inside/outside beauty

discipline & practice

As good health is essential to beauty, good eating and good sleeping are primary in the pursuit of loveliness. It is common knowledge, in Japan as elsewhere in the world, that without eating nourishing, purifying food in the proper harmonies and correct amounts, and that without sleeping long and well enough each night, not only will vitality and strength diminish but the skin, the hair, and the nails will suffer, growing dull, rough, and lifeless. In eating and sleeping, indulged in as pleasurable rituals essential to life, the application of discipline must be present as well, for balance. In the spirit of Zen training we can make use of these daily rituals as a means to a deeper, fuller link between mind and body.

"Eat this—it's good for your beauty" are words often heard in Asia. Food-knowledge seems deeper than in the West; everyone knows which foods give you beautiful skin or shinier hair, or slim you down, or purify your system of toxins, or encourage stamina, strength, and good blood.

In the Japanese cuisine, flavors are simple, presentation is stylish, but austere; the eating of the food takes far less time than its lengthy preparation. The aesthetic elements of the eating ritual—colors, shapes, compositions, harmonies between food and serving dish, between the ingredients themselves, and between foods and the season and occasion—are of the greatest importance. At a Japanese meal, the spirit is nurtured as well as the body.

The act of eating, for women, is also an exercise in grace. 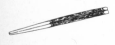 Foods are presented so that mouthfuls may be small and dainty, and the chopsticks are manipulated with care—held with the proper form and a light touch. Women lift food to the mouth elegantly, avoiding the lips so as not to mark the chopsticks with lipstick, then chew with unobtrusive tiny movements. While eating, the posture is perfect: back straight, arms close to the sides, all movements quiet, soft, and contained. There is an air of relaxed stillness to the body, and it is the result of training that begins in childhood.

Underlying the fulfillment of the three most basic human needs—eating, sleeping, and protection from the elements—is a sense of the need for discipline. Buddhist monks undergo the deprivation of these basic needs to strengthen the spirit, and even ordinary people may pursue such spiritual hardening at times. Simply applying one's attention to one's actions is another way of achieving the same result.

The Japanese regard exposure to cold as wonderfully strengthening to both the physical and spiritual being. An ice-cold dousing of water outdoors in the wintertime, walking barefoot through snow and ice, spending the winter in an unheated room wearing little more than one might wear in July: such practices, while not overwhelmingly popular, do claim a large number of devotees.

Improvement in circulation, stronger, more resistant skin, and a generally tougher, well-tempered organism are said to be the results of these practices that expose one to the cold. And with the physical discipline comes a spiritual discipline that arises from the victory of endurance. Each is one side of the coin in the quest for a purer, stronger self.

A spirit of discipline may be put to the service of beauty in many ways, not only in eating properly and sparingly, in sleeping right, and in learning to endure discomfort, but in the many areas where conscious cultivation may be useful: the way one moves, speaks, and interacts with others, the expression on one's face, the feelings and thoughts that inhabit the mind and heart. It is in this last area that beauty is determined.

medicine foods & teas

True beauty comes from within.

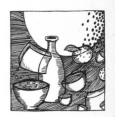

While we may interpret this as referring first and foremost to character, to the gentle luminosity of one who has what in Shinto is termed " a polished heart," there are actually several layers of meaning to the old saying. Also of importance in beauty are one's state of mind and the condition of one's health. Depression, high stress, lack of energy, and a diet deficient in certain essential nutrients will all act as very effective barriers to beauty.

In Japan, China, and other areas of Asia, specific medicinal foods have long been incorporated into the diet for their tonic, curative benefits. In beauty, the holistic approach is the traditional one: to effect a treatment, active substances are taken internally and applied externally, with the regime a long-term one of several months.

This ancient wisdom is so integral a part of the Asian beauty/health tradition that it is taken for granted. In examining one's diet with beauty in mind, first determine whether certain important basic nutrients are present.

Recommended for beauty: essential fatty acids, along with vitamin E; magnesium; zinc; manganese; copper; and selenium; folic acid; vitamins A and B. Ideally these elements are present in our daily diet. One should consider a basically well-rounded and nutritious diet—consisting of whole foods and little in the way of processed items—as fundamental to any successful beauty/health regimen. Let's have a closer look at what is needed and why.

Unsaturated Fatty Acids: Most of us don't get enough of this nutrient, especially dieters, who often restrict their intake of fats. The fatty acids are most commonly encountered in the form of liquid vegetable oils. A deficiency will be seen in the skin: dryness, loss of elasticity, thickness, and poor resistance. The hair will show a similar diminishment in healthy appearance.

If taken as a supplement, the fatty acids should be combined with vitamin E at mealtimes. Some nutritionists recommend two hundred mg of fatty acid with 100–200 IU of E as a daily dosage. Even simpler, include fatty acids in your diet by eating wheat germ, lecithin, sesame seeds, or a cold-pressed vegetable oil such as safflower, soy, or corn. A daily salad with an oil dressing or a couple of spoonfuls of lecithin or wheat germ on cereal will supply the necessary nutrients. There is no such thing as a toxic overdose, though excessive amounts of these oils will certainly lead to weight gain and possible metabolic disturbances.

Vitamin E: A deficiency will result in a shrinkage of collagen, among other things. Even if vitamin E is present in your diet, it may be destroyed in the body if you drink chlorinated water and breathe polluted air.

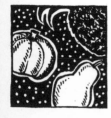

This vitamin speeds up skin healing, hunts down the dreaded "free radicals" and helps to destroy them (in the process counteracting premature skin aging and wrinkling), speeds up the formation of new skin cells, and gives elasticity to your skin.

Recommended dosages vary from 12 IU to 400 IU daily, and individual needs should be considered in determining proper dosage. There is some danger of overdosage; those with high blood pressure or chronic rheumatic heart disease must be very cautious. The best way to include vitamin E in your diet is to take wheat germ, cold-pressed vegetable oils, whole raw seeds and nuts, or soybeans on a regular basis.

Zinc: one of the most important elements for the human body. A deficiency is responsible for skin lesions, a breakdown of connective tissues, and the weakening of collagen and elastin fibers. Zinc speeds up the healing and scarring process in wounds and acne, gives tone to the muscles, and improves skin pigmentation. It can prevent stretch marks.

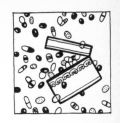

White marks in your fingernails, a dull complexion, or dull, limp hair may all be signs of a lack of zinc. A deficiency in zinc (and vitamin E as well) is often partially due to the flour-milling process; in order to eat pure white bread we sacrifice a huge number of beneficial elements. If you take zinc supplements, beware of an overdose: too much can result in nausea, vomiting, and diarrhea. Between 15–50 mg a day is the usual recommendation, the precise dosage to be determined by a nutritionist familiar with one's individual needs. To include zinc in your diet consume protein, whole grains, brewer's yeast, wheat bran, wheat germ, pumpkin seeds, soy lecithin, soybeans, and a variety of other foods.

Magnesium in proper quantities can delay the signs of aging—the loss of skin tone, loss of hair, the weakening of nails, bones, and teeth. This nutrient is also useful in preventing the infection of pimples. There is said to be no risk of overdose; 550 mg–2 g may be taken daily. Fresh green vegetables, raw wheat germ, soybeans, milk, whole grains, seafoods, figs, corn, apples, and oil-rich seeds and nuts contain magnesium.

Folic acid, part of the B complex group, plays an important role in cell multiplication. This nutrient will delay the appearance of gray hairs and prevent skin dryness. Folic acid is present in green leafy vegetables but is easily destroyed by heat and light. Liver and brewer's yeast are good sources. (Dried liver tablets are an easy way to get folic acid. If taken as a supplement, 2–4 mg daily is a common recommendation.) Other sources include barley, brown rice and other whole grains, dates, split peas, lentils, root vegetables, salmon, and tuna.

Thus, if you wish to obtain the ingredients essential to beauty by eating the right foods, you might include the following in your diet on a regular basis: wheat germ, seeds (sesame or pumpkin), vegetable oils (safflower, corn, or soy), liver, whole grains, green leafy vegetables, dried legumes, seafoods, and seaweed. Simultaneously, undertake a reduction in those foods that contain nothing but fat, sugar, and empty calories. (Remember to consult your doctor or nutritionist before embarking on any new nutritional program.)

In Europe, the big beauty thrust in recent years has been the development of beauty capsules, tablets, and pills. The idea of internal beauty is at the vanguard and is even considered revolutionary. The concept—that inner beauty is the foundation of outer—is acknowledged as a great new advance in the devising of potential anti-aging treatments, sun protection products, and products for the beauty of skin, hair, nails, and body contours.

A look at the labels of the European beauty pills reveals

ingredients like beta carotene, wheat germ oil, rice bran oil, salmon oil, fish bone, soy oil, and other alimentary substances. Many of the active ingredients are found in the average Japanese diet but not in the average European one; they are said to possess anti-aging, anticancer, and hair- and skin-strengthening properties.

That the effectiveness of the active elements has been firmly established through scientific research would come as no surprise to a Japanese grandmother.

What are some of the Japanese medicinal foods specifically taken as beautifiers?

Starting at the top, with hair, we can make it healthier by faithfully consuming seaweed, sesame seeds, shrimp, and *shiso* (perilla). The last two foods are thought to be helpful to those who have a falling hair problem, and they also improve the circulation and health of the scalp. Seaweed and sesame are generally useful, giving hair luster, moisture, thickness, and vigor.

The complexion will benefit from *genmai* (brown rice), *hatomugi* (pearl barley), *kuromame* (black soybeans), garlic, *daikon* greens, *shiitake* mushrooms, tofu, *soba* (buckwheat), and *renkon* (lotus root), among others. While all of these foods will contribute to skin beauty, some are indicated in the treatment of specific problems as well.

Hatomugi may be eaten daily as a specific complexion-beautifying food. Garlic—with its antibacterial properties—is recommended for the treatment of blemished skin.

The other foods listed contribute generally to the skin's health by providing important vitamins, encouraging the elimination of wastes and toxins, stimulating metabolism and circulation, and supplying moisture.

While any of the foods mentioned here can be eaten on a regular basis with no ill effects, it is always important to consume a variety of foods within a well-balanced diet. Do not eat inordinate amounts of one particular food over a period of time.

With the modern prevalence of overly refined and processed foods, even the world's traditionally healthful diets have been corrupted. It has become difficult for people to eat in a balanced way, and the huge popularity of sweet and starchy nonfoods has led to weight problems, even for the proverbially slender Japanese.

Unfortunately, there is no food that will directly cause weight loss. About the best you can do is eat less and better, choosing fiber over refined starches, fruits over sweets, unsaturated over saturated fats.

There are some Japanese foods, however, that are thought to be helpful in weight regulation, to the extent that they improve the efficiency of the metabolism, supply high protein with low calories, or offer high fiber content for healthy appetite control.

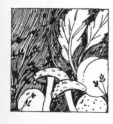

The *shiitake* mushroom is a food renowned for its health benefits; in the realm of weight loss, it is thought to help the body regulate weight and eliminate toxins by quickening the metabolism. *Shiitake* is delicious and low in calories.

Burdock, rich in iron, is said to improve the functioning of the kidneys, acting as a mild diuretic. Burdock is thought to normalize the various body functions and speed the elimination of wastes and toxins.

Dieters appreciate tofu for its low calorie count and high nutritional value. With high calcium, B vitamins, and protein, it is a very beneficial food for health. Tofu is said to improve digestion and quicken the metabolism.

Lotus root, seaweed, *konnyaku* (devil's tongue root), walnuts, cabbage, and brown rice are other foods that may be helpful to those who wish to control their weight.

The Chinese herbal medicine tradition offers the following wisdom to those who would lose weight and diminish a tendency to put it on: warm, hot, and pungent spices (e.g., licorice, nutmeg, black pepper, red chili, cloves, star anise, dried orange peel, cinnamon, the white heads of green onions, and fennel) should be consumed in order to render the system more yang. Fat should be avoided, but when consumed should be accompanied by green or black tea. Soups will encourage a feeling of fullness and discourage overeating.

Small red beans and pearl barley are effective diuretics, along with corn and corn silk, soybeans, and garlic. Ginger, cinnamon, and dried orange peel contribute to warming the body to induce perspiration. The yang tonics that will lend warm energy to the body include kidney, liver, shrimp, mussels, dried unripe raspberries, yams, walnuts, chive seed, and the seed of bitter gourd. But remember, no amount of *shiitake* or small red beans will help you if you can't stay out of those devilishly tempting *patisseries*....

While green tea is indisputably the queen of Japanese beverages, there are numerous other "teas" that are not only enjoyable to drink but may also contribute to health and beauty.

Pearl barley tea, or *hatomugi-cha*, is thought to be beneficial to the skin, clearing the complexion of flaws, freckles, warts, and moles. To prepare this tea is easy: using 60 g/ $1/4$ C of roasted pearl barley per liter (about 1 quart) of water, bring the grain and water to a boil and simmer for 5–10 minutes. Strain.

Kombu-cha is tea made from *kombu*, or kelp seaweed. This seaweed tea restores vitality and is said to be relaxing to the nerves. Drinking it regularly will give strength and vigor to the hair and nails. The easiest way to prepare *kombu-cha* is to use powdered *kombu*, available in most grocery stores in Japan and in health food stores elsewhere. The powder is simply stirred into

inside *(foods encouraging weight control)*

shiitake

burdock

tofu

lotus root

seaweed

devil's tongue root

walnuts

cabbage

brown rice

licorice

nutmeg

black pepper

red chili

cloves

star anise

dried orange peel

cinnamon

green onions

fennel

green tea

black tea

small red beans

pearl barley

corn

corn silk

soybeans

ginger

garlic

a cup of hot water. However, the purist may wish to make *kombu-cha* by boiling a piece of *kombu* in a liter/quart of water for 15 minutes. The tea has a pleasantly subtle ocean fragrance, and looks lovely served with a small strip of *kombu* drifting in the bottom of the cup.

The popular *mugi-cha* (roasted barley tea) is prepared in the same manner as *hatomugi-cha*, and when chilled is a delightful summer drink. Aside from its value as a no caffeine-free refresher, *mugi-cha* is thought to help eliminate fats from the body. However, its somewhat laxative properties mean one shouldn't overindulge.

Shiitake mushroom tea is known to be useful in lowering cholesterol levels, in helping to regulate high blood pressure, and in relaxing one who is nervous. To prepare, boil one large sliced *shiitake* in $1/2$ liter (about $1/2$ quart) of water for 15 minutes. A little salt or soy sauce may be added to taste. The tea should be taken in small amounts.

Any of these "teas" will certainly contribute more to your health and appearance than a cup of coffee … though it might be somewhat difficult to convince a devoted espresso-drinker to switch to seaweed or mushroom for the morning wake-up!

Those who wish to receive their beauty-nutrients in supplement form might consider the following, available in health food stores or Chinese apothecaries. (Many of the Asian ingredients are found now in products sold in well-stocked Western natural foods stores; read labels.)

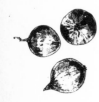

Chlorella is a "miracle" supplement that has taken the West by storm. Chlorella is an ancient microscopic green algae. Packed with nutrients and rich in nucleic acids, it is said to protect the human organism from pollution by binding and removing toxins from the system.

Essence of young barley grass: sold in the West as well, this supplement is exceptionally rich in nutrients, enzymes, amino acids, and chlorophyll.

Sea products: seaweeds in tablet and tea form, powdered pearls and oyster shells, extract of freshwater clams.

Native herbs and *kampōyaku* (Chinese traditional medicines): ginkgo, ginseng, pearl barley, *dokudami*, and many more. There are honeys, and vinegars made with curative herbs; energy drinks; and teas that eliminate fats and toxins. There exist many interesting *kampōyaku* tea combinations, tablets and granules that may be used as general tonics, tonics for men or for women, and curatives for specific needs. Consult an expert.

The traditional Japanese diet relies heavily on foods that have medicinal or curative properties—these foods are generally cleansing, balancing, or strengthening to the system. Small amounts of many different kinds of food are eaten at each meal, and the body is not subjected to overwhelming amounts of fat, sugar, or heavy meats. The Japanese diet is a complete system, of course—to truly experience its full benefits you can't do it halfway. But it is possible to begin by incorporating some of the most important foods into your diet.

sleep

Sleep is one of the basic requirements for health—both physical and mental—and also for beauty. During sleep, skin replenishes itself, renews texture, replaces tissue; cells divide and are renewed. These regenerative processes are always occurring, but it is during sleep that they are most active.

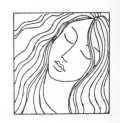

That is why a bad night's sleep shows on one's face the next day. (But do not think that conversely, sleeping a huge amount will make you look 10 years younger—too much sleep causes fluid to collect temporarily in facial tissues, making skin look puffy. Don't routinely oversleep, and use a pillow to keep the head elevated.)

Almost everyone has experienced sleep difficulties at one time or another—there is nothing more frustrating than wanting to sleep and not being able to, especially when there is no apparent external factor causing the problem.

If you have chronic insomnia, the first thing to do is to examine your environment and lifestyle for possible causes. Where insomnia might be associated with physical or mental illness, a doctor must be consulted.

Insomnia commonly accompanies asthma, diabetes, heart disorders, and depression. Among the causes of ordinary insomnia there may be external ones: noise, light, an uncomfortable bed, heat, cold—and internal ones: anxiety, tension, faulty digestion, stimulants in the diet.

If there are external causes, deal with these first. Try earplugs, dark curtains, a different mattress or pillow, heavier or lighter bedcovers. Make your bed inviting and comfortable, and avoid overheated, drying air in the bedroom—a little fresh air is good for the skin during sleep.

If your diet is high in stimulants such as alcohol, sugar, salt, coffee, tea, or soft drinks, eliminate or cut down. Don't go to bed on a full stomach. If sleeplessness is the result of tension and stress, establish a relaxing bedtime ritual: the proverbial glass of warm milk (milk contains tryptophan, much touted as a sleep-inducer), a warm bath, soft music, massage, meditation, and herb tea. Vitamins B-complex and C may be helpful in some cases of insomnia.

The Japanese *ofuro*, or hot bath, is a wonderful way to induce relaxation—to the bath you might try adding a herbal essence such as chamomile, melissa, orange blossom, hops, bay, or a mixture of these. In lieu of the essence, an infusion of the herbs may be used; there are also commercial bath products containing "sleepy herbs."

A Japanese remedy meant for internal consumption is green *shiso* (perilla) leaf in *shōchū* (distilled spirits), taken at bedtime. Western herbal teas include chamomile, anise, dill, elderflower, fennel seed, hops, lavender, lemon balm, marjoram, and thyme. Infuse one herb alone or a mixture of them; drink in moderation at bedtime.

One pleasant herbal sleep-inducer is the sleep pillow. Prepare a small silk pillowslip or drawstring bag, and into this place a combination of soporific herbs: hops, lime blossom, chamomile, lavender, bay, fennel, rosemary, jasmine. Choose a mixture that appeals to you, but do try to include the first two herbs in the list—they are especially effective in inducing sleep.

The sleep pillow should be placed inside your usual pillow. The fragrant potpourri is remarkably relaxing; for some people who are sensitive to smell, sleep will come easily and quickly. This is a nice technique to try with children who are restless at bedtime.

The expertise with which people sleep is one striking aspect of the Japanese way of life, one that is worth developing. Traditional wisdom passed on from parent to child has always stressed the importance of sleep. To go to bed early, sleep a long time, and rise early are rules that encourage both beauty and discipline. To sleep on one's back is the preferred posture; to keep legs straight and together is the feminine model of modesty in repose. Despite the seeming restrictedness of this sleeping position, it does ensure the avoidance of wrinkles caused by the nightly squashing of the face into the pillow.

The Japanese pillow, so oddly rigid-seeming to Westerners accustomed to billowing feather pillows, was in earlier times wooden or ceramic; these days the small supports are stuffed with beans or grain husks, allowing air to circulate around the head during sleep.

It seems that lately the whole world is sleeping on *futon* or variations thereof, but in many cases the full pleasure of the traditional Japanese sleep experience is missed due to the absence of *tatami*. The resilient firmness of rice-straw *tatami* provides the perfect underlayer to a luxurious futon with silken quilts.

The streets of Japanese residential neighborhoods darken early, village-like. There is a comfortable warmth to the dark streets; one senses the familial, communal abandon to sweet slumber behind the *shōji*. During the day babies riding on their mothers' backs sleep and doze intermittently; adults nap publicly everywhere. Sleep seems less separate from the waking state than in the West.

outside

sleep-inducing baths

sleep pillow with herbs

inside

perilla shōchū drink

soporific herbal teas

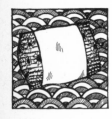

The following traditional rules for sleeping well were gathered from a variety of Japanese grandmotherly sources—surely among these suggestions an insomniac will find at least one solution to sleeplessness. Those in pursuit of true beauty would do well to emulate the Japanese readiness to sleep, with its wonderful benefits to the complexion, the disposition, and the spirit.

advice for a good sleep

Before going to bed, have a long soak in a hot bath.

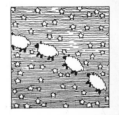

Alternate hot and cold baths—or follow hot bath soaks with ice-cold showers or bucket dousings—over a period of 15–20 minutes. Spend about 1 minute in each to improve genera health and circulation and encourage a deep sleep.

A small amount of alcohol, sipped as medicine to improve circulation and facilitate sleep, may be taken at bedtime. Because one will sleep soundly, the skin will become beautiful. However, too much alcohol will have the opposite effect, and in general drinking and smoking are bad for beauty and health.

If you have difficulty in falling asleep, drink a little *shōchu* with minced fresh green perilla leaf in it just before going to bed.

Eating peanuts makes you sleepy; eating dried sardines will wake you up.

When you can't sleep, slice an onion, wrap it in gauze, and put it under your pillow. Or—why not?—simply inhale crushed onion slices in a jar while you relax in bed.

Sleep in a room that has fresh air circulating, but no breezes or winds. Never sleep with a fan, air conditioner, or heater on in the room. Traditional Asian medicine links hot or cold winds during sleep with a weakening of the body.

Sleep on a thin board laid upon *tatami*, with nothing more than a light blanket for a covering, even in midwinter. Use a cylindrical wooden pillow. (Obviously, this is one of those spirit-hardening practices.)

In the summer, don't use an ice pillow except when absolutely necessary. The Japanese feel the head must be cool in order for sleep to be sound and healthy. To keep your head cool, make a pillow stuffed with old *azuki* beans: Sew a cotton rectangle and fill it tightly with the beans. Every now and then, lay the pillow in the sun to dry it. The *azuki* bean pillow will keep air circulating around your head.

On the hottest summer nights, you can make an ice pillow by filling a hot-water bottle with ice and wrapping a cloth around it.

You should go to bed by 10:00—midnight at the latest—and sleep for eight hours.

Sleep on your back with your legs together neatly. You'll get wrinkles on your face if you sleep on your stomach or side.

Don't lie with the feet pointing west. This is unlucky, because it is the direction of the Pure Land, where the spirits of the dead abide.

There is no beauty without health, and fundamental to good health are regular exercise, good nutrition, and good sleeping habits. Too little sleep or poor-quality sleep will lead to a multitude of problems, including a lack of vitality and strength in skin, hair, and nails. The inner balance that is so important to beauty is impossible without the deep relaxation and regeneration of truly deep, dream-rich sleep.

a sip of tea

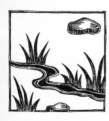

Allow it to, and life fills up with urgent meetings, deadlines, and too hectic schedules. It's the way we all seem to live. This reality may be the commonly accepted one, but I'm sure we all realize it's not a healthy one. It's not complete. We're missing out on the kind of relaxation that comes from doing nothing. Just *being* has become a rare luxury.

True health and true beauty can exist only when one is in tune with the body/mind, and it is difficult to be aware of inner rhythms when the external clock is ruling our days. One who does creative work of any kind learns to be respectful of the being's occasional insistence upon doing nothing. There are periods when a kind of quiet lull must be observed, following which one moves on into a time of productive activity. It is a natural cycle.

As an experiment, try giving in to languor when the mood comes upon you. To bring about that sleepy, indolent state of mind, you might look up the word "inactivity" in your thesaurus. I did just now, and a cornucopia of lazy, torpid, languorous words nearly rendered me supine with sleepiness. As an antidote, since I am meant to be in the deadline-conscious condition imposed by publishing schedules, I consulted the opposite word "activity" and found there enough vital effervescence to wake me right up again. Try peppy, snappy, zingy, verve, moxie, oomph, and pizzazz: words with a high caffeine content.

Many women in non-Western cultures and in some Western ones seem to possess a natural restfulness that is an integral part of their charm. I remember an Italian friend—she is both indolent in manner and a powerful high-achiever—mentioning that men tell her they are drawn to her by her air of dreamy quiescence. In Latin countries, this slowed-down take on life allows for a fuller, more sensual appreciation of existence. In the East, a certain relaxation of spirit (always accompanied—balanced—by prodigious energy and efficiency) brings a welcome feeling of ease, a refreshing quality. Her restful presence is an important element in the Asian woman's beauty. It is a worthy goal, the achievement of this ability to just be.

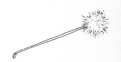

Setting aside time for oneself is something that should be a habit for all of us. Solitary relaxation is essential to well-being. The results of regular relaxation may not be immediately or tangibly apparent, but they can be much more important than other, more material rewards.

Relax, be lazy, be alone and do nothing (is it possible?). Try establishing a relaxation ritual, setting aside a regular time for this practice at whatever rhythm suits your lifestyle, but no less often than once a week.

During this time, concentrate on relaxing the physical being; the mental being will follow. Have a quiet rest, with no possibility of interruption. Meditate, stretch slowly, get a massage, take a bath, or swing in a hammock. Contemplate beautiful music or a landscape or a thundering rainstorm. Do nothing that will bring a tangible result. Slow down, breathe.

A sense of oneself as a separate, whole being, with the inner radiance that comes from self-love (very different from selfishness or self-indulgence), is a fundamental element in true beauty. To achieve this, one must devote some time to quietly deepening the connection with self. When I think of the truly beautiful women and men I have known, each of them has emanated this inner quality, which is seen as a kind of luminosity.

To aid in relaxation, try the following, culled from the plant traditions of East and West:

THE BATH

The bath is the perfect relaxation device; one is induced to let go and breathe more deeply by the steamy atmosphere, the lulling waters, and the heat. The addition of bath salts, hot-spring minerals, herbs, or oils can intensify the relaxing, regenerating effects. The following ingredients are known to bring about relaxation: linden, sage, burdock, comfrey, violet leaves, pansies, spearmint, roses, vervain, camomile, peach leaf, rice bran, milk, *sake*.

outside

relaxing herbal baths

relaxing milk or sake bath

relaxing scents

Prepare as for any herbal bath, infusing plants first, then adding the liquid to a warm bath. Milk and *sake* may be added as is; rice bran must be tied into a muslin bag.

SCENT

Aromatherapists recommend the inhalation of particular essential oils to achieve specific mental, physical, or emotional results. You may use the oils in the bath, on the skin or for massage when diluted with carrier oil, or to perfume the air in a room. For relaxation, try basil, bergamot, sage, thyme, lemon, lavender, camomile. Burn incense or scented candles; arrange fresh flowers that fill the air with fragrance.

TEAS

A tea interlude, taken alone or with friends, can be a time to pause, "do nothing," refresh one's being amid the fast pace of a day. To this end, Japanese green tea, light and limpid green, is certainly more conducive than coffee. But the beverage itself is less important than the act of preparing it (or being served it), the time taken to appreciate it, and the feeling of a small "time out" from all else.

For relaxation, the following teas may be tried: basil, camomile, dill, hyssop, lavender, lemon balm, marjoram, mint, rosemary, sage, thyme, *kuki-cha* (twig tea), *kombu-cha* (*kombu* seaweed tea), powdered pearl, *shiitake, mekabu* (root of *wakame* seaweed).

Prepare as you would any herbal infusion or tea. To make the *shiitake* and *mekabu* teas, first soak the item until soft, then boil for 10 minutes. (No more than one *shiitake* per day!) For powdered pearl tea, stir a teaspoon of pearl-dust into a cup of hot water.

From *The Book of Tea*, by Okakura Kakuzo, originally published in 1906:

> Meanwhile, let us have a sip of tea. The afternoon glow is brightening the bamboos, the fountains are bubbling with delight, the soughing of the pines is heard in our kettle. Let us dream of evanescence, and linger in the beautiful foolishness of things.

MASSAGE

Shiatsu massage can provide deep relaxation and melt away body-held stress. The technique has for one of its goals the reestablishment of the proper circulation of energy, and while in Japan it is most often practiced as a treatment for some specific problem, it may also be employed preventively.

There have been innumerable devices created for the massage of the feet—though a hand-done massage is fine—and a good foot massage will deliver benefits to the entire body.

Walking barefoot is a daily relaxer. A walk in the rain on a summer evening, a stroll through green gardens, a visit to a mountain retreat—there are many ways to relax and escape the stresses of modern life.

Stress has a bad image these days, but in fact a certain amount of stress is necessary for efficiency, energetic accomplishment, enthusiasm, and drive. It is when one is operating above or below one's "optimum stress level" that problems arise: too much stress and challenge lead to tension and serious physical problems, while too little stress results in lethargy, lowered resistance to illness, depression, and boredom.

The answer is to live a life of balanced stress: You must control the amount and type of stress you live with, and when that is impossible (everyone has those times!), you must learn to handle a stress-overdose wisely.

Because the stress response is largely physical, the body is alerted for action even in mentally or emotionally stressful situations where no direct action is possible (such as a communication problem at work, or worries over family problems).

What happens when the stress message to the brain is not followed by "fight or flight"? Large amounts of stress hormones, along with released fatty acids (cholesterol), begin to circulate in the bloodstream. A rush of nervous energy is felt. Breathing is faster and shallower; muscles tense; anxiety increases; fists clench; the heartbeat rises sharply. Internally, the body is hard at work: digestion processes stop; subcutaneous fat is released for energy; the liver releases sugar into the blood; salivation slows; muscles let go of lactic acid; the temperature falls; and the adrenal glands release hormones.

The often prolonged and psychological stresses of modern life rarely allow us to act on the immediate, physical stress response. Over a period of time, the resulting tensions place a huge burden on the body and can result in digestive problems, heart disease, and decreased resistance to illness.

One of the best things you can do to handle this free-floating stress is to exercise; a good workout when you're feeling angry can be a great antidote. Over the long term, too, regular exercise can make you more physically resilient, better equipped to handle stress.

A breathing discipline or meditation practice can also provide a way to regain inner balance. Whatever means works for you is the appropriate one.

purification ritual

A clean slate, a blank page: sometimes it's good to start over fresh! The whole idea of this is to instill existence with renewed consciousness, to purify oneself, to free mind and body from the weight of the past, to claim and establish a new identity or cultivate new habits. How exciting this is! And the interesting thing about such rituals of purification is that they are practices shared by many cultures.

How can we undertake purification? In actuality, the process of cleansing is the first—some say the most important—step in achieving health and beauty. An organism that is not burdened by toxins is able to function properly. The skin, that barometer of the physical condition, functions first and foremost as an agent of elimination. What follows are some suggestions for purification; any of them could become beneficial regular habits!

—Try a cleansing drink to start the day. A cup of warm water with the juice of a fresh lemon squeezed into it will help to purify the system. Your skin will benefit.

—When you've had too much to eat, or eaten the wrong foods, drink several cups of *ban-cha* or oolong tea with an *umeboshi* stirred in, then take a hot bath. But don't stop there—wrap yourself in quilts for an hour afterward to encourage a sweat. Then get back in a tepid bath for a rinse.

—When you're feeling susceptible to fatigue, viruses, and germs, take a ginger bath. Grate two big pieces of fresh ginger, squeeze through cheesecloth to obtain juice, then add the juice to a hot bath. Soak: you'll be warmed as well as purified.

—Add some lemons, tangerines, or oranges (cut in quarters) to your bath. This is a great way to encourage toxins to depart. All that vitamin C will enhance your complexion into the bargain!

—To eliminate residues on your hair, add a little vinegar to your final hair rinse after shampooing. Conditioners and styling products can cause quite a buildup on the hair, so try to make the vinegar rinse a routine treatment.

—Instead of coating your fingernails with polish, try buffing them with the little Japanese-type buffing kits that leave the nails natural, rosy pink, and shiny.

—See your dentist for a comprehensive tooth-cleaning and scaling. Keep your teeth in good condition by flossing daily.

—Try eliminating these substances from your diet to whatever extent is possible: white flour; sugar; alcohol; processed foods; preservatives; heavy meats.

—Think about increasing your intake of whole grains, fruits and vegetables, and good pure water.

—Make green tea a daily habit. Green tea has wonderful cleansing, astringent, and curative properties.

—To cleanse the skin from inside and out, make use of raw *daikon*. Eaten grated as a condiment or mixed with rice flour as a pack for troubled skin, *daikon* will reward you with translucent skin.

—To cleanse the skin of layers of dead cells, practice regular skin scrubbing with a brush as stiff as you can stand. Remember to use the brush gently and with respect for soft surfaces, and it will reward you with vital-looking, smooth, soft skin. An abrasive towel will serve the same purpose.

—For do-it-yourself acid exfoliation, rub fruit peels over your freshly cleansed face, leave as is for 20 minutes, then rinse. Pineapple or papaya work wonders.

—Take a day off from food if you're in good health—or try having only freshly made fruit and vegetable juices. Before undertaking any fast, first consult your doctor. The benefits from fasting are extraordinary, if you can do it safely. If you must eat, try raw fruits and vegetables, sprouts, and almonds for 24 hours. (And lots of water!)

—Take a day off from make-up. If you must use something, leave it at powder and lipstick.

—Get into the wilderness. Breathe fresh clean air, take hikes, bathe in hot springs. Wash your face in cold water. Eat simply. Learn about purification from the earth, by existing in harmony with nature.

botanicals

W hy botanicals? It is possible to design a simple beauty routine that is both pure and natural without ever going near an actual plant. There are many companies with good products on the market; by reading labels carefully one may choose astutely to find the products that most closely suit one's needs and predilections. And perhaps it seems ultimately simpler to buy ready-made products than to make one's own from scratch. But I would venture the suggestion that to brew a tea with which to silken one's skin, or to grind a bean to powder with which to cleanse it, are, after all, small and easily achieved rituals that may offer certain clear benefits:

—instead of a plethora of chemicals and preservatives, one applies to one's skin or hair only the active ingredient, simple and pure

—one acquires a degree of self-sufficiency

—is there not an undeniable difference between home-baked bread and the manufactured kind? Between tea brewed from a bag and tea brewed in a pot, from loose leaves? Is not "soul" present in what is done by the hands?

—expertise in healing is an ancient feminine heritage, and in this domain are mingled the arts of magic, medicine, beauty, and food; there is a depth of satisfaction to be found in enacting the rites, of creating the elixirs that bring beauty

—the recipes themselves have been drawn down through centuries; they are women's wisdom

—if one works directly with the plants, one comes to know them. If one grows and tends the plants, the working of the garden awakens another aspect of the feminine: the old rapport of woman with Earth

—there is, in the act of making these teas and powders, the natural arising of a meditative state

The next section of the book invites you to grow a garden, to harvest the flowers and leaves, and to concoct lotions, potions, and elixirs by which to cast spells of beauty of every sort.

the beauty garden

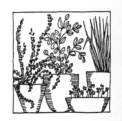

The herb garden is one of the most gratifying of gardening endeavors. The plants are generally appealing to the eye and fragrant in growth. You may snip the fresh leaves and blossoms as needed for cooking, teas, the bath, health care, and beauty care. They take up little space, and so are particularly suited to planting in the odd corner of a tiny garden, Japanese or otherwise.

For women, tending a garden of medicinal plants is a way to reclaim the ancient feminine magical-medical role, a way to engage in relationship with the earth. Gardening lends itself to a settled, meditative state of being.

Easy to grow, herbs will thrive in garden soil, pots outdoors or indoors, or in window boxes. Most herbs (but not all) need soil with good drainage (such as loam) and a sheltered spot that gets lots of gentle but not glaring sun. If you plan to dry herbs, your garden should include several plants of each variety, but for fresh use one or two of each is adequate.

Popular Western plants you might consider growing are basil, lavender, fennel, violet, mint, jasmine, rosemary, thyme, sage, marigold, chamomile, vervain, and yarrow. A crosscultural herb garden could include such Japanese standards as aloe, *wasabi*, *shiso* (perilla), *shōga* (for ginger shoots or ginger root), and *dokudami*. Any of the other *yakusō* mentioned further on in this section might be included as well.

Plant herbs as you would any other plant. Tiny herb seeds may be mixed with sand before sowing to ensure even spreading. Seedlings are simpler to grow—the major mistake made by novice herb gardeners is to plant them in soil that is heavy and slow to drain. Many Western herbs are native to warm, dry climates and cannot survive waterlogged roots. Another dampness-related problem, especially for mint, is mildew. Sand, peat, or gravel added to heavy soil will help drainage; don't put plants in the shade.

Care of herb plants involves attentive weeding and watering. Peat placed around the plants will help retain water and hold back weed growth. Since herb leaves are intended for consumption, your gardening methods should be organic; don't use chemicals. A soap-and-water solution can be sprayed on plants to kill aphids.

Plants grown for their leaves should have flowers removed before they bloom. Herbs may be cut fresh for use as needed, but if you plan to dry plants, you should harvest just before flowering, when the flavor is strongest. Harvesting should be done with sharp scissors on a warm dry morning. Handle leaves carefully. To dry, hang plants upside down indoors in a warm dry spot that receives a constant flow of air. (For detailed instructions on harvesting and storing herbs, see appendix.)

The Japanese word for herb is *yakusō*, and while until the recent past the Japanese medicinal plants were still widely known and used for this and that, during the '70s and '80s they were eclipsed by modern pharmaceuticals. "Granny's strange old remedies," people would say.

Fortunately, however, there has been a strong revival of interest in the native *yakusō*; over the past few years the plants have begun to acquire a new, more positive image. One need only stroll through a well-stocked Japanese pharmacy or even a good tea shop to see proof of the change: elegantly packaged *yakusō* for teas or the bath, the special tea pots in which they are brewed, even canned drinks of *dokudami-cha*, a traditional detoxifier and tonic. Like the herbs of the European tradition, the Indian tradition, the African, or any other, Japanese herbs may be used in a wonderful variety of ways: as gentle but effective illness remedies, as restorative teas, as external treatments for skin, hair, and body, or added to the bath to benefit circulation, skin tone, or the nervous system.

The most easily found herbs in the Japanese tradition are the following: *dokudami* (*Houttuynia cordata*); aloe (*Aloe vera*, *Aloe aborescens*): *tōki* (*Angelica sinensis*); *kumazasa* (bamboo grass, *Sasa veitchii*); *soba* (buckwheat, *Fagopyrum esculentum*); *hakobe* (chickweed, *Stellaria media*); *kuko no mi* (Chinese wolfberry, *Lycium Chinense*); *tampopo* (dandelion, *Taraxacum officinale*); *uikyō* (fennel, *Foeniculum vulgare*); *sugina* (field horsetail, *Equisetum arvense*); *seri* (double dropwort or meadowsweet, *Filipendula vulgaris*); *biwa no ha* (loquat leaf, *Eriobotrya Japonica*); *kuwa no ha* (white mulberry leaf, *Morus alba*); *kaki no ha* (persimmon leaf, *Diospyros kaki*); *shiso* (*Perilla frutescens*); *hatomugi* (pearl barley, Job's Tears, *Coix lacrymae Jobi*); *ōbako* (plantain, *Plantago major*); *benibana* (safflower petals, *Carthamus tinctorius*); and last but not least, *cha* (tea, *Thea sinensis*) in its many forms. The plants listed here are the ones sold for general use; there are many more Japanese herbs, of course, but they are less available outside apothecaries. Many of the herbs in the above list come in premixed form for use as healing teas, often with a base of *hato-mugi* or *dokudami*.

Although the *yakusō* are now easily available in Japan, they generally carry no accompanying directions for usage or information about effects. While most of the *yakusō* are mild and safe when used properly, no medicinal plant should ever be taken without full knowledge of its properties and proper preparation.

The general rules for working with herbs apply: store them tightly sealed—the Japanese traditionally recommend wrapping herbs in paper to avoid the moisture and mildew that can accumulate when they are stored in glass, especially when they've been improperly dried; shelf life is 6 months for leaves, 1 year for bark and seeds; when preparing herbs use only enamel or glass pots, pans, and bowls and only wooden utensils—no metal ever. Use pure water.

Here is one small, wonderful, sublimely easy beauty tea to serve as an introduction to *yakusō*: the green tea face pack. Whip up some *matcha* as for tea ceremony (using about 3 tsp per cup of water), allow it to cool, then apply the green froth to the cleansed face. Leave for 10 minutes. The green tea pack will cleanse and tone, calm the complexion, and lend whitening and cooling benefits to the skin. For further exploration, move on to the teas and baths described next.

outside

the green-tea pack for face

herbs for the inside

For the kind of glowing beauty that comes from within, from a healthy body and a serene mind, develop a herbal tea habit. Just as caffeinated, carbonated, or alcoholic drinks can upset the body's balance and thereby be harmful to one's appearance if taken too frequently, so can herb teas help gently to restore physical harmony, health, and beauty.

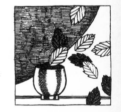

An herb tea can be enjoyed purely for its flavor and aroma, but since almost every herbal preparation has specific effects on the body, it is useful to be aware of what these can be.

A tea's effects can range from the subtle to the dramatic, and while many herbs are mild and generally beneficial, there are some that can be hazardous if ingested in large amounts or by those with certain health conditions (pregnancy is one condition that calls for caution).

In all cases, large doses and frequent or prolonged use of any particular herb should be avoided. Of the herbs mentioned below, for example, rosemary and sage are two that can cause adverse reactions if taken over a period of more than a few weeks or in immoderate amounts. Peppermint taken too frequently by a nursing mother may cause an allergic reaction in her baby. So use herb teas wisely; if you have doubts or questions about a particular herb, consult your doctor or any good book on herbs. (And note that essential oils are far more concentrated than herbs, and thus should not be used interchangeable.)

I introduce below some of the common herbs of East and West that may be used for teas; as we are interested here in those that contribute to a healthy beauty, I do not include the many herbs that are employed for more serious medicinal purposes.

CHAMOMILE: calming; relieves stomach problems and indigestion
LAVENDER: stimulating, a good "wake-up" beverage; relieves headaches and fatigue
LEMON BALM: relieves pain of menstrual cramps and headaches; calming, sleep-inducing; helps alleviate indigestion, gas
ROSEMARY: aids circulation, digestion; relieves headaches; stimulating (combine with lavender)
SAGE: calms anxiety, aids depression; reduces perspiration; stops the milk flow in nursing mothers
PEPPERMINT: relieves insomnia, nervousness; helps alleviate abdominal pain, nausea, heartburn, colds, headaches
ROSE HIPS: general tonic; diuretic; the vitamin C relieves colds
LINDEN: sedative
ELDERFLOWER: calming; relieves colds; promotes perspiration
DOKUDAMI: detoxifying; tonic; said to cleanse the system
PEARL BARLEY: diuretic; skin beautifier; rids the skin of warts and moles
BAMBOO GRASS: diuretic; calming; astringent
DANDELION LEAF or ROOT: skin beautifier; tonic
PERSIMMON LEAF: relieves and prevents colds; skin beautifier

inside

herbal teas for beauty & health

A herbal tea is commonly prepared as an infusion. The method for preparing an infusion is as follows: pour boiling water over the herb (300 ml/1 1/4 C per 2 T of the herb), steep for 10 minutes, then strain. Proper infusions employed as part of a curative regime are generally drunk cold or at room temperature taken 2–3 times per day.

herbs for the outside

Bathing with herbs is a very pleasant way to get acquainted with them. It is difficult to go seriously wrong when experimenting with herbal baths, but the following guide will help you choose the herbs that best suit your needs.

Stimulating/Tonic
Eucalyptus, Sage, Lavender, Pine, Peppermint, Thyme, Comfrey, Marigold, Rosemary, Patchouli, Savory, Vetivert

Calming/Sedative
Linden, Rose, Vervain, Chamomile, Peach Leaf, Violet Leaf, Pansy, Spearmint, Mistletoe, Passionflower, Burdock, Balm, Meadowsweet, Angelica, Yarrow, Bamboo Grass, Jasmine

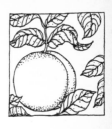

Astringent
Rose, Lemon, Strawberry Leaf, Lavender, Witch Hazel, Borage, Elderflower, Rosemary, Aloe, Yarrow, Green Tea

Diaphoretic (Cause Sweating)
Linden, Chamomile, Borage, Elderflower, Pennyroyal, Burdock, Marigold, Buckwheat

Deodorant
Rose, Orange Flower, Sage, Thyme, Witch Hazel, Lemon, Perilla

Healing/Skin Softening
Comfrey, Peppermint, Aloe, Borage, Pearl Barley

Soothing to Sore Muscles
Comfrey, Mugwort, Sage, Burdock Root, Sassafras Bark, Ginger

Aromatic
Peppermint, Pine Needles, Jasmine, Orange Peel, Rose, Lemon Peel, Lavender, Perilla

Cooling/Refreshing
Peppermint, Aloe, Pine, Peach Leaf, Elderflower, Lavender

And for specific skin problems, the following: **Acne:** Lavender; **Aging skin:** Comfrey; **To exfoliate dull skin:** Chamomile, Rosemary; **Dry skin:** Comfrey, Patchouli, Rose, Ginseng; **Oily skin:** Lemongrass, Lemon Peel, Pansy, Peppermint, Witch Hazel; **Heat rash:** Comfrey, Peach Leaf.

Any of these herbs may be used singly or in combination with others. Confirmed herbal bathers often have a "personal mixture" that they have developed to suit their particular needs and favorite scents. From the Western tradition you might choose, for example, a mixture of lavender (aromatic and stimulating), peppermint (tonic and refreshing), and rosemary (tonic and astringent) for a regenerative wake-up bath, or a combination of linden (sedative), chamomile (relaxing and diaphoretic), and vervain (calming) for a "serenity" bath.

To prepare any herb bath, the best method is to place 115 g/ 1/2 C of herbs in a covered nonmetal pot of water and simmer for 15–20 minutes. Strain, and add the liquid to the bath, where you should spend at least 20 minutes soaking. (You can tie the discarded herbs into a cheesecloth bag and use them as a scrub if you like.)

outside

herbal baths for beauty & health

the communal bath

I once had the pleasure of taking a bath with three very old Japanese women. It was a public communal bath fed by a hot mineral spring, a simple big bathing chamber of the usual type—steaming water flowed over the big smooth rocks that surrounded the brimming tub. A row of faucets with buckets and stools, a fogged-up window, a wet tile floor. The greenish water smelled of the depths of the hot earth.

When I arrived, two of the old women were soaking, immobile and peaceful as rocks. The third old woman was having her back vigorously scrubbed by a woman of about my age. My sudden appearance in the bathing room caused a momentary disturbance of the ambiance; I had the feeling that a conversation had ended in midstream. Wishing not to create further ripples of discomfort, I went about my scrubbing with businesslike enthusiasm, as is customary. I hadn't brought shampoo, so I did everything but wash my hair. It seemed that no one was taking any notice of me, but silence still reigned. The old woman who was being scrubbed was now having her long gray hair carefully shampooed.

After rinsing I got up to enter the tub, and at that moment the younger woman came over to me and handed me a bottle of shampoo, another one of conditioner. Surprised, I thanked her and sat down to shampoo, and the conversation started up again. At first the talk did not include me, but after a while someone asked me a question, then another and another, until finally everyone in the room was engaged in lively discussion.

The talk at first centered around bodies—I being a foreigner, differences and samenesses were a matter of major interest. One old woman complained about her sagging breasts, another about her round stomach. They were all proud of their long hair, and they talked about how often one should wash hair (every two days in one's twenties, every three days in one's thirties, every four days in one's forties, etc.; with summertime shampoos being more frequent). We talked about beauty, cooking, bearing babies, work, life with men, all in an easy, laughing atmosphere. I learned that the younger woman and the woman whose back she'd been scrubbing had only just met in the bath. They were all local countrywomen, and this is where the three old women met every day, soaking in the bath for an hour or two. By the time we were all leaving, they knew the story of my life and I knew theirs.

Thinking about the experience later, I realized how similar had been my communal bathing experiences in other parts of the world, among women of diverse cultures. In a steam bath among Bedouin women in the Sahara, in an Arab *hammam* in Paris, in the Russian baths in New York City's Lower East Side, in a river lagoon in Botswana, in an outdoor sulphur bath in Taipei, in a California hot spring, a sauna in Malta: in all the places where I had bathed among women, there had been the same camaraderie, the same straightforward intimacy. And the impetus for conversation had almost always been the sharing of a bar of soap or some shampoo or some more mysterious concoction for cleansing or beautifying the body.

These days, even in cultures where communal bathing is not customary, women belong to sports clubs and health clubs; women journey to spas, beauty retreats, and health ranches. In all these places, the communal bath provides the meeting ground, a comfortable melting pot. To carry out the beauty ritual in the company of other women, whether strangers or friends, would seem to be a ritual that knows no cultural boundaries.

the beauty medicines of east & west

Many of the substances presented here are drawn from the Japanese and Chinese traditions. The European herbal tradition is woven through, and in quite a few instances the plants belong to the traditions of both East and West. There is a sprinkling as well of the plants and recipes of India, Russia, Polynesia, and the Middle East. The selection might be seen as a kind of "world beauty" potpourri with a distinctive Asian character.

I choose to focus strongly on the Asian botanical tradition for several reasons:

—Japan—whose botanical tradition, though drawing on the venerable Chinese medicine system, has, over the centuries, developed a direction of its own—is a culture that has devoted great attention to the pursuit of beauty, feminine beauty not excluded.

—While Westerners have long assumed that the Japanese woman is genetically blessed with porcelain skin that does not seem to age, thick shiny hair, and a natural tendency to slenderness, if one compares a middle-aged Japanese woman who has grown up in a traditional way with one who has grown up outside Japan and lived a modern Western lifestyle, one often sees an astonishing degree of difference in regard to skin, hair, and silhouette. The visible signs of aging are usually more pronounced in the woman who has lived a nontraditional lifestyle. While there are with certainty genetic differences—straight black hair, for example, tends to be thicker, with a coarser shaft, and less vulnerable to damage than fair hair—I believe that the medicinal Japanese diet, the practice of *shiatsu*, and the avoidance of the sun result in the promotion and preservation of the attributes of beauty. Further, in Japanese teenagers, who have begun to follow more modern ways (sun exposure and a junk-food diet), one can now see the appearance of beauty problems that are identical to those found in the West: cellulite and overweight, unhealthy hair, and troubled skin. If the test of beauty is whether it endures, then of all the countries I have had occasion to spend time in, the Japanese tradition presents the most efficient means by which this may take place. Nowhere else in the world have I seen 80-year-old women with such fine, luminous skin or such sylphlike physical grace. As well, the inner aspects of beauty are an essential part of the Japanese teachings. One encounters, in this system, a holistic joining of the spiritual with the physical, the body with the soul, the mind with the outward appearance.

—This book is written for the English-speaking reader, and thus it is assumed that most readers will be somewhat familiar with the Western botanical tradition. It is for this reason that I present more detailed information on the Eastern botanicals. The Eastern plants will round out your pharmacopeia, much in the same way that the food you eat not only incorporates the foods of the world but takes inspiration from the new possibilities in combination.

🌿

a note on safety

In choosing which plants to experiment with, the first rule is undoubtedly to select those to which one is intuitively drawn. For any particular need, there will always be a choice of several possible botanical solutions. Further, pay careful attention to any contraindications. While the list below names plants that are known to elicit allergic reactions in some people, and plants that may be toxic if taken too frequently or in too large a quantity, there is always the possibility that one might suffer an adverse reaction to any herbal substance. The nature and benefits of these cures and plants have been in most cases empirically understood and thus they should all be handled with a degree of caution. It is important to remember that often the very constituent of a plant that heals can be toxic when overadministered.  Essential oils, which penetrate the skin rapidly and affect the internal organs, must never be applied to the body undiluted. Also, be aware that almost any essential oil can be fatal if taken neat internally, and this applies to dosages as small as 1 ounce! While contraindications given in the ingredient guide supply information on recognized cautions for each substance, almost any herb or botanical substance is a potential source of allergy or irritation in those susceptible, and certainly when misused. Do consult a medical expert whenever embarking upon a treatment program involving substances with which you are unfamiliar. In addition, the "patch test" may be conducted to check for possible sensitivity. Mix the substance under investigation with water to make a paste, then apply a small amount of the mixture to a patch on the forearm near the crook of the arm. Cover with a bandaid and leave the paste in position for 24 hours. If any redness, irritation, or other adverse reaction is seen, use of the substance is not advised.

Recommended dosages for all herbs must be respected.

Aloe: as a powerful emetic, do not overdose; pregnant or lactating women abstain

Apricot: the fruit pit is highly toxic; the fruit can provoke allergic reactions

Azuki Bean: high in saponins, which can be toxic in overdose

Bitter Orange (Neroli): abstain during pregnancy

Black Pepper: avoid essential oil in direct application to skin

Buckwheat: causes allergic reactions in some

Chamomile: some possibility of allergic reaction; avoid essential oil when pregnant

Cherry: the cherry pit contains a powerful poison

Cinnamon: avoid during fevers or when pregnant; avoid essential oil in direct application to skin

Citrus: avoid essential oils in direct application to skin

Clove: avoid essential oil in direct application to skin

Cucumber: may cause allergic reactions in some

Daikon: avoid overuse of greens in bathing for their effects on reproductive system

Dandelion: do not apply stem sap to normal skin, but only to warts; children should not take dandelion internally due to diuretic action

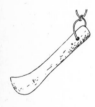

Dokudami: observe caution in dosage

Fennel: in pregnancy, no more than a couple of fennel seeds daily; avoid overdosage and avoid essential oil for danger of convulsions

Field Horsetail: taken internally, may reduce menstrual bleeding; consult herbal practitioner before ingesting

Ginger: may cause inflammation in large dosages or concentrated external application; avoid when stomach ulcers are present or in early pregnancy

Ginkgo: the nuts and leaves can be extremely toxic if taken in large amounts or too frequently; the outer skin may cause contact dermatitis or inflammation

Ginseng: overdosage may lead to high blood pressure, depression, insomnia; exercise caution during pregnancy or in cases of hypertension

Iris: toxic if taken internally

Japanese Yew: highly poisonous, can be fatal; not to be taken internally

Jasmine: may cause allergic reactions in those susceptible

Lavender: pregnant women abstain

Lemon: used externally, may cause allergic reactions in some

Licorice Root: not only the plant but also licorice candy is dangerous in overdosage; abstain in pregnancy or if suffering from
high blood pressure or kidney disease

Mint: avoid overdosage; children and babies and lactating women
abstain

Mugwort: avoid overdosage or continued use; pregnant women
abstain; avoid essential oil

Mulberry: may cause allergic reaction in those susceptible; avoid
overdosage

Mylitta lapidescens: mildly toxic when taken internally

Nutmeg: over 7 g/$^1/_4$ oz taken at one time may cause convulsions
or palpitations

Orange: used externally may cause allergic reactions in some;
nonorganic oranges may contain pesticide residues on the skin
so do not use in recipes calling for orange peel

Peach: the fruit pit is highly toxic

Perilla: diuretic and laxative; not to be consumed in large doses
or taken as a cure by children

Plantain: may cause allergic reactions

Plum: the fruit pit is highly toxic

Red Chili: the seeds are toxic; overdosage may lead to liver damage or gastroenteritis; not to be taken during pregnancy or lactation; direct application to the skin may cause blistering; do
not allow contact with eyes or broken skin

Safflower: pregnant women must abstain from the herb

Sassafras: avoid essential oil

Sage: epileptics and pregnant women must abstain

Strawberry: may cause allergic reactions

Tea: limit dosage during pregnancy and lactation; avoid if stomach ulcers or cardiac irregularity are present

Thyme: abstain during pregnancy

Ume: the fruit pit is highly toxic

Vervain: abstain during pregnancy

Yarrow: avoid internal overdosage; external use may cause allergic reactions; abstain during pregnancy

aloe

Although the aloe plant is not native to the Far East, it has long
played an important role in the Asian herbal tradition. Many fami-
lies grow it as a potted plant; it is useful as an on-hand remedy
for burns of all kinds. Aloe is valued in most parts of the world for
its healing and beautifying properties—Cleopatra herself is said
to have used it as a complexion treatment. More recently, aloe
has been shown to be remarkably effective in the healing of
burns caused by nuclear radiation.

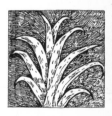

Aloe, an evergreen perennial, is known as *Aloe vera, Aloe*

barbadensis, or *Aloe aborescens* in Latin, depending on the variety; in Japanese, *rokai* or *aroe*; and in Chinese, *lu hui*.

Aloe is available in several forms: as the living plant, the bottled leaf extract, and the desiccated leaves, used for making tea.

For external use, the living plant or the extract may be used in several ways. An efficient moisturizer, aloe also possesses antiseptic properties. The long, thick, fleshy leaves contain a gelatinous sap that heals burns. When applied to the skin, aloe acts to immediately cool and soothe the burns or irritations, then forms a transparent protective seal that allows rapid healing to occur. This sealing property makes aloe an ideal moisturizer for skin types that do not take well to oil-based creams. Recommended for sunburnt skin and oily or dry complexions, aloe has no contraindications for external use.

While many people are familiar with aloe's external uses, in Japan the sap is also popular as an internal health remedy. Internally, aloe acts to cleanse the system, encouraging the elimination of wastes and toxins. However, because of its laxative, purgative properties, aloe should not be taken indiscriminately. More than a spoonful a day is too much. Pregnant women should avoid aloe entirely as an internal remedy.

Following are some of the ways aloe is used in Japan:

ALOE POULTICE: Slice leaves and apply gel side directly to the skin for sunburn, chapped skin, dermatitis, and eczema.

ALOE MOISTURIZER: Apply a few drops of gel to the freshly cleaned face with fingertips. This treatment stimulates cell metabolism, softens and refreshes skin, soothes sunburn and skin irritations, and encourages the healing of blemishes.

ALOE JUICE DRINK: A spoonful of aloe gel may be added to a blend of freshly made juices—e.g., lemon, parsley, carrot, and apple.

ALOE LIQUOR: Wash 300 g/10 $^1/_2$ oz of leaves or a 6–7 cm/ 2 $^1/_2$-inch piece, then place in a clean bottle with 100 g/3 $^1/_2$ oz of rock sugar and *shōchū* to cover. Place the tightly sealed bottle in a cool, dark place. After three weeks remove the aloe leaves, then return the bottle to the same place for another three months. Take $^1/_2$ a *sake*-cupful (about 2 T) every day as a tonic.

ALOE EYE COOLER: Slice two leaves and apply gel side to the closed eyelids for a soothing, cooling treatment for tired eyes. Lying down for fifteen minutes is an important part of the treatment!

ALOE TEA: Prepare as for ordinary tea, using the dessicated leaves.

bamboo

While it is in early spring that bamboo pierces the earth with its tender edible shoots, or *takenoko*, it is in late summer that I most appreciate this ancient Asian tree. When the weather has reached a peak of heat and heavy wetness, the sight of a bamboo grove is a gift of coolness. The sway and swish of the long trees in even a slight wind is soothing to both eye and ear.

Any good medicinal Asian garden will be planted with bamboo, both the *Nandina domestica*, or sacred bamboo, and the *Phyllostachys nigra*, or black bamboo. This latter is the common bamboo, a familiar sight in the Japanese or Chinese landscape.

The bamboo is a temperate evergreen perennial that may grow to a height of 10 meters or so, and whose growth rate can be as rapid as 20 cm a day. The stems begin green and turn to brown-black in old age. The leaves are long and narrow and pointed; it is said that the bamboo may occasionally flower, but that is rare. The uses of bamboo are many—in Japan the blonde wood makes appearances in bamboo fences, bamboo work in homes, bamboo baskets, musical instruments, toys, brush handles, cooking utensils, and tools. Japanese cuisine often features *takenoko*, a delicious medicinal food that detoxifies the body and is safely diuretic.

The Chinese medicine tradition ascribes to bamboo many properties. Roots are astringent, antipyretic, and styptic, employed for fever relief in babies. Leaves are antipyretic and diuretic; decoctions are employed in the treatment of coughs and colds. The epidermis of the shoots is sedative and antiemetic. The juice taken from the stem is sedative and antipyretic. Further, the siliceous concretions termed *tabaschir* found inside the joints of the bamboo stem are employed as antipyretic and antispasmodic remedies for a variety of serious illnesses.

Also associated with bamboo is an interesting medicinal fungus known in Latin as *Mylitta lapidescens Horan.*, a *Polyporaceae* that grows underground with the roots of the bamboo. It occurs in globules of various sizes that dry to form hard, shriveled, brown-grey nodules, which are ground to a powder for medicine. The medicine is somewhat toxic and acts as a powerful vermicide. This evocative description of the potent subterranean fungus dates to 16th-century China: "*They are produced by thunder and the metamorphoses of the subtle vapors of plants; they have the power of destroying worms and driving out evil spirits.*"

Tabaschir, the siliceous concretion mentioned above, is *Bambousa arundinacea* in Latin; one company markets the substance in Europe in capsule form, under the name of Bamboosil. *Tabaschir*—the name is an East Indian one—is used in beauty treatments as an internal strengthener for the skin, hair, and nails; those who suffer from breaking or thinning hair and weak nails undergo 3-month cures. Rich in silica, *tabaschir* is also used as a tonic for the entire organism; it is highly regarded for its ability to reinforce the cartilage and all connective tissues of the bones and skin, and is considered useful in treating osteoporosis

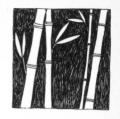

inside

*bamboo shoot medicine
   food*

tabaschir *tonic (skin,
   hair, & nails)*

bamboo grass tea

and joint pains. As an anti-aging tonic *tabaschir* is justly appreciated. (Another Japanese herb valued for its absorbable organic silica is the field horsetail, known as *sugina* in Japanese, *Equisetum arvense* in Latin.)

A popular herb tea in Japan is made from *kumazasa* or bamboo grass, *Sasa veitchii* in Latin. This plant offers a range of benefits similar to bamboo's—astringent, styptic, antipyretic, diuretic, and sedative properties are attributed to it. Prepare as you would an ordinary infused tea, using nonmetal containers and pure water.

Bamboo and its associated substances offer an extraordinary variety of medicinal riches. To undertake a bamboo beauty cure, one could daily sip *kumazasa-cha* (bamboo grass tea) and take tonic doses of *tabaschir*. With these two in tandem, one would be detoxified, calmed, and beautified by smoother skin, thicker hair, and stronger nails. And one might even try to emulate that graceful tree: its vitality in growth, bending flexibility, great strength, winter greenness, and its delicate lyric beauty.

bean

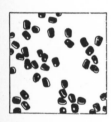

outside

bean powder face wash

Among favorite old-time Japanese beauty secrets, a face wash made from *azuki* bean powder ranks high. This has been used in Japan since the 8th-century Nara period, which makes it a venerable tradition of 1,200 years. The longstanding success is understandable: *azuki no kona* is effective, inexpensive, and simple to use. Pale pink, delicate, and silky, it is practically poetic, utterly Japanese in spirit.

While *azuki* beans' medicinal properties and pink hue make them the most popular of the bean-powder cleansers, occasionally soybeans or a dried green variety of bean are used. In every case, the beans are roasted briefly to remove moisture, then stone-ground into flour and finely sifted. The powder is so fine that when water is added it forms a cream with which to polish and cleanse the skin.

There are several ways to apply the face wash. The simplest is with the hands: moisten them, put a little bean powder and some warm water into the palm or on the fingertip, then massage the face with the frothy cream. Rinse well and that's it!

The ancient aristocratic version entails tying *azuki* powder into a small silk bag, which is then moistened and used for scrubbing. The cotton bag is a plebeian variation—less luxurious but just as effective.

Still another method is to mix together equal parts rice bran and *azuki no kona* in the *nukabukuro*, or rice bran bag. *Kurozatō* (so-called black sugar, or the least refined of brown sugar) may also be added.

Azuki no kona may be used daily in place of soap or make-up remover. It will cleanse, whiten, smoothe, exfoliate, stimulate, and improve your skin's circulation and metabolism.

black sugar

Sugar for beauty? We are so well versed in the evils of sugar that it may seem surprising to hear there's anything beautifying about it. Mind you, I'm not suggesting a daily diet of éclairs or the use of white-sugar face packs. The sugar that's good for you is whole sugar—what's known as black sugar, or *kurozatō*, in Japan. Residents or visitors will enjoy discovering black sugar's uses in beauty.

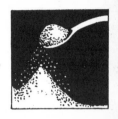

outside

black sugar calming lotion for skin

honey face massage

inside

blackstrap molasses skin tonic

Kurozatō is the active ingredient in Japanese sugar soap, or *kurozatō sekken*, easily found in many Japanese stores. It's a dense, dark brown chunk that cleans the skin—especially benefiting oily or blemished skin—and soothes itchiness. You can also make your own *kurozatō* lotion to calm rashes and acne: dissolve some of the sugar in warm spring water and apply where needed, then rinse.

Blackstrap molasses, which is what remains after the sugar-refining process, can be a potent internal cure for troubled skin, stress, hair damage, and anemia. One tablespoon supplies iron equivalent to that in nine eggs and as much calcium as a glass of milk, and thus a daily tablespoon can be especially beneficial for women.

The other important sweet thing for beauty is honey. Honey acts as a humectant, drawing moisture from the air to the skin, and is very useful for aging or dry skin.

There are many ways of incorporating natural honey into your beauty routine—the easiest is simply to apply honey after a face wash or steam, then gently pat and massage for five minutes. Rinse well.

This quick treatment really "wakes up" the complexion—your face will feel warm as the honey revs up the circulation. Afterward your face will look toned and smell sweet.

Honey is very gentle, but it is reputed to cause delicate exfoliation and to clear up blemishes and help eliminate blackheads. It is known to have antibacterial properties.

A gentle liquid honey-soap is made in Japan, recommended for babies and those with sensitive skin. Look for *hachimitsu sekken*. My three-year-old refuses to use any other soap—perhaps part of its appeal is its luminous honeyish way of trickling slowly out of the bottle onto the sponge.

buckwheat

I have a Russian friend who now and then follows a traditional Russian blood-purification regime, a program that consists of eating nothing but buckwheat in any form over a period of ten days. Is this buckwheat ritual Konstantin's secret source of vigor and glowing skin? At 60, he's in better shape than many 30-year-olds. When he told me of the regimen I was immediately reminded of the Japanese uses for this seed. Buckwheat is known as a blood-purifier and general strengthener of the system in the Japanese tradition as well. Both *soba* and *soba* tea are good everyday medicinal foods.

Buckwheat, in Latin *Fagopyrum esculentum*, is considered a cleansing and stimulating plant in both Eastern and Western traditions. As an external treatment, buckwheat acts as an acid astringent, purifying and cleansing the skin with immediate and visible results. Taken internally, among other various benefits is that same ability to beautify the skin. A generous dose of amino acids and sulfur gives skin a gloss and vitality when buckwheat is included in the diet on a regular basis. Japanese tradition also shows buckwheat to be useful in the treatment of some allergies and in the improvement of lactation. The presence of rutin, an active principle of vitamin P, makes it beneficial when accompanied by vitamin C. In Italy, a mixture of buckwheat and polenta (corn flour) is said to be a detoxifying food.

Attention however! Despite buckwheat's many lovely properties, there are those who are allergic to it. You may be one who finds *soba* indigestible—if so, avoid further use of the substance, whether internally or externally. Allergies to buckwheat are common, so if you don't know your reaction to it, try the patch test described at the beginning of this section.

To use buckwheat externally as a complexion toner, try mixing a European-style face pack with finely ground *soba* flour and a little warm spring water. Apply the creamy mixture to a freshly cleansed face and leave for 15 minutes before rinsing. This simple pack will deep-cleanse the skin and leave the face a tingling rosy color.

An original variation of this pack is what I call the Three Powder Pack, in which the flours of buckwheat, rice, and soybean are mixed with water and applied as above. Those who like a moisturizing pack may add a bit of honey, black sugar, or even a few drops of camellia oil. This pack, recommended for tired skin, will stimulate, soothe, tone, nourish, astringe, cleanse, and strengthen it. Use weekly or as needed.

Another way to use buckwheat externally is to apply an infusion of it to the skin as a rinse. This treatment draws out poisons and is said to have specific benefit in the case of streptococcal skin infections. To make the infusion, steep 10 g/2 tsp of the roasted, coarsely ground kernels in 240 ml/1 C just-boiled pure spring water. Two or three minutes of steeping, and the tea is ready. (Cool before applying to the skin.)

The same buckwheat tea is the thing to take when you need a gentle toning and strengthening of the entire system. If you drink this traditional Japanese tonic tea on a regular basis, over time you will feel the benefits in your body and see the effect on your skin. The flavor is lovely and smoky and the tea is entirely enchanting to drink.

Now, I'm not sure whether scientific studies have been done on the Russian purification program, but I hear that one not only becomes cleansed but also amazingly slim after the ten-day diet. Is that because one can eat only so much buckwheat, I wonder? (Check with a medical practitioner before embarking on this diet, of course.)

the beauty that is inside

Feminine beauty, say the Japanese, is not found on the surface. It exists between things: between the wrapping and what the wrapping conceals; between nature and artifice; between the manifest and the hidden; between the image and the observer. The greatest beauty is that which is not fully seen. Because truly poignant beauty must intimate depth, must arouse a perception of the inner nature, the container for this spiritual essence must be simultaneously unobtrusive and suggestive of an interior presence. The gentle surface beauty, entirely reduced and subdued, controlled by artifice, serves to tightly concentrate and contain the ephemeral essence within, rendering palpable what a too-prepossessing surface beauty might obscure.

burdock

The humble *gobō,* a root vegetable ubiquitous in Japan, is a very useful plant for beauty. In the West, it is known as burdock and is less commonly known but it has there an equally ancient reputation as a potent beauty aid.

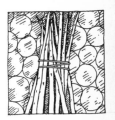

There are many ways, both internal and external, to use *gobō.* Eat it regularly and you will be rewarded with clearer skin and rosier cheeks; the root aids in slimming, as it is a diuretic, and it encourages perspiration and the elimination of wastes and toxins from the body.

The high iron content will help those who are pale, anemic,

and lacking in vitality. Used either internally or externally, burdock's general effects are to purify, normalize, and to increase vitality.

Make a decocted tea from the root or leaves by simmering one part burdock (the root must first be scrubbed, chopped, and soaked) to 10 parts water for 10 minutes. The tea may be taken regularly to clear up skin problems or aid the body in recovering (as after childbirth or surgery or prolonged illness). The seeds may be infused for a rinse or made into a tincture (see appendix) for local application to blemishes or other skin irritations, such as eczema or heat rash.

The decocted root tea may be added to the bath as a diaphoretic and skin-purifier or used in a facial steam for blemishes … a picturesque plant for a picturesque you!

bush warbler

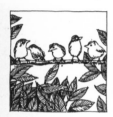

The bush warbler, otherwise known as the *uguisu*, is the source for that most classic of the traditional Japanese beauty treatments, *uguisu no fun*, commonly translated as nightingale droppings but actually the droppings of the bush warbler. Unlike the nightingale with which it is confused, the bush warbler sings during the daytime, most often from a perch in a blossoming plum tree, during the very earliest days of spring.

Uguisu no fun is without a doubt the most exotic of the Japanese natural beauty treatments. It is also extraordinarily effective; due to the action of enzymes contained in the substance, the skin washed with bush warbler droppings is both thoroughly exfoliated and measurably lightened. As this is a chemical process, the skin's rough, dead skin cells are removed without the necessity for rubbing or scrubbing. The lightening action is substantial as well—*uguisu no fun* started out centuries ago as a bleach for fabric; in Korea, it was used to draw white designs upon colored silk. Women of the time, ever desirous of a means of rendering the skin pale and fine, put two and two together and decided to see what would happen if they used the stuff on their complexions. As we see, it worked remarkably well, and *uguisu no fun* became the standard skin beautifier for Japanese upper-class women, geisha, and courtesans.

Uguisu no fun is still made commercially in Japan by a company called Mimiran. It may be found in natural beauty specialty stores, some drugstores, and in the traditional cosmetics shop in Asakusa, Hyakusuke. (See appendix for information.) The package is labelled "Nightingale Droppings," and it contains a fine, pale green powder that is meant to be mixed with a bit of warm water—and soap or cleansing cream if you like—and massaged into the face. If the substance is being used as a lightener, don't add soap and allow to remain on the skin for 5 minutes or so. Some sensitive skins may experience an allergic reaction to bush warbler droppings—if any irritation is felt, rinse immediately and discontinue use. The powdered droppings sold commercially will stay in good condition indefinitely if kept dry and sealed.

camellia

I live in a house with a camellia tree in the garden. The rich and delicate flowers surprise me by blossoming with the first chill of fall. One by one the buds open into frothy pink-edged white blooms, warm yellow at the center.

outside

camellia oil hair dressing

camellia oil moisturizer for hair & skin

I feel honored to have in my presence such a lovely *tsubaki* tree, for not only does it bear glorious flowers but its nut is the source of a most venerable Japanese beauty oil, *tsubaki abura.*

Though camellia oil has traditionally been used for a variety of purposes (lamp oil, furniture polish, cooking), it is best known as a dressing for the hair. The light, odorless oil, which is cold-pressed from the camellia fruit or nut, has been used in Japan for centuries and continues to be popular today. It is a nondrying oil, very high in oleic acid and low in lineolic and linolenic acids. That means it not only has generous moisturizing properties but it also possesses stability—it's less likely than others to deteriorate.

To condition and control hair, camellia oil should be applied a few drops at a time and massaged gently into the scalp and hair ends. Comb through to give your crowning glory a luxuriant sheen. This treatment may be used daily as a health-giving moisturizer for hair and scalp. Applied to the skin it will soften, nourish, and moisturize.

There is something poetic and feminine about the camellia tree—it is fitting that such a tree should give a gift of beautifying oil for women to use in their hair.

carrot

The *Daucus carota* may be utilized in its entirely for health and beauty: the greens are cleansing, diuretic, and carminative, while the root vegetable, source of beta carotene, is attracting immense scientific attention for its antioxidant, anticancer properties. The beauty field sees in the carrot an anti-aging component of the first order; in Chinese medicine the carrot has long been employed not only against the effects of aging but for skin purification and protection, as a treatment for stress, high blood cholesterol, anemia, rheumatism, and allergies, and as a stimulant to the production of red blood cells. In simple terms, it appears that the carrot is good medicine indeed.

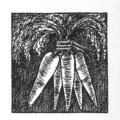

inside

carrot medicine food

outside

carrot juice face pack

Scientific studies suggest that high levels of beta carotene in the bloodstream will protect against UV damage as well as improve skin pigmentation problems. Against cancer, this substance appears to discourage tumor growth even when the process has already begun. Japanese studies show that beta carotene boosts the immuno-surveillance system.

Beta carotene, by the way, can be found not only in carrots but also in sweet potatoes, winter squash, and green leafy vegetables. Along with the beta carotene in carrots come many other carotenoids, and scientists conjecture that it is in the mixture of these hundreds of substances that the secret of the cure is held. Whether some other of the carotenoids performs the miracle is unknown—but it is clear that by consuming the vegetables listed above, along with cabbage, broccoli, brussels sprouts, spinach, kale, and other dark green leafy vegetables, one will improve one's health to a stunning degree.

Drink raw carrot juice, then, and have raw carrots frequently; you may also apply the juice to your skin for a toning treatment pack that will leave you with a luminous glow. When going to a sunny place, prepare your skin by eating plenty of carrots in the weeks prior—not only will you possibly reduce your risk of sun damage, but you will acquire a subtle golden skin tone! (But eat too many and you'll be bright orange! Don't overdo it....)

cherry

The Japanese cannot think of cherry blossoms without being reminded of fresh feminine beauty. The pale pink flower is the symbol of all that is pretty, precious, and quick to pass.

When one looks more closely at the cherry tree, one finds an array of other, less fleeting assets—this tree may be enjoyed both for its many phases of loveliness and for its many uses in health and beauty. There is no part of the cherry tree that does not serve us, if we wish to so avail ourselves.

Shall we start with what's in season in summer? The bark of the tree is a hair-smoother. The time to gather good bark from the tree is golden midsummer, when the sap is rich. Used to bathe the hair, this substance is a supreme de-tangler and silkener. To make conditioner, bring 60 g/2 oz of chopped bark and 600 ml/ 2 1/2 C of pure water to a boil in a nonmetal pan; lower heat and simmer 30 minutes. Add water to bring final volume to 300 ml/ 1 1/4 C, then cool at room temperature. Filter through gauze. Refrigerated, the decoction will keep for three days. Use as a conditioning rinse after every shampoo. This treatment need not be followed by a clear-water rinse.

The bark of the cherry tree can also be used as a darkening rinse for the hair. Follow the above steps for making a decoction, but add walnut hulls and reduce the amount of bark: 30 g/1 oz of cherry tree bark, 30 g/1 oz of walnut hulls, and 600 ml/2 1/2 C of

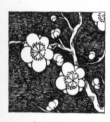

outside

*cherry bark hair-
conditioning rinse*

*cherry bark & walnut
hair-darkening rinse*

cherry leaf bath

inside

*cherry-tail cleansing
tea*

*salty cherry blossom
tea*

pure spring water. The rinse will give deep rich tones to brown or black hair. Its soothing and healing properties make it an ideal rinse for a sensitive scalp, damaged hair, or hair that needs smoothing and toning. It should not be applied to fair hair, although some may wish to try it for darkening greying locks. The application process is identical to the preceding recipe.

Another cherry tree ritual is the cherry tree leaf bath, for stimulating the circulation and cooling inflammations. It is beneficial for all skin types and can alleviate rashes and prickly heat. To make it, add several handfuls of fresh or dried cherry leaves to a tepid bath. The leaves may float loosely or be wrapped and tied in a large square of gauze. As this spring or summer bath is one that is meant to refresh and cool, the water temperature should be kept rather low. Do not rinse after bathing.

In *Golden Secrets of Mystic Oils* by Anna Riva, a handy little book of magic and spells, the essential oil of cherry blossom is prescribed for making the wearer cheerful, gay, lighthearted, and good-humored. Worth a try!

One who wishes to eliminate toxins and excess fluids from the body may do so by consuming the so-called *queues de cerises*—the tails of cherries, also known as the stems. This is an ancient diuretic remedy known in many parts of the world; I came across it in France. A cherry-tail decoction safely and efficiently cleanses the system in cases of hypertension, cystitis, and edema. (Always check with your medical practitioner before embarking on any such program.)

And as the Cat in the Hat would say, that is not all—no, that is not all! You may perhaps want to celebrate a moment of joy by drinking cherry-blossom tea. To make this beguiling Japanese beverage, pour 120 ml/1 1/2 C of just-boiled spring water over 2 or 3 salt-preserved cherry blossoms (available in Japanese markets) in a festive cup, then sip with delight. What to celebrate? Why not the many phases of feminine beauty? There is so much more to it than just that poignant brief blossoming!

chickpea

The East Indian beauty tradition has given us the charming chickpea. Try the following chickpea powder pack for skin-cleansing and toning treatment (you can find chickpea powder, or *chana besan*, in an Indian market): mix a couple of spoonfuls of chickpea powder with the juice from half a lemon and a little yogurt. Apply the light creamy mixture to the entire body. Let it stay on for 20 minutes, then bathe. This delightful body pack leaves the skin amazingly fresh and vibrant-looking.

Taken internally, the chickpea benefits the blood by helping to reduce cholesterol levels. High in potassium, calcium, iron and

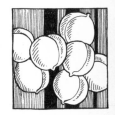

outside

*chickpea & lemon &
yogurt body pack*

vitamin A, and a low-fat, high-protein source of nourishment, the chickpea is a good addition to a vegetarian diet.

chinese wolfberry

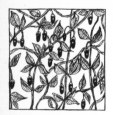

Don't you love the name of this plant? Perhaps in ancient forests the little red berry was nibbled by wolves and wild dogs, and maybe the healers of those early times saw that the fruit was a kind of medicine for them. Whatever the case, the Chinese wolfberry enjoys a strong and central position in the traditional Asian pharmacopeia.

The plant *Lycium Chinense Mill.* (*Solanaceae*) is known particularly for its berries (these are called *gou qi zi* in Chinese, *kuko no mi* in Japanese). The berry is used in Chinese medicine as a nutrient kidney and liver tonic, but it is popularly prized as well for its role in sexual rejuvenation, beauty, and longevity. The berry may be incorporated in dried form into everyday cuisine or taken as a decoction or tincture. The root skin is medicinal as well. The orange-red berry ripens in late summer or early fall and is a native of China and Japan.

As a tonic for the blood and bodily fluids, the Chinese wolfberry is designated a yin tonic. Conditions treated by the berry include diabetes and tuberculosis, while the root skin is antipyretic and employed as a cough remedy in tuberculosis. In Ayurvedic medicine this type of substance is said to encourage moisture and soothe an excess of fire and wind. Dry skin, menstrual irregularities, lethargy, pallor, and weakness are among the conditions commonly treated by the wolfberry. An herb associated with earth in the Chinese classification system, the *gou qi zi* is a sweet, neutral herb, with affinity for stomach, liver, kidneys, mouth, and muscles.

The root skin (*di qu pi* in Chinese), is used also as a tonic, with an affinity for lungs and kidneys. This part of the plant is prescribed for asthma and coughs, blood in urine, and fevers due to yin-deficiency; as well, the fresh root also lowers both blood sugar and blood pressure.

Rich in vitamin A and iron, the Chinese wolfberry is associated with beauty, and is indicated as a remedy for hair loss or to restore hair's natural pigment. The skin too is treated by this herb, which is said to soften wrinkles and eliminate age spots or other pigment-related problems. For men, the berry will nourish semen, and for both sexes it will act as a sexual tonic. A Chinese friend includes the Chinese wolfberry in her family's diet on a regular basis to ensure the long-lasting beauty of both skin and hair. Here is one of her recipes:

sex & beauty meal

ingredients: 200 g/7 oz chicken wings
3 T/1 1/2 oz Chinese wolfberries
water
5 *shiitake* mushrooms
1 yam cut into bite-size cubes
a handful of chopped bamboo shoots

preparation: Place chicken wings and Chinese wolfberries in a heavy pan with water to cover,
then simmer gently for 30 minutes.

Add *shiitake*, cubed yam, and chopped
bamboo shoots. Simmer one hour, then add
seasonings as desired (e.g., soy sauce and
spices).

chrysanthemum

October is the month that brings lovely warm blue days and early-
darkening nights, the month when we remember that winter is to
come again. But before the coming of the cold weather, we enjoy
the changing leaves, chrysanthemums, the first good apples; we
begin to appreciate hot baths again, the soak that takes the chill
from early autumn evenings.

To combine two of autumn's special pleasures, take a bath of
floating chrysanthemum blossoms. This bath is called *kiku-yu* or
shungiku-yu and is a most Japanese experience. Chrysanthemums in Japan have a traditional symbolic association with
longevity, and devotees believe that soaking in a chrysanthemum
bath ensures a long and healthy life.

Along with the unique fragrance of chrysanthemum wafting in
the steam, the bather may contemplate the visual charm of yellow blossoms drifting in the hot water, inspiring autumn thoughts.

Aesthetic and sensual appeal aside, the chrysanthemum-blos-
som bath will bring health benefits as well. As an antibacterial
agent, the flower can help to heal wounds and skin irritations,
banishing bacteria and germs.

Although autumn is the natural season for chrysanthemums,
summer is a good time to add both flowers and leaves to the
bath. The astringent, purifying, healing whole plant benefits skin
that is sensitive to heat and humidity, skin that gets irritated,
bumpy, and unpleasant in response to summer.

The edible chrysanthemum is the one you want to use for
either seasonal bath; buy the yellow flowers and the fresh, pun-
gent-smelling greens at a Japanese vegetable store or pluck
them from your garden. Wash the plants carefully, then wrap a
generous bunch of blossoms and greens in a big gauze or muslin

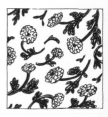

outside

*chrysanthemum flower
and leaf bath*

inside

chrysanthemum tea

square and tie it closed. Plunge the bundle into a pot of boiling water, remove from the fire, then let it steam for 30 minutes, covered. That done, toss the whole lot into the freshly drawn bath and then you get in, too. There you will soak for 20 minutes or so, making sure to apply the water to your face as much as possible. You may nibble the petals if you feel the inclination.

Chrysanthemum tea offers cleansing, astringent, and liver-toning benefits: prepare with greens as an infusion.

citrus

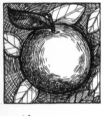

outside

citrus peel bath

neroli skin moisturizer

inside

citrus medicine food

The ordinary everyday citrus fruit holds some surprising qualities within its juice and rind. Take, for example, *Citrus reticulata blanco* (a type of tangerine, or *mikan* in Japanese): the rind of the unripe fruit—*qing pi*—is used by the Chinese to mobilize *ki* energy; the rind of the ripe fruit—*chen pi*—is used to mobilize *ki* and also to aid the digestion, calm a cough, and generally tone the organism. The Japanese bathe in the powdered rind of the ripe tangerine, and also with *yuzu*, or citron. The circulation and the skin benefit from this practice, the latter becoming more silky, more fine, more glowing—more beautiful in all respects. The vitamin C in citrus helps to protect against sun damage, lighten the skin, and fight the signs of age, whether the fruit is taken internally or applied externally. Female rice farmers in Japan know that to rub the fresh rind of a citrus fruit over the face will beautify it. (Do not apply just prior to sun exposure, however, as the vitamin C may then increase photosensitivity. Bergamot should be avoided for the same reason.)

The orange tree originated in China but became a beloved source of medicine among Arab physicians in the Middle Ages. The flower of the bitter orange, the *Citrus aurantium*, yields the exquisite essential oil neroli, and the bitter orange itself is used in China for the mobilization of *ki*, to stimulate digestion, and as a sedative for the nervous system. The oil is both sedative and antidepressant; used in greatly diluted form externally, neroli softens dry skin. (Add a tiny drop to a pot of face cream or to a small bottle of camellia oil.)

To try the medicinal magic of the citrus family, buy organic tangerines (clementines or mandarins will do, just as well) and citrons. Don't discard the peels when you eat the fruits, but hang them up to dry or let them dessicate on the windowsill, then use them in the bath as is or in a cloth bag for *ki* and beauty. Whole citrons may also be floated in a hot bath to wonderful effect.

cucumber

A more refined version of the basic cucumber-slice face pack, traditional Japanese cucumber tonic is made by soaking chopped cucumbers in good *shōchū* for a month or so. What you get is a cucumber tincture that will cool hot or sunburnt skin, heal inflammations, relieve pain, and correct excess oiliness. Cucumber tonic used daily will lighten the skin considerably. Other pleasant effects: skin is smoothed and wrinkles are softened. And if you want to lighten freckles, this is the way to do it.

To make your own cucumber tonic, wash and dry fresh cucumbers and chop or grind well. Place in a sterilized wide-necked bottle with *shōchū* or vodka in a 1:3 ratio. Seal the bottle and let the mixture stand undisturbed for two weeks to a month. Strain and rebottle when the tonic is ready; store in the refrigerator.

During the summer months, the traditional Japanese beauty applies cucumber tonic lotion in the morning and loofah-vine water at night. Neither lotion is rinsed after application. This practice is thought to ensure skin that is delicately pale, clear, fresh-looking, and smooth.

For painful sunburn, make a pack by grinding cucumber finely and mixing with rice flour and water to a creamy consistency. Apply to a clean face, leave on 15 minutes, then rinse well with cool water. Pain and redness will diminish. Cucumber juice or purée is used as a full body pack in Thailand, where it's prized for its effects on skin texture.

A note for those with very dry skin: cucumbers are astringent, so avoid excessive use. Instead, stick to loofah-vine water, which has moisturizing properties.

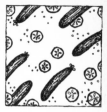

outside

cucumber facial tonic

cucumber sunburn pack

daikon

With the chilly days of late fall return some special pleasures: in Japan, ripening persimmons glowing vivid orange on their branches, the low steam-whistle sound of the sweet-potato vendor, the warming luxury of the Japanese bath.

For "body-heating," an old-time Japanese favorite is the *daikon* greens bath—a cold-weather bath that is thought to stimulate the metabolism and warm the body.

To prepare the leaves (which may be of *daikon*, radish, or turnip), hang them up indoors away from the light. When they are thoroughly dried, boil several bunches in a large pot filled with water for an hour. The water is then added to a preheated bath.

The *daikon* greens bath may be taken once a week or so; more frequent use is advisable only for medical treatment of certain health conditions. (This bath is used particularly in the treatment of problems involving the female reproductive system, and for poor circulation. However, it must be prescribed for these purposes—do not use it frequently unless a specialist has advised you to do so.)

Another, simpler method of preparing the *daikon* greens bath

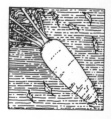

outside

daikon *greens bath*

daikon *face pack or lotion*

is to wrap a few dried daikon leaves in cheesecloth and add this to the bath. You will enjoy similar benefits, but not to the degree offered by the first method.

Though the *daikon* greens bath is known in Japan as a "woman's bath," anyone may use it occasionally with good results. Along with its benefits to the metabolism, it will deep-cleanse the skin, freeing it of toxins and odors. A note: the *daikon* greens bath should not be reheated or saved for another day, a common practice in Japan where bathtubs often have reheating systems.

In the summer, *daikon* may be applied in slices as for a face pack, or grated and squeezed for juice, to be applied as a lotion. These are soothing remedies for summer skin aggravation.

dandelion

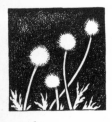

outside

dandelion sap wart remedy

inside

dandelion root tea for beauty

dandelion greens medicine food

The beloved *tampopo* of Japan is a plant valued worldwide for its uses in health and beauty care. Known as *Pu gong ying* in Chinese and *Taraxacum officinale* in Latin, the charming weed we call dandelion is important in herbal traditions everywhere.

The most useful part of the dandelion is the root or rhizome, which is sold in dried, chopped form in tea shops, well-stocked pharmacies, and *kampōyaku* apothecaries in Japan, where it goes by the name *tampopo-cha*. (While one may certainly harvest the fresh root for home-drying, the process takes a long time; also, improperly dried roots can easily grow moldy and mildewed.) The fresh sap is also occasionally of use as an external remedy for a wide variety of skin problems; the sap is best gathered directly from the stem of a living plant.

Known in both European and Asian traditions as a potent purifier, the root of the dandelion is taken internally as an infusion or decoction to improve liver functions, aid in the elimination of toxins and wastes, lower cholesterol levels, treat female hormone imbalances, and encourage more efficient digestion. Dandelion root tea is thus useful for one who consumes alcohol or nicotine in excess, overindulges in highly processed or high-fat foods, experiences stomach problems or chronic constipation, or suffers from kidney stones. The dandelion may act as an anticandida agent, according to some sources. Due to its purifying properties, the vitamin A-rich dandelion root will clear and beautify the skin—relieved of some of the burden of toxins improperly processed by a sluggish liver, the skin becomes translucent and vital-looking. Dandelion root tea is known in Japan as a beauty tea.

A diuretic tonic, *tampopo-cha* may be taken daily over a period of several months to effect a gradual cure. Because it is a diuretic, no more than 2 cups per day are advisable, and still the diet should include plenty of pure water. Unlike most diuretics, this tea helps the body to replace potassium. Japanese grandmothers attest that it encourages the production of breast milk in lactating mothers. Children should not drink this tea.

Tampopo-cha is most often prepared exactly as one would prepare ordinary tea—that is, by steeping approximately a teaspoonful of the herb in approximately 1 cup of just-boiled water, then straining. An alternative way to take *tampopo* is as a coffee substitute or even a coffee additive like chicory. For this purpose, one can purchase roasted and ground dandelion root; the substance is steeped, lightly boiled or percolated, or infused by the drip method, either with coffee beans or without. A final way to take dandelion internally is to toss the greens into a salad.

To use the plant externally, one merely plucks the flower; the watery sap contained in the stem may be applied to warts or eczema daily for a gradual improvement in the condition. It is said as well that the sap is an effective antitoxin in cases of snakebite—however, if I were bitten by a slithering serpent, I think I'd prefer to resort to something slightly more dynamic! But it is worth remembering that the humble little dandelion is a poison-fighting purifier whether used inside or out.

dokudami

Dokudami (*Houttuynia cordata*) is one of those traditional "miracle" plants, used in Japan for centuries to treat everything from dry skin to liver spots to rheumatism. The leaves of *dokudami* may be used in shampoo, in tea, to flavor vinegar and honey (and supply medicinal benefits to those foods), as a facial rinse, and in the bath as a curative.

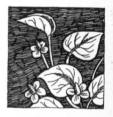

outside

dokudami *tea*

dokudami *treatment for skin & hair*

dokudami *bath*

inside

dokudami *tea tonic*

These days in Japan, in good drugstores, health food stores, and natural beauty shops, you can buy *dokudami* honey, *dokudami* tea, *dokudami* vinegar, *dokudami* food supplement tablets, *dokudami* soap, *dokudami* skin lotion, and *dokudami* bath salts. As this is a healing plant that has survived the centuries with its reputation intact, it may be worth a little exploration by those who are so inclined.

Dokudami is one Japanese medicinal plant that appears not to be common elsewhere. Thus, experiment with this one when on Japanese soil.

As far as I have been able to gather, *dokudami* acts as a general tonic. Traditionally, it has been taken internally to improve the condition of the skin, helping to cleanse it of toxins and to remove such imperfections as liver spots. In fact, people I have talked with about this plant (those ever-knowledgeable grandmothers) claim it will cure just about anything, and that it will strengthen the body against illness if taken as a preventative, as a tea or in honey or vinegar.

External treatments are thought to be good for such skin problems as eczema, dry skin, prickly heat, and poor circulation. Those who suffer from neuralgia, rheumatism, lumbago, muscle aches, or poor overall condition may benefit from the *dokudami* bath. As a hair rinse or shampoo, it strengthens and purifies.

Dokudami is a rapidly propagating creeping perennial that grows weedlike all over Japan. Recognize it by its heart-shaped leaves (see illustration), its small, white, four-petaled blossoms, and by its utterly overwhelming bitter-pungent fragrance.

The traditional recipe for preparing *dokudami* tea (which is ingested, applied to skin or hair, or added to the bath) is as follows: Wash 30 *dokudami* leaves. Mash in a mortar and squeeze through muslin to obtain plant juice.

Note: because extreme caution is always advised when treating oneself with potent medicinal plants, I do *not* recommend making the tea from scratch for drinking—it is too easy to mistake amounts. But do make the tea for external use, always diluting before application. If you are new to *dokudami*, the best approach is to buy the ready-made products and follow the directions carefully.

egg

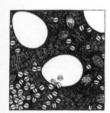

inside

*egg-*sake *tonic & cold remedy*

Tamagozake, a hot, sweet, egg-and-*sake* drink, is a popular home remedy in Japan, to be taken at the first sign of a cold or when one feels chilled and run-down. This drink warms the body and causes sweating. It is said to improve circulation, and the alcohol will certainly encourage sleep.

To prepare *tamagozake*, you will need *sake*, sugar, and an egg. Beat the egg, and when it is frothy, add sugar to taste. Set aside. Pour the *sake* into a ceramic *sake*-serving container, set into a pan of water that has been heating over a low flame, and heat for a few minutes. Slowly add the *sake* to the egg-sugar mixture, then set alight if desired. (A little flamboyance raises the spirits, too.)

As we've said, there is an area of interface between beauty and health, and very often the two realms are inseparable. A cold certainly leaves one feeling unglamorous! So I will call this a beauty cure, no question!

eggplant

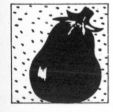

I asked the assistants at my Japanese dentist's office about charred-eggplant toothpaste, and I got cries of what seemed like dismay that I had discovered such a thing still existed. Giggles, admonitions not to use it, and even disbelief greeted me.

However, this toothpaste does exist and is marketed by several companies in Japan. It is gloriously *black*. The toothpaste, *yakinasu no hamigakiko*, is traditionally made from the charred tops of eggplants, which black substance is then ground to a powder and mixed with salt. Nowadays you can buy tubes of it; the principal ingredients are the same, but other substances have been added to make it more tasty and toothpastey. The stuff is said to be wonderful for the gums, and in fact it feels and tastes very much like the old salt-and-baking-soda tooth cleanser my father used to swear by for healthy gums.

I have tried several brands sold in Japan—the most palatable was Binotomo Dentifrice Jet Black, found in the health corner of many department stores. Health food stores outside Japan some-times carry eggplant toothpaste. It's very salty, and the taste seems odd at first, but it does seem to clean well. If you like that minty aftertaste you get with regular toothpaste, just follow up with a second brushing using your usual brand.

Eggplant toothpaste is perishable; keep it out of the light. Also, it may stain clothing, so brush neatly. Close the cap tightly after use. The toothpaste is said to eliminate smoking stains and bad breath. I don't know if that is true, but I do love the way my teeth gleam so whitely after a jet-black brushing! (The recipe for charcoal powder tooth-and-gum cleanser—a similar dentifrice— is found in many areas of the world, and is still used in parts of the South Pacific.)

outside

black eggplant tooth cleanser

---

eggplant toothpaste

Perhaps you want to make your own black toothpaste? You'll need some fresh baby eggplants and some sea salt.

First pickle the eggplants by placing them in an earthen-ware pot with hot water and sea salt, 1 part salt to 5 parts eggplant, water just to cover. Use a heavy stone as a weight on the press-lid (the lid can be any flat nonmetal disc, placed directly on the eggplants).

Let pickle for at least 3 days.

Remove eggplants from the brine, then detach the stems with the calyxes (the bit where the stem connects to the vegetable); string the stem-and-calyxes up to dry in an airy, shady location.

When dried, roast in a covered heavy skillet over a very low fire for a long time—until black and powdery.

Pulverize the black powdery charred eggplant tops com-pletely in a mortar and pestle.

To store this black toothpowder, place in a sealed glass or ceramic container away from moisture and sunlight.

Use as any toothpowder, by applying an adequate amount to a moistened toothbrush for brushing teeth and gums.

Note that this toothpowder is somewhat abrasive, so brush gently. If teeth and gums are sensitive, use only occasionally.

fennel

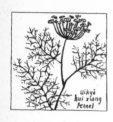

outside

fennel seed eyewash

fennel bath

inside

fennel seed tea

Fennel, *uikyō* in Japanese, *hui xiang* in Chinese, and in Latin *Foeniculum vulgare* (*Umbelliferae*), is one of those plants that has a worldwide reputation as a health and beauty herb. Roman gladiators consumed fennel in large quantities to achieve ferocious strength and maintain health; Roman women of that ancient time ate fennel in an effort to control their weight. Anglo-Saxons believed fennel had the power to combat evil, and in A.D. 812 Charlemagne pronounced fennel an imperative imperial garden plant. Fennel today adds flavor as a culinary spice to many of the world's cuisines.

In Asia, fennel has had a long tradition as a healing plant and is one of the more common of the *yakusō* sold for home remedies. Though it is the seeds that are most commonly used, every part of the plant may be consumed: root, stem, seed, leaf, and flower. Its aromatic seeds make *uikyō* a cherished plant in the Japanese incense tradition; in both East and West the seeds are chewed as a breath-sweetener. While the plant is basically safe for both internal and external use, excessive doses must be avoided (i.e., when taken as a tea, no more than 1–2 cups per day).

Taken internally, either infused for tea or sprinkled into foods during or after they are prepared, fennel seed is said in Japan to improve the general condition, balance and regulate *ki* (vital energy), improve the condition of the stomach, regulate weight, increase mother's milk, and subdue pain. (The Western herbal tradition recognizes the same properties.) Pregnant women are sometimes advised to take small amounts of fennel seed as an inducement to lactation and as a prechildbirth strengthener, though large amounts may be harmful.

As for external uses, in Japan an eyewash made from the infused seeds is said to relax and cleanse the eyes. In both West and East, a bath using the whole plant is said to warm, stimulate, deep-cleanse, and soothe. Basically a relaxing bath, the fennel water will also act to soften and smooth the skin. The bath may be taken daily if desired.

To prepare an infusion of the seeds, boil 240 ml/1 C of water, remove from flame, and add one teaspoon of seeds to steep ten minutes or longer. Remember to use pure water and no metal containers in the preparation. To prepare the bath, chop fresh fennel stalks and leaves, tie into a gauze square, then suspend the bag from the faucet; fill the bath first with hot water only, in order to infuse the plant. Later, add the appropriate quantity of cold water to achieve a comfortable bathing temperature. (Dried fennel may be used in the same fashion.)

field horsetail

Going by the old Japanese solar calendar, which originated in China and which divided the year into 24 seasonal segments, one begins looking for the first shoots of *sugina*, or field horsetail (*Equisetum arvense*), in *Keichitsu*, or the End of Insect Hibernation, which falls in early March.

A medicinal, edible plant that grows in humid areas, *sugina* may be found in forests, mountains, gardens, and vacant lots. It is also an internationally available packaged herb.

Another of the plants used in both Asia and the West for its medicinal properties, field horsetail stems are infused into a tea that may be employed externally or internally. In Japan, the plant is also cooked as a vegetable in season.

Extraordinarily rich in minerals, especially potassium and silica, field horsetail is considered a "remineraliser" and regenerator whether used inside or out. When applied as a hair treatment, it stimulates hair growth and eliminates dandruff; when used for the face, it can remedy pimples and "unhappy skin." A stimulant to the complexion, *sugina* improves the texture and tone of aging skin, and restores skin's moisture balance.

Both the hair treatment and the complexion treatment are prepared in the same way: add a handful of fresh horsetail stems ($1/2$ the amount if the substance is dried) to 300 ml/1 $1/4$ C of just-boiled water in a nonmetal pot, cover, and allow to steep until cool. Remove solids by straining through gauze; it may be necessary to strain the remaining liquid twice. (This liquid may be stored for a maximum of 3 days if transferred to a sterile glass bottle and refrigerated.)

For use on the face, apply with cotton to a freshly cleansed face; do not rinse. As a hair rinse, the field horsetail liquid may be massaged into the hair after shampooing, then either rinsed out or left in, as desired. (Field horsetail possesses cleansing properties, thus it was used in the Japanese tradition as a gentle, curative hair wash.) Both the skin and the hair treatments may be used on a regular basis for any type of skin or hair.

Taken internally, field horsetail infusion will reinforce the general constitution, and thus it is particularly useful for fatigue. The plant acts as a diuretic and thus stimulates the liver, improving that organ's functioning.

Sugina has the ability to strengthen bones, cartilage, and tendons, making it an important remedy for athletes, those with broken bones, or those suffering from joint problems. Not only does this plant encourage the regeneration of connective tissue and the reconstitution of cartilage but it increases the suppleness of tendons and vascular walls. Those whose tendons are under stress—tennis players, cyclists, and runners—may take *sugina*

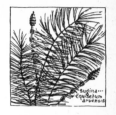

outside

field-horsetail-tea skin & hair rinse

inside

field horsetail tea

tea daily as a preventive remedy. Those who suffer from tendonitis may take the tea as a cure. For the drinking infusion, prepare as above but use only one teaspoonful of plant substance per 240 ml/1 C of water, and steep five minutes then strain. Take one cup per day for maintenance, 2 or 3 cups daily during a 2-week period for curative purposes.

fruit

Grapes, melons, peaches, and berries of summer—who can resist the luscious colors? Frosty purple, golden pink, cool green, crisp white, scarlet … August is the perfect time to try these fruits in beauty treatments. The European natural beauty tradition and the Japanese as well make much of fruits in season—they can be used as facial tonics, packs, scrubs, and in the bath. Their benefits are many.

In summer, skin is overheated, stressed from pollution, prone to irritation and sunburn, and if oily or sensitive, inclined to behave in unattractive, unruly ways. Summer skin needs cooling, protecting, soothing, and refining.

In choosing your fruits, follow these general guidelines: Peaches and melons are good skin-texture refiners; berries are softening and astringent; grapes are tonic, cooling, soothing, and nourishing. Normal skin types will benefit from grape, canteloupe, watermelon, and peach; oily skin from Persian melon, watermelon, canteloupe, peach, grape, strawberry, or cherry; dry skin from honeydew melon, watermelon, canteloupe, and grape. The mashed fruit of peach is especially good for soothing extremely irritated skin.

Fruit packs are used to refine and deep-cleanse the skin, and to tighten and stimulate the complexion. To prepare, mash the fruit and drain excess juice. Apply fruit pulp to a freshly washed (or preferably, steamed) face, then relax for 15 minutes before rinsing.

For a facial scrub—a superlative way to stimulate and cleanse—mash fruit and mix with cornmeal, ground oatmeal, or almond meal. Use gently as an exfoliating massage; rinse with water.

Fresh fruit skin tonics are simplicity itself: after washing the face, pat the skin with a slice of the fruit. Don't rinse, just pat dry. Melon slices are effective compresses for tired eyes, or eyes with bags or dark circles under them.

Tropical fruits are also rich in beauty benefits. From the South Pacific's wealth of fruit, flower, and nut beauty secrets, the fruit treats that follow are derived.

Papaya is an amazing fruit, full of enzymes that can tenderize meat, help digest proteins, and exfoliate dead skin. Papaya juice

outside

fruit face pack

fruit facial scrub

fruit facial tonic

melon eye compress

papaya juice peel

papaya face pack

papaya purée body pack

pineapple juice facial rinse

pineapple face scrub

coconut oil hair pack

monoï & sand exfoliant

coconut milk & honey face pack

monoï for skin & hair

applied occasionally to the skin for just a few minutes will effect a gentle peeling, ridding your skin of those dulling, complexion-clogging dead skin cells we all despise. A pack of mashed ripe papaya will gently do the same, smoothing the skin while it combats oiliness. In Thailand, a body pack of papaya purée is applied to refine skin to a state of velvety perfection. Use papaya only once a week, and always on a freshly washed face; rinse well.

Pineapple juice is another remedy for too-oily skin; you can use it daily as an astringent rinse, diluted with pure water. The mashed fresh fruit can be used as an exfoliant scrub.

Coconut oil makes a wondrous oil treatment for hair: apply the warmed oil copiously to hair and scalp, then cover head with a plastic shower cap and hot towels and relax in a tub or sauna. Shampoo twice and your hair will be luscious—thick, and glossy.

A simple but effective skin treatment from India also utilizes the coconut: mix a little coconut milk with some honey to make a very nourishing face pack. As might be imagined, this treatment results in luminous, milky, honeyed skin! Coconut milk is said to possess gentle cleansing properties as well. The next time you're stranded on an island in the South Pacific, you'll know what to use to remove your make-up.

Monoï, a beauty treat made in Tahiti from coconut oil and fragrant flower essences, is the ultimate tropical indulgence for skin and hair. Tahitian beauties mix *monoï* with fine sand as an exfoliant for the skin of the entire body. *Monoï* is easy to find in French-speaking parts of the world.

garlic

Garlic is so universally respected as a healing plant, and the subject of so many recent studies, that it seems almost redundant to bring it up. The Japanese do everything imaginable to make use of garlic's powers, including bathing in it. It's the inside/outside cure par excellence.

The Egyptians prescribed garlic to the builders of the pyramids, and evidently with good reason. Garlic is now recognized as possessing a remarkable ability to reduce blood cholesterol and diminish the risk of heart attack in those susceptible. Further, garlic stimulates the immune system and shows impressive results in controlling allergic reactions in laboratory animals. Garlic has been used as a medicinal agent for about 5,000 years; almost everywhere in the world its antibiotic and antifungal properties have long been recognized.

A dab of garlic juice on a pimple will speed the bump on its way, and garlic included in the daily diet will do a lot to improve resistance to infections. Although odorless forms of garlic and garlic tablets are available, the authentic, aromatic fresh garlic

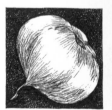

outside

garlic juice for pimples

garlic bath

inside

garlic medicine food

clove is by far the most effective medicine.

To bathe in garlic (if you dare): crush quite a few cloves of garlic and squeeze the juice for adding to the bath. This is an ancient recipe for health, beauty, and longevity, although you might conceivably regret the loss of social life that could ensue, unless you could convince all your friends to garlic-bathe as well....

ginger

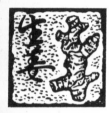

outside

ginger bath

ginger flower juice for skin

ginger flower & coconut oil for skin

inside

ginger tea

ginger medicine food

What can you do when you're tired, feeling run-down, and just not looking your best? Take a ginger bath, of course.

An Indian yoga teacher first recommended this ancient Asian treatment for beauty and health to me. She knew of nothing better for eliminating toxins or soothing sore muscles after exercise. Ginger is an important ingredient in Japanese folk remedies for fever and colds, and a member of Chinese medicine's panoply of star botanicals. Concoct a tea from fresh ginger by grating some into a cup of hot water, or simply add a few root slices to your customary cuppa.

How to try a ginger bath? Grate two large pieces of ginger root. Squeeze the grated ginger in cheesecloth until you have about a cup of ginger juice. This zesty elixir is then added to your hot bath. Relax in the bath at least long enough to perspire freely, as you would in a sauna.

A good soak in the ginger bath will rejuvenate and stimulate, and it's a lovely way to combat aches and pains, tension, fatigue, and colds. Ginger is warming, aromatic, and invigorating—can you think of a nicer, spicier way to chase a malaise?

In Tahiti, a sunburn remedy is made from the ginger flower; squeezed juice from the petals is said to soothe and heal burns. And in nearby Palau, the same flower juice mixed with coconut oil is used to prevent and treat stretch marks. Combined with ginger's ability to aid in weight control, warm the body, and stimulate circulation and local metabolism, these skin-saving benefits make the root an all-around beauty treasure.

ginkgo

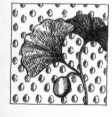

I have always delighted in the shape of the ginkgo leaf—it is like a tiny Japanese fan. On Japanese city streets in autumn—when the ginkgo leaves turn yellow—there are thousands of the delicate bright fans fluttering in the breeze. The ginkgo nut is also something to appreciate: in Asian cuisines it is prized for its sweet mild flavor and creamy texture, and in Asian natural medicine it is treasured for its benefits to health and beauty. Western scientists are exploring the ginkgo nut's potential efficacy as an anti-aging component, employed externally, and scientists on both sides of the globe have been studying its benefits to the cardiovascular system for the past 10 years.

The Ginkgo Biloba is an exceedingly old tree. It belongs to the order Ginkgoales, and can be traced back 200 million years to the Mesozoic Era. Originally from Asia, where it flourished in temple gardens and perhaps survived the centuries for this reason, the ginkgo arrived in Europe in 1730, where it enjoyed a prestigious position as a favored ornamental. The ginkgo can reach a height of 35 meters and exists in male and female forms. It is the female tree that bears the nuts. Both leaves and nuts are used medicinally.

In regard to the nuts, it is important to know that they become yellow when ripe and then begin to fall from the trees. In Asia in autumn, if you watch, you will notice scores of housewives and gourmet cooks out searching the ground under the trees; join them and pluck some of these little treasures for yourself!

A word of warning here: the nuts, described in botanical terms as foul-smelling and drupe-like, must not be retrieved with the bare hands, for the outer layer that encases the good part is not only odoriferous but irritating to the skin. Handle these nuts carelessly and you'll have not only hands that stay smelly for days but probably a good case of contact dermatitis. The usual way is to pick them up with a handkerchief.

When you get the nuts home, don rubber gloves to remove the fleshy orange outer layer—this is the nasty part—while running cold water over them. After washing and draining the nuts, gently crack the middle layer—a whitish shell—with a nutcracker. The third and final layer is a brown skin that is removed by immersing the nuts briefly in hot water. The skin can then be easily peeled away.

Lacking access to fresh nuts—but look around you! the trees are everywhere!—purchase fresh precleaned nuts in any food store in autumn. Various components of the ginkgo plant are available in *kampōyaku* apothecaries, but do consult a specialist for appropriate dosages and applications. And while the nuts themselves are taken safely as food and are generally benign when applied externally, in both internal and external use quantities must be kept low. Large amounts or repeated use can be extremely toxic, leading to convulsions, skin reactions, headaches, and other adverse reactions.

In Chinese medicine, the ripe nut (known as *bai gou*) is macerated in oil for 100 days and employed internally as a treatment for tuberculosis. The ginkgo is thought to act directly upon the lung and kidney meridians. The nut taken as a medicinal food is said to offer astringent, sedative, antitussive, and anti-asthma properties, and the outer pulp is employed as a vessicant. The

outside

ginkgo leaf tea for varicose veins

ginkgo nut skin treatment

inside

ginkgo nut medicine food

leaf is used in Western herbalism for circulatory problems; it appears that the leaf enacts a powerful effect on severe cardiac problems, causing dilation of blood vessels and stimulating blood flow. Externally, a tincture or infusion of the leaf applied to varicose veins and hemorrhoids soothes and ameliorates those conditions. Western herbalists see the ginkgo as an important tonic, with special impact on the mind, emotions, and memory.

While it is clear that the ginkgo has extraordinary powers, for any of the truly medicinal uses always, always consult a specialist! If you wish to add the ginkgo nut to your diet as an occasional treat, you will be getting some of the benefits without the dangers. However, there are two topical recipes that may be tried for those so inclined. From Europe, this recipe for varicose veins: apply a strained infusion of 50 g/1 3/4 oz of dried leaves to 50 ml/1 3/4 oz of water regularly to varicose veins. An easy way to do this is to pat the tea on with a saturated gauze pad. And from the Japanese folk medicine chest, this recipe for soothing, protecting, and purifying the skin: grind freshly peeled ginkgo nuts very fine using a mortar and pestle, massage gently over a well-cleansed face, then rinse. Practiced weekly, this ritual will clear and enrich the skin. Again, if you tend to have sensitive, allergic skin, don't even try it. And do a patch test on your arm first if you're not sure. While the leaves are thought to be benign, if there is any sign of inflammation, immediately discontinue use.

ginseng

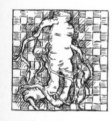

inside

ginseng tea

outside

ginseng tea rinse for face and hair

Panax ginseng is a root of great power. This Eastern medicine is used as a tonic against fatigue, as a remedy for stress, and to promote endurance. Ginseng is generally prescribed for specific periods of short duration. The root is known as *ren shen* in Chinese, a word that translates as "man-root." Ginseng is an adaptogen, simultaneously sedative and stimulating in effect, regulating and balancing body functions like blood pressure and blood sugar levels, and lowering cholesterol. A general revitalizer, ginseng has long been acknowledged in the Chinese tradition as a longevity aid and sexual tonic.

A combination of ginsenosides (also known, in Russia, as panaxosides, these are eleven or so hormone-like saponins), vitamins B and C, essential oils, amino acids, and estrogens work together against problems like loss of vigor due to aging, impotence, lassitude, energy deficiency, weakness, hypertension, insomnia, and sluggish physical and intellectual performance. In Chinese medicine, an energy tonic such as ginseng is often employed in tandem with blood nourishers, prescribed when *ki* is deficient. Together, these substances stimulate blood production as well as its circulation. Persons of normal health should not take ginseng for periods longer than three weeks; persons who are depressed, anxious, or who have inflammatory illnesses should not take it at all.

An occasional cup of ginseng tea will calm and tone the nervous system, and one may use the same tea as a facial or hair rinse to stimulate, strengthen, and tone. Were good ginseng not so costly, I would even advise a tonic man-root bath now and then! If you've got ginseng growing in your garden, by all means indulge.

---

the beauty that disappears

The greatest beauty dies young, goes the old Japanese saying. The rich sadness of perfect beauty, beauty that is at its fullest blossoming, lies in the knowledge, aroused in the observer, that it is destined to disappear. It is the delicate beauty of a young girl, the pale pink splendor of the blossoming cherry, the radiant magnificence of the moon behind a wisp of cloud. Beauty lasts but a moment. The emotional instant when simultaneously are felt the mingled sensations of aesthetic delight and the realization of its impermanence, beauty and sadness, is *mono no aware,* a deep and exquisite melancholy. True beauty is felt in the heart, where it resonates with quiet poignancy.

---

grape

The grape and its wine have been a delectable source of medicine since antiquity. The Egyptians and the early Greeks made use of the fruit and the beverage in rites and rituals, and in more recent times the French, Italians, and others have vigorously carried on the noble tradition of the vine. Native Americans are said to have employed the grape for its powers of purification, and in Chinese medicine the grape is used as a tonic to fortify the constitution and nourish the blood. Modern researchers find grapes full of promise for their antiviral, antitumor properties, and grape juice appears to kill bacteria and slow down tooth decay. Wine also destroys bacteria and viruses, and to consume a glass of it per day is said to help increase the beneficial HDL blood cholesterol by 6–8%. Because of wine's stimulating effect on the metabolism, it can be a help in a weight loss regimen—if it is consumed within reason, of course. (However, a model of my acquaintance avoids drinking even a little wine the day before a photo shoot—she says it shows up on her face the next day as pallor and puffiness. If you need to look your best, it might be

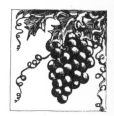

inside

grape medicine food

wine medicine food

outside

grape juice facial rinse

*mashed grape face
pack*

*grape leaf bath (wine
optional)*

wiser to have water the night before the big day.)

To benefit from the antianemic, antihemorrhagic, antiseptic, astringent, diuretic, laxative, stimulating, tonic, vaso-constrictive properties of the grape: indulge in the fruit as a sweet snack. Apply a grape juice facial rinse when troubled by blemishes, or try a pack of mashed grapes for its nourishing, toning benefits. A bath made with vine leaves (use fresh or dried leaves wrapped in cloth) lends astringent, restorative qualities to the soak, and if you add wine to the water it will sterilize it.

the beauty that is wrapped up

The country of the wrapped gift; the gift itself is less important than the meaning it encloses, the harmony of the wrapping. Woman, too, is wrapped, not so often now in the elaborately draped, tucked, folded, knotted, and tied kimono and *obi* bow of times past, but wrapped nonetheless, in grooming so impeccable and clothing so fashionably perfect, so apt for the season, so appropriate for the occasion, so seemly for her status and role that the woman herself, the individual, is indiscernible. The natural self is hidden—presented by a carefully wrapped exterior, but not known by it. The Japanese woman's clothing does not serve to externalize her but to make her blank, a mystery, in the same way that her make-up is not meant to accentuate but to erase, neutralize, reduce.

honeysuckle

June is the month of weddings and the summer solstice, and in Japan, of plum rains and honeysuckle bathing. What could be more romantic: sweet-smelling flowers in a warm bath, evening moonlight, the Japanese mists of early summer….

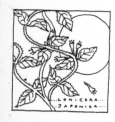

LONICERA JAPONICA

In Japan, the honeysuckle bath, or *suikazura-yu*, has traditionally been used for both its medicinal and aesthetic properties. The infused water of honeysuckle blossoms is thought to improve circulation, regenerate and renew the body, cure prickly heat and other irritations, and tone and nourish the skin.

In the European herbal tradition also, we find honeysuckle water, prescribed for the care of delicate skin and as a topical application for headaches. Honeysuckle syrup is used as a gargle for sore throats and asthma, and an oil made from the bark of the honeysuckle vine is reputed to remove wrinkles if applied regularly.

To prepare your summer *suikazura-yu*, begin to gather honeysuckle leaves and flowers—these you will dry in the sun (if you can find any errant rays during the *tsuyu*, those delicate, elegant rains that fall in the time between warm golden May and steamy hot July in Japan) and then infuse by steeping in just-boiled water for 20 minutes.

Add this to the bath and then soak sybaritically, thinking dreamy thoughts amid the honeyed fragrance and steam.

iris

The iris bath is meant to be taken on Children's Day (also known as Boys' Day), celebrated on the 5th of May, but I don't think it would be improper to take it anytime during the spring. This bath is a fleeting, one-season pleasure: iris leaves are scarce when spring is gone.

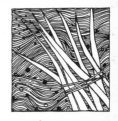

outside

iris bath

This traditional Japanese iris bath has powers: it expels evil from mind and body! If you need something more mundane, be assured—an iris bath will cure your sprains and strains, soothe your skin imbalances, and smooth your worried brow.

The iris is a member of the *Iridaceae* family. While the Japanese blue, white, or violet-flowered *shōbu*, sometimes referred to as sweet flag, is the type used for the bath in Japan, the leaves of various species of iris may be employed for bathing.

The *shōbu* closely resembles the *Iris versicolor*, also known as blue flag or flag lily; the dried root of this iris has traditionally been used by Native Americans to purify the blood and ease skin problems. (As a detoxifier, the root of blue flag, like other irises, is powerful—undoubtedly the purported magical benefits of the *shōbu* were inferred when early healers observed the potent cleansing action of the plant.) When iris root is used in medicine, it is always prescribed in tiny doses and used in dried form, for the fresh root is poisonous. Iris root is beneficial for digestive problems.

Another type of iris, the *Iris florentina* or *Iris germanica*, known commonly as orris, has been part of the European folk pharmacopeia since ancient times. The Greeks and Romans used the violet-scented dried orris root in powdered form as a perfume and fixative, and during the 18th century the same substance was used to powder the hair. In later periods, the dried root was used as a dry shampoo. This root, like its relative described above, acts to cleanse and purge the body of toxins. An expectorant and diuretic when taken in small doses, the root causes violent vomiting and diarrhea if taken in overdose or in fresh, undried form. Clearly, the iris is not a substance meant for self-administration internally; such dangerous herbs must never be used without strict medical supervision.

A bath in iris leaves, however, is a treatment you may indulge in safely. If you are tired, *shōbu-yu* will rest you. If your blood moves slowly, the iris bath will speed it up. If your hands are clammy and your feet are cold, take an iris bath to heat those cool extremities. To prevent a cold, to have skin that is satin-soft, and to ease the spirit, take an iris bath. With all these curative powers, you might expect such a bath to be medicinal in feeling, but no! The *shōbu-yu* is not only picturesque, it is wiltingly fragrant....

To indulge in this sublime bath and banish evil from your being, simply gather iris leaves, tie them in extravagant bunches, and float them in your hot bath. Celebrate the ascendency of good as you soak in the healing, beautifying water....

loofah

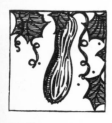

outside

loofah-vine water

The cooling water of the loofah vine brings to mind the long hot Japanese summer—so high in humidity that nothing ever seems dry—with the sun-beaten farmlands, the new green of the rice fields, the sound of the cicada, and the twinkle of fireflies in the evenings. Loofah water, or *hechimasui*, is used to comfort, refresh, and cool the complexion during this sticky season.

Are you planting a garden this year? If so, you might consider putting in a couple of loofah plants, to experiment with making your own loofah-vine water in the time-honored Japanese way.

Hechimasui is one of the stars of traditional Japanese beauty lore. It has been used for centuries and is still a favorite among women all over Japan. *Hechimasui* is not difficult to make, but these days it is available commercially from many companies. Whether you make it or buy it, such a venerable beauty secret is worth trying.

This beautifying water is simply the sap from the *hechima* vine, sometimes with a little *sake* or other preservative added. If you have your own loofah plant—which, by the way, is the same plant that gives us the lovely loofah scrubbing sponge—you can make loofah water yourself. Cut the loofah vine 2 or 3 meters away from the root, place a container (traditionally a *sake* bottle) under the cut end, and wait for the sap to collect. (Do this in mid-September, when your vine is mature.) You may add some *sake* to help preserve it and provide extra skin benefits. Divide the liquid among several small bottles and store in the refrigerator. Note: even commercially made loofah water must be refrigerated if it is the very pure type.

Hechimasui, though it's associated with summer, may be used year-round to smooth, calm, and lighten the complexion. The water helps the skin to maintain a healthy moisture balance without the use of any oils.

Hechimasui should be patted onto the face after washing, like a tonic. Do not rinse. This water is recommended for all skin types, but it is especially appreciated by those with wrinkles or freckles, for it is said to make both less noticeable. Use loofah-vine water daily for best results.

loquat

Japanese folk medicine gives the evergreen leaf of the loquat tree an exalted position, one that it holds in the Chinese medicine tradition as well. This is one of those plants that seems to be good for almost anything. My initial acquaintance with the medicinal tree began thus: the first house I inhabited in northern Japan had a leafy little loquat tree in the side garden, next to the kitchen. One day I looked out the window and saw the old landlord creeping about under the tree. He picked leaf after leaf and stuffed them into a canvas bag. What was he doing? Over a period of several days he carried out the same ritual, until finally the tree was picked almost bare. I never asked him what he was up to, and he never offered to explain.

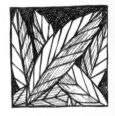

outside

loquat leaf bath

loquat leaf facial water

inside

loquat leaf tea

When some time later I began my research into folk medicine, I understood. It was the loquat leaf that held pride of place in many peoples' stories about healing plants. The *biwa* leaf is hoarded by those who know it, for it has the ability to improve internal and external conditions of a wide variety.

The loquat is an evergreen tree that reaches a height of 6 meters. It is known in Latin as *Eriobotrya Japonica*, in Japanese as the *biwa*, and in Chinese as *pi pa ye*. The officinal leaf can reach a length of 30 cm and a width of 8 cm or so. The tree flowers in late fall; the fruit ripens in June. This is a tree of Asia—southern China, Japan, Vietnam, India, Malaysia—and of southern Europe.

The loquat leaf has a bitter taste. The young leaf contains saponins. The seeds are poisonous and should be avoided. In the Chinese tradition, the dried leaf is used internally as a cough remedy and an expectorant. In Japanese folk medicine the leaf is infused for tea or made into a liquor, both of which may be taken internally to treat fatigue, cough, loss of appetite, or skin problems.

Used externally, the infusion of loquat treats rashes, acne, and blemishes. It is added to the bath to tone the skin, destroy bacteria, stimulate the circulation, and soothe and warm the body. An eyewash of loquat is said to remedy eye fatigue.

The leaf of loquat may be gathered from the tree, if you get to it before my old landlord does. The *biwa no ha* is also available as a tea in dried packaged form in good pharmacies and health-minded tea shops in Asia, and of course you can find it in Chinese medicine apothecaries. If you pick the fresh leaves, right after harvesting you must scrub them well with water and a vegetable brush to remove leaf-down. Next, dry them in the sun for 10 days, then store them wrapped in paper in a cool dry location indoors.

Once you have the leaf, here's what to do with it. The basic proportion for tea is 10 g/2 tsp of the dried leaf to 600 ml/2 1/2 C of pure spring water. Bring water to a boil in a nonmetal pan, then add leaves and simmer until the liquid is reduced by 1/3. Filter the liquid and discard leaves.

This tea may be taken internally to calm the skin, counter fatigue, and improve the appetite. It is not a tea for daily use, but one to take for relief from specific symptoms like rashes or signs of allergy in the skin. The amount gained by the above method supplies enough tea for one day, to be warmed for drinking and taken in small doses throughout the day.

The same tea may be added to the bath to soothe skin problems externally or to boost circulation—an effective action in the battle against cellulite. The loquat leaf bath is to be soaked in for 20 minutes and should not be followed by a rinse.

As a facial water, loquat leaf tea will purify, heal, destroy bacteria, and eliminate a variety of unsightly blemishes and inflammations. Splash or pat the cool tea onto the face after cleansing; don't rinse. It may be used daily until skin condition improves.

marigold

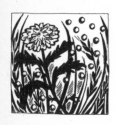

outside

*marigold-petal-tea face
pack*

marigold petal bath

*marigold-petal-tea
facial rinse*

inside

marigold petal tea

Among the many glorious flowers that bloom in the early summer, the marigold is a medicinal treasure. Many will know this orange-gold flower with the pungent aroma as the calendula. *Calendula officinalis* is one of the great healers of the homeopathic and Western herbal traditions. Ancient Egyptians, well versed in health and beauty herbalism, used the calendula as a rejuvenator. Taken internally in infusion or tincture form, the flower improves liver functions, soothes the pain of menstrual cramping, and stimulates the flow of lymph and cleanses it.

The infusion or diluted tincture of calendula applied externally is a potent healing antiseptic. Its regular use prevents scarring. The herb is antifungal, antiviral, and antibacterial. Like the strawberry, this flower carries powerful purifying and healing medicine within its beautiful presence.

Dried marigold petals may be powdered and used as a delicate skin-soothing body powder; for a newborn baby, such a powder makes more sense than an artificially fragrant, chemical-laden talc.

For soothing inflamed or irritated skin, an infusion of marigold flowers applied as a daily rinse after cleansing will do wonders. The same infusion applied to the hair will lighten and brighten the color, while a hair pack made of the infused and strained petals can offer significant red-gold lights to hair that is brown or blonde.

Calendula acts as a gentle stimulant and diaphoretic to the skin and thus may be used to great benefit in the bath or in face packs. To make an infusion for internal or external use, simply add a teaspoon or two of the dried petals to a cup of just-boiled water and allow to infuse several minutes as for tea. For a bath infusion, add a big handful of petals to a liter/4 C of spring water and allow to infuse for 30 minutes, filtering out solids before adding to the bath.

An essential part of the beauty ritual is to enjoy the entire process—out picking berries and blooms, fill a basket with them and appreciate the new life blossoming forth in the garden at the start of summer. At the vegetable store, have fun noticing all the recently arrived vegetables and fruits of the season—taking in all that color is tonic to the soul! And when you prepare your infusions, concoctions, and fruit-and-flower beauty medicines, use your favorite bowls and utensils. Set aside plenty of time to indulge peacefully in creating your own harmony with the season....

milk

In the old days, only the wanton privileged few could bathe in milk, smear their skin with honey, and otherwise squander—all in the name of beauty—the foods that lesser subjects toiled for.

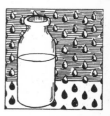

outside

milk bath

herb & fruit & milk bath

turmeric milk body pack

Now that the milk bath has become a somewhat more afford-able indulgence, we can all join the ranks of historical beauties and discover the skin-smoothing powers of milk, not to mention the exquisite pleasure of partaking in such mildly decadent behavior.

The milk bath is a classic among beauty baths, perfectly sim-ple and basic and luxurious. For those who have never tried it, the milk bath is a superb way to smooth and moisturize skin; it not only softens but seems to rejuvenate and relax and replenish, too (applied on the face, it eases tiny lines and signs of tension).

Use either milk powder or fresh milk, the more the better—pour as much as you like into a preheated bath. Rinse well after-ward, and do not reuse this bath.

A lovely variation on the basic milk bath is the herb/fruit milk bath. Three or four hours before bathtime, mix a handful of your favorite herb (chamomile, jasmine, rose, linden) into some warm milk. When you are ready to bathe, add the mixture to the tub. (A few drops of an essential oil can replace the milk-herb infusion if you like.) The fruit is optional and can be strawberries or peaches or melon or papaya—crush the fruit and strain the juice, adding it to the bath along with the herbal milk.

From India comes a traditional milk-based pack: this ceremonial beauty treatment employs turmeric powder (called *haldi* in India), which is mixed with cream skimmed from freshly boiled milk. The orange-colored mixture is applied to face, arms, legs, and breasts, where it will remain for twenty minutes before it is rinsed off, leaving the skin luminous, with a subtle golden glow. Interestingly, turmeric is a medicinal spice, known in Europe as such since the Middle Ages. In Indonesia *temoe lawacq* (turmeric) is a well-known liver tonic. Of the same family as ginger, *Zingiberaceae*, turmeric is antibacterial, with a reputation as a tonic of particular benefit to the digestive system.

mint

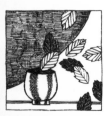

outside

mint oil skin wash

mint bath & steam

mint & rosemary vinegar for hair

mint massage oil

mint & jasmine face pack

inside

mint tea

Whenever I taste mint tea I remember the time I was offered a tiny glass of the sweet sugared tea by a Bedouin in the Sahara. He brewed it with ceremony, boiling water in a tin can over a very small fire made from 2 or 3 sticks. He had only one teaglass, so first he brewed a tea for me. When I'd finished mine, he brewed one for himself.

The universally appealing flavor and fragrance of mint, and the widespread use of the essence in everything from toothpaste and gum to soaps and cigarettes, might make it seem to be no more than a palate-pleasing, nose-tingling little leaf. In fact, the mint plant enjoys a long history as a medicinal herb in the East as well as in the West. As a cosmetic herb, mint is employed as a restorative stimulant for the complexion and scalp; in healing, mint is an important digestive tonic, a calmative and tonic for the nervous system, and is useful in a myriad of ways for minor illnesses. "*If a man can name all the properties of mint, he must know how many fish are aswim in the ocean*," wrote Wilafried de Strabo in the 12th century. It is worth getting to know the plants of the *Mentha* species, for they are easy to grow and use fresh, and you will likely find that the fragrant leaf will soon become a staple herb in your quest for beauty and health.

The mint species belong to the *Labiatae* family, within which we find the peppermint, or *Mentha piperita*, herb beloved in the Occident; and the *Mentha arvensis*, also known as Japanese mint, a medicinal mint favored in the Chinese botanical tradition. A common garden mint is the *Mentha spicata*, otherwise known as spearmint. There are more mints than this, but here we shall concern ourselves with the first two, as they are the most useful and most available.

Peppermint is a digestive antiseptic and an antispasmodic, useful in the treatment of nausea and the digestion of fats. The Chinese designate peppermint as a cooling herb, especially good for detoxification of the liver. Peppermint also acts to benefit the respiratory system. Painful menstrual cramps, anxiety, hysteria, and migraines will all respond to the soothing peppermint leaf taken as a tea.

To make the tea, steep 1 tsp of mint in 230 ml/1 C of just-boiled water for 3 minutes. Precautions include the following: Don't use more often than three times a day. Never give mint to a baby. For children, limit a mint-tea course to one-week periods to avoid irritation of the mucous membranes. Don't overdo essential oil inhalation, and be wary of mint if you are a nursing mother, for this herb can reduce the flow of milk.

Used in essential oil form (always diluted in a carrier oil!), peppermint will act to improve local circulation, digestion, and skin ailments caused by fungus and parasites. Peppermint oil relieves fatigue when added to the bath, and will beautify the skin by purifying and calming the complexion. Ancient European belief holds that it restores the memory. Inhaling the scent of mint will relieve nasal congestion. Use the oil (2 drops to 10 ml/ 1 $^1/_2$ T of pure water) in a wash for the treatment of skin irritations, itching, minor burns, cold sores, and to repel insects.

Aromatherapists employ peppermint oil for concentration, stimulation, and wakefulness. The menthol fragrance that seems so cooling is interesting, because it actually warms as well. (Spearmint does not contain menthol, so it possesses slightly different qualities. In aromatherapy spearmint oil is used for energizing.)

Mentha arvensis, or Japanese mint, will promote the mobilization of liver-blocked *ki*, according to the Chinese. Further, this mint may be used in many of the same ways as peppermint, with benefits for the digestive and respiratory systems.

Any mint added to the bath (tie a bunch of fresh or dried leaves into a muslin bag and let the hot water run through it, just like steeping tea) will restore and stimulate, strengthening nerves and muscles. The local circulation will be revived, and the whole being will be imbued with a refreshing feeling of being toned and alive.

Dandruff? Make an herbal vinegar of rosemary and mint and use as a rinse after every shampoo. Dry skin? The mint bath will soothe and gently moisturize with its precious mint oil. Enlarged pores? Steam the face over a basin full of hot water and mint leaves. Aching muscles? Add 5–10 drops of mint to a 250 ml/8 oz bottle of almond oil and massage with it. (The same mint oil will relieve a headache and a fever.)

And finally, my favorite beauty pack in all the world is a minty one from India, a delightful concoction of mint leaves and jasmine blossoms. Place these two items fresh in a small bowl of pure water overnight, then in the morning mash the mixture using a mortar and pestle. Apply to the face and leave on for 30 minutes, then rinse. Guaranteed: a luminous, intoxicatingly sweet-scented complexion.

mugwort

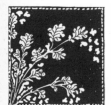

outside

mugwort bath

inside

mugwort medicine food

mugwort tonic tea

Don't you love that witchy, Shakespearean name? In Japanese it's *yomogi*, in Latin *Artemisia vulgaris*; whatever one chooses to call it, mugwort is everywhere. Know what you're looking for, and you're likely to find it in the empty lot next door, or even growing vigorously in your own garden. You'll also find dried leaves sold for tea in any good tea shop in Japan, or in an herbalist's elsewhere.

Mugwort is a perennial leafy herb that grows 7–12 cm/ 3–5 inches tall, with an indented, midgreen leaf that is silvery on the underside. The stem is hairy, ridged, and reddish. The plant is in season from approximately late June to September in Japan, depending on latitude. It grows in semiarid and temperate regions, as do the other plants in the *Artemisia* species. The aromatic and bitter-tasting leaves of mugwort are officinal. If you're going mugwort-hunting, find a color photograph in a herb guide and carry it with you for identification.

Mugwort is one of those deceptively humble-looking wild plants that is so potent medicinally, it has been used in all parts of the world for centuries. In Japan, *yomogi* shows up in *mochi* rice cakes, in soup and other foods, and it's a staple tonic tea as well. In Chinese medicine, mugwort is used as a hemostatic and stomachic, and in both Japan and China mugwort is the main ingredient in moxas. In Europe, mugwort has been used since pre-Christian times as a strengthening and purifying agent.

In every part of the world, this plant has been associated with magic! So the witchiness in the name is appropriate…. In the ancient European "Lay of the Nine Herbs," mugwort appears in the first incantation as the "mother of herbs." In Japan, *yomogi* is one of the traditional herbs picked ritually at the start of the new year for protection and purification.

What to do with your mugwort, once you've gathered it? An "herb lady" friend of mine puts it into little plastic bags—the kind with hundreds of tiny holes in them—and hangs it all over her house to dry. Follow her example: in an area that's cool, shady, and breezy, tie a string to your ceiling and suspend your mugwort from it for a few weeks. Not only will you have nicely dried mugwort that you may then pack away for year-long use, but you will cleanse your house of evil spirits into the bargain.

Mugwort tea is good for lactating mothers and anyone who needs a little fortifying. Prepare as for ordinary black tea, (i.e., shred the leaves and put them in the teapot, about 1 tsp per cup) with a brief infusion in a nonmetal container. Mugwort may be mashed when fresh and applied to blemishes as a spot pack. Cover the pack with a whole fresh leaf, rest peacefully for 20 minutes with your leaf on, then rinse.

A mugwort bath is a magical strengthener. Add generous handfuls of fresh young leaves to your bath for a refreshing seasonal ritual. Dried leaves may be used if fresh ones are unavailable. Here is what the bath will do for you: exfoliate your dead skin cells, soften rough skin and calluses, refresh and warm you, improve your circulation, calm skin inflammations, soothe pains in joints and muscles, and soothe heat rash.

Here is the magical incantation, for those who wish to use mugwort as a charm of protection:

> Have in mind, Mugwort, what you made known,
> What you laid down, at the great denouncing.
> Una your name is, oldest of herbs,
> Of might against thirty, and against three,
> Of might against venom and the onflying,
> Of might against the vile she
> Who fares through the land.

mulberry

The mulberry is the fruit of the goddess Minerva, deity of wisdom, the arts, and the trades. The tree of the white mulberry is where silkworms weave their luxurious cocoons. While the curious source of silk was once a secret closely kept by the ancient Chinese, the medicinal properties of the tree were common knowledge in various parts of the world in earlier times.

Morus alba, the white mulberry, is the dawn-tinted sister of the blackish berry known as *Morus nigra*: juicy little yin-yang medicine-fruits. The *Morus alba* grows naturally in China, Southeast Asia, the Philippines, and Japan (known as *kuwa* in Japanese). The *Morus nigra* originated in the Near East, from whence it was transplanted to Europe, finding favor in antiquity with Greeks and Romans who grew enamored of the fruit. And in both the *nigra* and the *alba* the medicinal parts are the root skin, leaves, branches, twigs, and fruit. The berries of both trees ripen in summer.

In Europe in the 16th century, the black mulberry fruit was used against inflammations and bleeding; the root skin to relieve toothache; and the leaf as a snakebite antidote. In Chinese medicine, coughs, bronchitis, and asthma may be treated with the skin of the white mulberry root; the fruit is taken as a yin tonic, with benefits for hypertension and insomnia; the leaf is antipyretic and is prescribed as a sedative to the liver.

The white mulberry and the black mulberry fruits are related

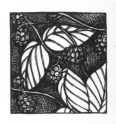

outside

*mulberry juice gargle
  or mouthwash*

*mulberry & hemp &
  sesame treatment oil
  for hair*

inside

mulberry medicine food

*mulberry & elder-
  blossom & mint tea*

but somewhat different in appearance and flavor, though similar in healing actions. (The other parts of the respective trees are used differently for healing purposes.) Where the black mulberry is without peduncle and rather rounded, purple-red, with a sour-sweet taste, the white mulberry may be either pale and yellowish or purplish-red as well, of smaller, elongated shape, and very sugary in taste.

Both the white and the black mulberry are highly regarded as tonics—in China the white is generally used, and in Europe the black. The *sang shen*, as the white mulberry is known in China, is a yin tonic that nourishes both blood and *ki*; this berry exerts a gentle laxative action as well. The black mulberry is a traditional European folk medicine prescribed in convalescence or cases of chronic fatigue. This berry too is a laxative, and as such was taken in medieval England as a cleansing medicine. To benefit from these tonic berries, simply add them to your diet in moderate amounts (no more than 20 g/ 3/4 oz per day). As gargle or mouth wash, the juice of either berry will soothe a sore throat and help heal canker sores.

The leaf of both trees possesses antibacterial and expectorant properties. The black mulberry leaf has an ancient reputation in Europe as a fever remedy and an astringent, and it has been used for generations in the Balkans as an antidiabetic agent. In Chinese medicine the white mulberry leaf (*sang ye*) is used for colds with fever, headaches, or sore throats, and to cool the liver in cases where liver-related irritability or vision problems are noted. Recently in Europe, the leaf of the white mulberry has been adopted in the treatment of diabetes, found useful for its ability to stimulate the production of insulin. To warm the body or treat a cold, infuse equal quantities of mulberry leaf, elderblossom, and mint, then sip throughout the day.

To strengthen the hair and help preserve it where there is a hair loss problem, make a treatment oil from leaves of the white mulberry, hemp leaves, and sesame oil. Good for all hair types, the oil is made by crushing equal amounts of each type of fresh leaf, using a mortar and pestle or a food processor. This leaf pulp is then packed into a clean jar, adding sesame oil to cover. After sealing tightly, leave the mixture to macerate for two weeks, shaking the jar each day. At the end of this time, filter the liquid and discard solids, then add crushed leaves once again and repeat the entire maceration process. For a very potent treatment oil, carry the complete process out a total of 4 or 5 times. Filter a final time and transfer to an appropriate bottle. Keep well sealed in a cool location. This traditional Asian hair tonic may be massaged into the scalp daily.

The branches and twigs of the white mulberry (*sang zhi* in Chinese) exert an analgesic, soothing action especially useful in cases of rheumatism of the upper body. In the Chinese tradition a mélange of this substance with other herbs such as ginseng would be employed together in a decoction.

In Chinese medicine, the white mulberry root skin (*sang bai pi*) is decocted, usually with several other herbs, for use as an expectorant for coughs associated with fever and heavy phlegm. This remedy is an important asthma calmative. The root skin is sedative and diuretic.

oats

Oatmeal is a classic among natural beauty ingredients. It has been used faithfully in the West for generations, and continues today to find its way onto the face of many a woman. It is one of the most common and effective beauty treatments. The Western use of oatmeal as a beautifier is similar to the Japanese use of *nuka*, or rice bran. It is inexpensive, easy to get, does wonderful things for the skin, and can be used in the bath, as a pack, as a scrub, and as a food, all with beautiful results.

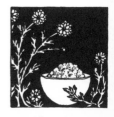

outside

oatmeal scrub

oatmeal bath

cooked oatmeal bath

oatmeal face pack

inside

oatmeal medicine food

Some of the oaty benefits derive from its texture: used as a scrub, the oatmeal gently exfoliates and stimulates the skin. Its other benefits are in its highly nutritious contents: silicon (which helps to counteract skin damage caused by pollution), B-complex vitamins, phosphorus, and calcium.

Let's look at some of the interesting ways to use those oats sitting neglected in your cupboard!

THE OATMEAL SCRUB: Add water to ground or flaked oats. Honey is a lovely addition, for its virtue as a humectant. Rub the mushy mixture on the face and body and then leave on for a few minutes, if you wish. Rinse. (Be careful not ot let this mixture clog the drain.) Your skin will respond to the scrub by becoming noticeably softer, smoother, and fresh-looking.

THE OATMEAL BATH: Fill a small cheesecloth bag with finely ground oats or oat flakes. You can add finely ground almonds and a few drops of vegetable oil if you wish ... then just let the bag float in the bath while you soak, or rub it softly over your skin. This bath will leave you glowing. Oatmeal seems to have a calming effect on skin, soothing inflammations and giving it a kind of baby-pure feeling.

THE COOKED OATMEAL BATH: Some people prefer to use cooked oatmeal in the bath. It requires a bit more preparation, but the cooked-oat-bath method may be the more potent in terms of treating skin irritations. Put cooked oats in a cheesecloth bag and add to the bath. This will be helpful for rashes, itchiness, and other common skin problems. It is wonderful for babies—the oatmeal's cleansing properties allow you to forgo the use of soap, and any diaper rash will begin to fade quickly with oat-water bathing.

THE OATMEAL PACK: Mix flakes or ground oats with warm water, yogurt, or milk. Apply this mixture to the face and neck and allow it to sit for 15 minutes or so. If your skin is dry, use whole milk, a few drops of oil, or some egg yolk in the mixture. If you have oily skin, you don't need the extra oil; the oatmeal mush will normalize your skin. The longer you allow it to work, the more it will seem to "pull" out dirt and toxins.

If your skin is very sensitive, use honey, and don't leave the pack on longer than five minutes or so. Best is to experiment. My favorite way is to grind oats and almonds together, add some warm water and honey, then rub my face gently with the mixture before applying it as a pack. My skin feels positively *new* after this treatment!

Finally, don't forget that oats may be eaten, raw in muesli or cooked for porridge—the combined effects of using oats both outside and in should make you most healthily beautiful! (Oats were a holistic health-and-beauty food long before oat bran became a Western trend; ask any European grandmother.)

peach

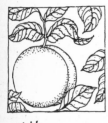

outside

*peach-leaf-tea skin
 lotion*

peach leaf bath

rice-bran-bag wash

In the hot season we are seekers of shade and iced drinks, fans and air-conditioned rooms, clothing that invites a flow of air, and relief for insect bites, irritated sweaty skin, and sunburn. Babies whine from heat rash. Children display exotic fungi acquired at swimming pools. We all wilt.

There are several traditional Japanese remedies for summer skin aggravation—these treatments are so popular and reliable that they are prepared commercially, but they are easy to make at home.

Peach leaf lotion, summer skin-cooler par excellence, is made by infusing peach leaves and cooling the strained infusion for application to the skin after bathing. (See "infusion" in appendix for measurements and directions.) The lotion will soothe heat-induced irritations of the skin: heat rash, blotches, inflammations, sunburn.

A peach leaf bath may be prepared by mashing leaves in a mortar—add a bit of water—then squeezing the green purée through cheesecloth to obtain juice. Add the juice to a bath that is rather cooler than usual, then soak. The bath is very good for children who have played too hard in the heat and sun.

For serious heat rash and other skin irritations, try washing with a rice bran bag instead of soap. Suffering babies will appreciate both the peach leaf bath and the *nuka* wash—cool, gentle relief.

pearl

Pearls are fashionable again, we hear—but have pearls ever been out of style? Classic and classy, their gentle luminous shine has always been attractive. But did you know that you can wear your pearls and eat them too? Wash your face with them? Condition your hair, massage your skin with them, or take them with tea to purify the blood? But wait! Before you begin to nibble away at your priceless Mikimotos, if you are in Japan you can buy powdered pearls at the drugstore; they are called *shinju no kona*. If you are elsewhere, try a Chinese herbal apothecary.

It's interesting to note how often the age-old beauty secrets contain an element of magic. With the pearl, which has been used for beauty and health in many cultures and throughout history, we see the sympathetic principle at work: Use a pearl to be like a pearl. (Won't a little of that opalescent beauty literally rub off on you if you wash your face with pearls?) Combine this primitive association with the pearl's aura of luxury—a genuine treasure from the sea that has monetary value—and its remarkable formation within an oyster, and you see the deep symbolic potency of the pearl.

Mothers in certain areas of Japan used to offer a little pearl powder to their infants before nursing them; this practice was thought to ensure their growth in health and beauty. Another folk technique employed pearls to beautify the eyes: a tiny pearl the size of a poppy seed was placed in the eye. When this irritant caused the eye to tear, the pearly iridescence was dissolved and released onto the surface of the eye.

In Japan and China, the pearl has long been used as a medicine to treat eye diseases and other illnesses. In self-treatment, the pearl is most often employed as a restorative and blood purifier. A little pearl powder taken with tea is thought to help the body eliminate toxins and animal fats. Also, like gold and silver leaf, the pearl is thought to have a tranquilizing effect when taken internally.

Some people use the pearl primarily for calcium, and they add a little to their daily rice before cooking. Oyster pills and pearl pills, both widely available in Japan, are taken for their superior combination of calcium and protein.

Pearls used externally are said to combine effective moisturizing qualities with pH-balancing and protection from sun damage. The pearl is thought to lighten freckles and liver spots and to activate cell regeneration. Used as a massage cream agent or in a wash, the slight abrasive action will exfoliate and stimulate the skin.

To experiment with powdered pearl at home, use *shinju no kona* as an ingredient for washing face and body by combining it

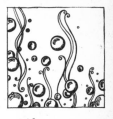

outside

pearl powder face
   wash

pearl powder face pack

inside

pearl powder medicine
   food

with a mild washing cream. Scrub very gently. A face pack may be concocted by mixing some pearl powder with yogurt and honey; leave on the face for 15 minutes and rinse well. Another technique is to mix pearl powder with water and leave on the face overnight as a skin beautifier.

And the next time you are entertaining at home, why not add some pearls, gold, and silver to the menu? A sure way to impress your friends and a novel way to offer health, beauty, and serenity.

pearl barley

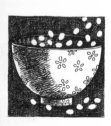

For beautiful skin, there is a Japanese tea made from pearl barley, also known as Job's Tears (*Coix lacrymae Jobi*), and the leaf of the persimmon. In Japanese, pearl barley is *hatomugi*. The tea is said to make the complexion clear and smooth, ridding the skin of toxins and, when taken regularly, diminishing moles and other growths.

inside

pearl barley & persimmon leaf tea

pearl barley tea

pearl barley porridge

It is possible to buy the ingredients for this tea in Japan in a store selling *kampōyaku*, or Chinese medicine. Ask for *hatomugi-cha* and *kaki no ha-cha*. Persimmon leaves and pearl barley are available in the West in Chinese apothecaries.

Mix the two ingredients, add to water in a 1:8 ratio, and simmer in a nonmetal pot for 10 minutes. (Some prefer to infuse the mixture as for ordinary tea. In that case, infuse the mixture in water for 15 minutes.) The tea has an interesting flavor and may be taken frequently.

The Japanese dietary approach to acquiring clear, luminous skin involves eating plenty of foods high in vitamin C, and a three-month regime of *hatomugi*. *Hatomugi* tea bags are widely available now in well-stocked Japanese natural/traditional pharmacies and many tea shops. The roasted seed in whole or ground form may also be found in the same shops or in *kampōyaku* apothecaries. Outside Japan, check herbalists or Chinese apothecaries.

The *hatomugi* regime consists of drinking the tea two to three times daily, prepared as an infusion, and for the truly dedicated, eating pearl barley porridge once a day. The porridge is made by stirring powdered roasted pearl barley into just-boiled pure water, enough to achieve a creamy consistency. (The powder may be made by any convenient grinding method.) The unroasted whole grain may also be cooked and eaten in the same manner as rice.

Such a diet is said to rid the skin of whatever problems may plague it. However, because the substance is a diuretic, it's important not to overdo things—paradoxically, if one drinks too many cups of *hatomugi-cha*, one could become dehydrated! As a diuretic, pearl barley is a useful supplement to a weight loss regimen.

the beauty that is unseen

Just as the Japanese garden is loveliest on a gloomy day or under a light rain, and the full-blooming cherry is most splendid by night, the beauty of woman is enhanced by darkness. What light there is should be dim, filtered, natural—faint light from a garden coming through the rice-paper screen, barely illuminating the woman as she sits in the darkened room, her face a soft mask of luminescence. The pale complexion gleams pearl-like in the dusky light, while the body recedes into the shadows, leaving the face to float on its own, an otherworldly countenance. The lunar, reflective beauty is lost when exposed to the bright light of day, its luster destroyed by sunshine, rendered invisible by perfect visibility.

perilla

By July the summer garden is rampant—growth is exuberant and wild, with perennial plants luxuriating in their usual places and new plants shooting forth their tendrils, vines, and blossoms. Many of the weeds that threaten to overwhelm the garden in midsummer are actually highly valued medicinal plants: dandelion, *dokudami*, plantain, field horsetail, bamboo grass, and perilla.

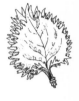

Shiso, the ubiquitous leafy accompaniment to raw fish, is known in Latin as *Perilla frutescens*, in English as perilla or the beefsteak plant, and in Chinese as *zi su zi*. In Asia its antibacterial and preservative properties are commonly recognized, thus its indispensability to the chef, especially in the hot season. Perilla's purifying presence may be utilized also in the realm of health and beauty.

outside

*perilla-tea rinse for
  skin & hair*

perilla leaf bath

The annual herb is native to Asia and grows with glorious abandon in hues of minty green and scarlet (the red leaf is used to tint *umeboshi*). In the Chinese medicine tradition, perilla leaves and seeds are documented as officinal, bearing a treasured essential oil of pungent taste and aromatic fragrance. Prescribed for their antitussive, antiseptic, expectorant, laxative, stomachic, antiasthma, and diaphoretic properties, the perilla leaf and seed are classified in this system as pungent and warm.

inside

perilla medicine food

perilla purifying tea

perilla breath freshener

In the Japanese folk tradition, perilla, which is brimming with vitamins A and C and minerals like calcium, iron, and phosphorus, is used both internally and externally for a variety of purposes. Eaten as a food condiment or prepared as a tea, perilla acts as a cold preventive, a stimulant to the circulation, a normalizer of metabolism, and a "brain food." Perilla will ameliorate an acid condition and benefit the stomach and bowels. By virtue of these balancing, cleansing abilities, perilla is said to bring beauty to skin and hair, retarding hair loss and preventing split ends and dandruff, moisturizing the skin and ridding it of imperfections. When it is cleansing and purifying that one needs, call first on the fresh green magic of perilla.

As with all Asian remedies, the holistic internal and external approach is employed for optimal results. Thus, any internal regime of perilla may be intensified by its external use in the bath or as a rinse for hair and skin. An infusion of perilla may be used as a final rinse for face and hair to combat dryness or skin or scalp problems. To prepare, place a handful of fresh or dried leaves in a pot of just-boiled spring water (use a nonmetal pot) and allow to steep, covered, for 15–20 minutes. The filtered tea may be stored in the refrigerator for up to 3 days.

Perilla in the bath is especially useful for encouraging a cold to depart before it's had a chance to settle in and take hold. The perilla bath will also ease tension, heal bruises, combat infection, aid rheumatism, and beautify the skin. All skin types will benefit from this bath, and it may be taken as frequently as desired. To prepare, wrap perilla leaves, seeds, and stalks in a gauze square and tie securely. Attach this to the hot water faucet and allow the plant to infuse while filling the tub. Leave the herb in the bath while soaking, which should be for 15 minutes in the hottest water one can stand. Because perilla is diuretic, it is wise to drink water or salty bancha before taking the bath.

For internal applications, along with eating the fresh leaf or dried *shiso momiji* (a blend of dried red perilla leaf and sea salt) as a garnish, a tea may be prepared by bringing 15 g/1 T perilla per 240 ml/1 C of water to a boil, then reducing the flame and simmering for 10 minutes before filtering. The tea may be taken daily over a prolonged period of time, but one should keep in mind that its diuretic qualities must be compensated for by drinking lots of pure water. (Note: children should not take this tea on a regular or prolonged basis.) Perilla tea is a remedy for troubled skin; its actions include the purification and moisturizing of the complexion, the elimination of imperfections like age spots and rashes, the stimulation of local metabolism, and the calming of skin sensitivity. Another use for the tea is as a gargle for cleansing the mouth and perfuming the breath.

Perilla grows free and wild in many parts of the world, and is available in food stores where Japanese ingredients are sold.

persimmon

October is the season of *kaki*, the Japanese persimmon. The radiant orange fruits linger in profusion upon leafless tree branches, and the *kaki* strung for drying sway from the eaves of farmhouses like giant necklaces of amber. You may buy the fruit for eating fresh, the sugary and chewy dried slabs, or the dried leaves for tea—*kaki no ha*. Beyond its obvious appeal as a delectable snack, the persimmon holds a special place in the Asian medicine tradition, with uses in both health and beauty.

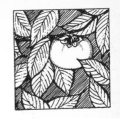

outside
persimmon fruit bath

inside
persimmon leaf tea

The *Diospyros kaki* is originally a native of China, Japan, Vietnam, Annam, and India, although the tree may now be found in many other parts of the world. The fruit's growth season is from August to November or so, with harvest time in Japan falling in November–December, depending on the latitude.

The fresh fruit is described as sweet-cold in the Chinese tradition, while the dried variety is sweet-neutral. The peduncle is bitter. Along with sugars, tannin, and carotene, the persimmon contains vitamins A, B, and C.

According to the Chinese system, the general action of the fruit is to reduce inner heat, and it is said that further benefits include the reduction of arterial tension and the improvement of blood circulation. The ripe fruit is said to be useful in cases of hypertension, constipation, diarrhea, and hemorrhoids. When the peduncle is prescribed, it is generally as a cough remedy. The juice of the unripe fruit is given for hypertension.

In the Japanese folk tradition, persimmon leaves are used extensively as a health and beauty tea. Sipped alone or with roasted pearl barley, *kaki no ha* tea or *kaki no ha-cha*, is thought to clear the complexion of imperfections: warts, moles, freckles, and blemishes. Taken daily over a period of months, the tea should smooth and refine the skin, encouraging the elimination of toxins and improving local circulation.

The recipe for persimmon leaf tea is simple. If you have a persimmon tree, gather your own leaves in the summer or early fall while they are green, wash them with clear water, remove the center pitch, then cut into tiny pieces. Steam the pieces for no more than 3 minutes, fan them for 30 seconds, then steam again for 2 minutes. Dry the leaves indoors in a shady cool spot. Once the leaves are dried, store them carefully to keep them free of moisture, as you would any herb.

In Japan the packaged dried leaves are easily found in any well-stocked traditionally minded pharmacy or tea shop. Outside Japan, one will find them in Chinese apothecaries and in good Oriental markets. To make the tea, pour just-boiled water on the leaves and steep for a few minutes before drinking. Some advocate boiling the leaves for several minutes. The tea may be taken 2–3 times a day for a period of three months as a complexion cure. Do not drink more often or give to children in large amounts as the tea is diuretic and could cause dehydration.

How about a picturesque persimmon fruit bath? This traditional bath is thought to nourish the skin, ease sore muscles, improve circulation, and lighten the skin—the latter effect may perhaps be attributed to the high vitamin C content. The bath is said to be good for older people's stiff joints.

For the bath, take two persimmons, either fresh or dried. Dried persimmons should be soaked in warm water for an hour beforehand. Add fruits to the hot bath and soak. Persimmon-purists advise not rinsing after this bath, so you don't lose any of the medicinal magic of *kaki*.

What else can the inimitable persimmon do for you? The beauty of the last fruit, vivid orange against a blue winter sky, is a certain balm for the soul.

pine

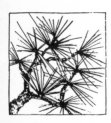

outside

pine bath

Here's a bath to welcome in the new year: *matsuba-yu*, the pine needle bath. You will soak peacefully in steamy water, fragrant with the forest scent of pines. The pine is not merely symbolic of renewal and freshness; used in the bath it also imparts such benefits to the body.

To indulge in the *matsuba-yu* bath is easy. Collect branches of evergreen and clip off a good quantity of "needle-bunches" (not individual needles). The fresh needles are always best, but you can also use needles that you have saved and dried.

Wash the needles well, then add to the hot bathwater as is or wrapped into a cheesecloth bag. If you are the sort who enjoys a picturesque bath, just let the pine needles float. You'll feel you are doing something quite special.

If you want to get the most out of the pine, to tap the fuller essence of the evergreen, the thing to do is to make a decoction from your needles, then add it to the bath. In a general ratio of one part needles to five parts water, simmer the water-pine mixture for 20 minutes or so. Strain and pour the liquid into the bath. (Toss in a few needles for effect.)

A long soak in the pine bath is said to benefit the skin by stimulating cell regeneration, along with encouraging purification through the elimination of toxins. The pine has antiseptic, soothing properties, so it will ameliorate skin problems such as acne, inflammations, and rashes. The skin is toned and somewhat tightened as well, making this a beautifying bath for those with aging skin, or for anyone with skin that is tired, sluggish, not looking its best. General body benefits include improvement in circulation and metabolism, resulting in a more efficiently functioning organism.

Because pine is so invigorating and refreshing, this bath is a good morning one, or one to take before a party to perk you up. *Matsuba-yu* will stimulate and soothe your skin, ease rheumatic pains and backache, get rid of tension in your muscles, warm you up, get your blood circulating more efficiently, and renew your energy. I don't know if it will help you keep your New Year's resolutions, but it's worth a try.

plantain

Ōbako: in English, plantain; in Latin, *Plantago major;* in Chinese, *che quian zi.* A common garden weed (as are many of the world's valuable medicinal herbs), the plantain is employed in European, Native American, and Asian traditions as a natural antiseptic and antibiotic.

Available growing wild in many palces—but as always when harvesting herbs, have an expert along for accurate identification—or packaged as dried tea leaves, *ōbako* is well known among the older generation in Japan as a bath herb or a curative tea. (A word of warning: *ōbako* is known to cause allergic reactions in some individuals, so those susceptible to such things are advised to steer clear of it.)

Used externally, the leaf of plantain may be applied to boils and sores or wounds as a poultice to purify, reduce inflammation, and speed healing. The Japanese plantain bath brings stimulating, cleansing, and soothing benefits to the skin, and is especially recommended for those with troubled skin or inflammations of any kind. The bath, which should be taken once or twice weekly, is prepared by infusing several handfuls of fresh or dried plantain leaf for 10 minutes in very hot water. Add this to the bath, then bathe for 20 minutes in the liquid. A bath temperature of around 39° C/102° F is optimal.

Even in a bath the plantain has diuretic properties, useful in toxin elimination. The same diuretic effect is encountered when the herb is taken as a tea. Other effects include antiallergic and anti-inflammatory actions. Because of its important expectorant and calming properties, plantain is indicated in the treatment of respiratory problems: asthma, sinusitis, rhinitis, bronchitis, pharyngitis, laryngitis, and simple colds and coughs. In Asian botanical medicine traditions, the plant is used to normalize high blood pressure, to tone the kidneys, and to improve the vision; aphrodisiac qualities are recognized as well!

To prepare the tea infuse a teaspoon of the dried leaf for 5 minutes in 240 ml/1 C of just-boiled water in a nonmetal container. For maintenance, the tea may be taken twice each day; as a remedy, three times per day at most. When on a plantain tea regimen, care must be taken to drink plenty of plain water to counteract the potentially dehydrating effects of the diuretic. Again, those prone to allergic reactions should avoid this tea or discontinue use if any untoward symptoms are noted. While some types of allergies are benefited by *ōbako*, others may be aggravated.

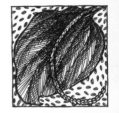

outside

plantain bath

inside

plantain leaf tea

For anyone who is in need of purification, plantain is the herb to try. The skin is the organ of elimination most obviously troubled by an overload of toxins. The plantain bath and maintenance tea regimen will result in a clearer, smoother complexion, a healthier beauty.

rice bran

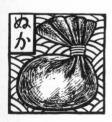

outside

rice bran wash

One can't go wrong with a classic. In the realm of natural beauty, the classic recipes are those that have survived unchallenged for generations, and those upon which women can still rely for solid results. Some of the Japanese classics date back to the 8th century! It is extraordinary that seaweed shampoo, bush warbler droppings, *azuki* bean washing powder, camellia oil, and rice bran washing powder are still available commercially, especially in the face of all the high-style, high-tech competition.

Of all the classic recipes, rice bran remains the quintessential Japanese staple.

Here's a bit of history. Back in the old days, when people washed their polished rice before cooking it (in just the way that they do now), they began to notice that the rice-washing water (rich in rice bran) had some special properties. The water was used for cleaning—and people who washed dishes with it found that their hands became not only clean but also soft and velvety. The wooden floors that were washed with *nuka* water not only were relieved of dirt but took on the soft sheen of the natural oil from the rice germ.

The bran water recycled for the bath beautified the skin and calmed skin ailments. Skin seemed to become moist, smooth, and fine. Rice bran cleansed the hair but did not remove natural oils—instead, the gentle dose of light rice germ oil nourished and protected the hair. It was in this way that the use of rice bran in the beauty ritual became widespread, and it is thanks to the incomparable effects of the bran that it is still popular today.

The best way to employ rice bran as a face wash is to use a rice bran drawstring bag or *nukabukuro*. In Japan one may buy the filled *nukabukuro* ready-made in good pharmacies, beauty boutiques, and health food stores. As an alternative to the bag, one may wrap bran in a muslin or silk square, tying it securely shut to avoid leaking. The right size for the face is a standard handkerchief square. For the body, or to soak in the bath, a larger bag should be made, big enough to hold a cup or two of bran.

An important note on the bran itself: if one does not buy the specially prepared beauty bran, which is purified and very fine in texture, one should acquire bran that is completely free of the materials used in the rice-polishing process and of any chemicals such as insecticide residues. Unless one has a trustworthy organic connection for bulk quantities, it is best to buy the commercial beauty bran. Store bran in a cool, dry location as it quickly becomes rancid.

So, once you have your little bag stuffed tight with rice bran, you will soak it for a few minutes in tepid water. Squeeze it a bit to soften it. When you see a white milky liquid seep from the bag, it is ready for use. Wash the face with it, or let it float in the bath and use it as a body scrub. After a bran bath, it's best not to rinse. For the face, it's up to you.

The rice bran wash is perfect for washing a baby's sensitive skin and will heal diaper rash. *Nuka* is excellent for any skin type, but people with sensitive skin, blemishes, dry skin, or any kind of rash particularly benefit. Rice bran may be used for every washing *instead* of soap.

After 2–3 washings, the contents of the *nukabukuro* should be discarded. Between washings, hang the bag up to dry. After emptying, launder it thoroughly and dry it in the sun prior to subsequent use.

rose

In the Western poetic tradition, the rose and the beautiful woman are so often linked that the two images seem almost synonymous. The English rose, the American long-stemmed beauty, the girl with roses in her cheeks … perhaps it is the combination of fresh sweetness and natural elegance that make this flower the perfect symbol of loveliness in woman.

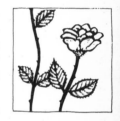

Too, the colors found in roses include all the pinks—from a delicately pale blush to a deep rich magenta—the true reds, the blue-reds, and the soft apricot and peach tones: all ideal hues for lips and cheeks, the colors of feminine beauty. And there is the fragrance of the flower, the velvet of its petals, the inimitable form of the bloom.

Historically, the rose has been the flower par excellence of love and beauty and inspiration. The power of the rose extends beyond aesthetics and literary metaphors, however. The rose is a healing plant as well. It is fitting that the rose was termed in ancient times "the gift of the angels."

Rosa in Latin, *bara* in Japanese, the rose that all the world is familiar with is a member of the *Rosaceae* family and grows as a flowering, thorny-stemmed shrub in temperate regions. It is said that the first roses were cultivated in Persia; the rose was believed to have sprung forth there from the blood of Adonis. In ancient Rome and Cleopatra's Egypt, roses were present at scenes of festivity and romance. Early Muslims used rosewater in a purifying bath. The rose has long been an important presence in ritual and myth.

In aromatherapy, essence of rose is employed as a sedative note in treatment oils, assuaging digestive problems, earaches and headaches, menstrual irregularities, nervous tension, depression, insomnia, and a variety of skin problems, and benefiting the circulation. Rose oil acts as a gentle antiseptic; it is the least toxic of all essences and thus is safe for use on children.

It takes approximately thirty roses to make one tiny drop of rose oil! The Bulgarian Otto of Rose is distilled from *Rosa damascena*; first extracted in 1612, this famous oil is now produced mainly in Morocco. The small amount of rose oil produced in France is derived from the process of making rosewater—the essential oil of rose floats in a thin film on top of the liquid and is skimmed off. Rose oil is one of the most fragrant of all essential oils, and it is by far the most versatile.

The rose has been an important component in love spells concocted by European witches and herbalists: worn as a "love oil," the rose fragrance is said to attract affection and love. Another use in magic is as a spell for bringing peace to the home: a container of dried or fresh petals and buds annointed with rose oil is placed in the abode and left undisturbed for three days. On the fourth day the contents of the container are sprinkled around the premises to the accompaniment of the recitation of the 23rd Psalm.

In Chinese medicine, several varieties of rose are used for healing. The Rosa rugosa and the Rosa Chinensis offer the flowers as *ki* and blood tonic and circulatory stimulant, while the rose hips of the Rosa laevigata are useful for *ki* as well as diuretic and laxative needs. *Rosa gallica*, the Apothecary rose, is the rose of traditional European herbal medicine.

How to enjoy the healing, beautifying rose? Try using pure rosewater as an astringent tonic for the face. This gentle antiseptic is the perfect soothing lotion for young and blemished skin. The Ayurvedic tradition employs rosewater compresses for this purpose, and to wake up dull skin. An infusion of rose petals will offer similar benefits, cleansing and purifying the complexion with utter delicacy.

A vinegar in which rose petals are steeping may be used as an antiseptic deodorant rinse. A decoction or infusion of rose hips is rich in vitamin C and will whiten the complexion when used regularly as a rinse or tonic. The dried petals and buds may be sprinkled in the bath for fragrance and skin benefits; in potpourri these will impart the characteristic rose scent to a room or linen closet.

Ghassoul, the hair and skin treatment that women of North Africa and the Middle East favor, is made from Tertiary-era clay mixed with ground cloves and rosewater.

Taken internally as a tea, an infusion of rose leaves will act as a tonic astringent, while that of rose hips will ward off colds and other ailments of winter. Why not brighten and sweeten the dark, chilly days of January with roses in everything? Try making rose wine as did the ancient Persians, Turkish Delight with rosewater, rose petal jam, rose petal pie; scatter rose petals on ice cream, salad, syrup, and sorbet. A red rose in your hair and a fluttering of rose petals in your path: what better response to winter?

safflower

Benibana: scarlet flower. The Japanese name is so lovely to intone that by comparison none of the other names seems quite suitable. *Carthamus tinctorius* in Latin, safflower, dyer's saffron, or American saffron in English, *hong hua* in Chinese: the bright red brush-bristle blossom of the plant is a staple of Asian medicine and has long been associated with women's beauty in Japan. The red dye produced from the tiny petals supplied women there for centuries with lip color, eyeshadow, rouge, and a wide range of hues for their silk kimonos. The glorious red of the flower is the color of the rising sun, the color that in Japan symbolizes woman, festivity, goodness, beauty, and life.

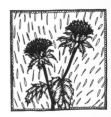

outside

safflower petal poultice

inside

safflower petal tea

The flower originated in China, Indochina, and Tibet but now grows in many parts of the world. The Yamagata region of Japan is famous for its mountain fields of cultivated, flowering *benibana*. While the Asian herbal tradition primarily utilizes the flowers for their medicinal properties, in other traditions the oil is extracted from the seeds for culinary, cosmetic, and medical purposes.

In the Chinese classification of medicines, the safflower is characterized as pungent and warm, with an affinity for heart and liver. The flower taken internally is said to promote circulation, dissolve blood clots, and act as an astringent. It is prescribed in cases of menstrual cycle abnormality, to ease bruises, stiffness, and pain in the joints, and for postnatal abdominal discomfort. Pregnant women are warned against taking the safflower blossom internally, although generally speaking the medicinal tea is known as a woman's tea, used mainly in treating women's disorders.

In the West, safflower oil has long been utilized in the formulation of a variety of cosmetic preparations. The same oil is used in the East for medical massages. The oil is of interest for internal use as well; due to its cholesterol-lowering effect, Western doctors advise an intake of the oil to protect the health of liver, gallbladder, and arteries. Note the correspondence to the ancient Chinese organs of affinity!

The flowers have been used medicinally in the West against jaundice, liver problems, and as a cleanser for the blood, especially in cases of eruptive illness like measles and chicken pox. In beauty care, the flowers are decocted (see appendix) for use as a poultice in the treatment of skin eruptions like pimples and blemishes.

What are the common, everyday uses for *benibana* in Japan? The packages of dried red-and-yellow petals are sold everywhere. While occasionally one sees an intriguing tea mixture made from safflower petals and *kombu* seaweed, most commonly one finds the petal alone. Safflower petal tea is made by steeping 2 1/2 g/1 T of the petals in 240 ml/1 C of just-boiled pure water for 30 minutes. The liquid is filtered to remove the solids, and sipped while still warm. This is a tea for occasional use, not to be taken daily. It is advised as a general tonic for women, both strengthening the system and improving the circulation. For chilly hands and feet, this is the tea prescribed to get the blood moving. Other benefits are a calming effect on the mind and the toning of the female reproductive system. Remember: this tea is off-limits to those who may be pregnant!

For beauty, an interesting drink is made from peach pits and safflower. A pinch of *benibana* is added to water in which 1 or 2 peach pits have been boiled. This is a traditional beauty medicine, a blood cleanser that will ward off age spots, liver troubles, and stress. (However, given the well-documented toxicity of the peach pit, I don't recommend trying this one without the aid of a medical specialist trained in Asian herbalism.)

So now you know what to do with bright red *benibana* blossoms. There is a poetic unity to the uses of the bloom: the flower-red dye that tints the kimono a brilliant red, the traditional lip-paint used by geisha, and a beauty tea designed to heal the female reproductive system are all derived from them. And I've always wondered whether the decocted petals would have a reddening effect on the hair … might be a lovely color if so!

sea

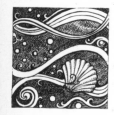

The balmy blue weather of early spring makes me think of the sea. The seaside is entrancing at any time of year, but there is something particularly appealing about it in spring: warm but breezy weather, refreshing salt spray in the air, whitecaps whipped up by the wind, and no people!

For well-being and beauty, there's nothing to compare with a couple of hours spent walking on the beach in the springtime—well, maybe a hot-spring soak comes close. In this luminous golden season, my beauty advice is: take a day off and pay homage to the ocean. (And wear a hat—the sun may not seem blistering but it still has enormous burning power, especially when reflected from sand and sea.) Why not combine the regenerative hot-spring soak with the invigoration of the ocean air by visiting a seaside spa? The best of two worlds.

If getting away from home is a too-remote possibility, maybe making an ocean in the bathtub is the answer. Invoke the sea by taking a sea-salt bath or a *wakame*-seaweed-and-sea-salt bath; both will make your skin silky and revive circulation and spirits. For these baths, the water should not be terribly hot. The salt may be added directly—a kilo or so is about right—but the *wakame* before it is added should be rinsed first if it's fresh, soaked for 20 minutes if it's dried. Use a couple of handfuls. Add it, step in, and soak amid the swirling green.

If you want to do more, try a salt scrub before soaking; this is a popular skin-rejuvenating treatment at the big spas. Simply rub coarse salt gently over your skin. Then, post-bath, a seaweed hair and body pack will polish your skin and hair to a fine sheen. All you have to do is imitate a green sea-monster for 30 minutes—but we all know that beauty has its price! For the body, just apply strips of *wakame* and relax for a while; for the hair, see the recipe in the "seaweed" section.

An even more charming means of invoking the sea in your bathing room is to adorn it with a full array of items oceanic: bath products, sea-scented pumice and sea shells, seaweed soap, candles fragrant with the ocean, sea sponges, and other deliciously marine bath-accoutrements. Apply color and symbol in whatever way strikes your fancy.

In your poetic reinvention of the ocean, you may find, perhaps, a sage-scented sea most pleasant…. you may strew your sea shells and pumice stones wherever the sight of them will please the eye…. you may annoint beach stones with eucalyptus oil for a windswept beach aroma.

Salts from the sea are good for toxin elimination, improvement of the circulation, and healing. Scrubbing with a big chunk of seaweed soap and a stiff-bristled bath brush will approximate the exfoliating, skin-polishing powers of sand. And after your scrubbing and soaking, use some mineral-rich marine-based moisturizer to nourish and soothe the skin.

An ambiance-tape of waves gently sighing upon the sand will make your private ocean complete….

Why is the sea so highly regarded in matters of health and beauty? Thalassotherapy—the use of seawater and sea plants for therapeutic healing—has long been practiced in Europe. In Japan seaweed has been used in the bath, for shampoo, and as a body scrub for centuries. Cultures in many parts of the world have traditionally employed seaweed as a preventive medicine and healing agent.

Extraordinarily rich in trace minerals, seaweed also contains many natural chemical agents that have been found in laboratory studies to be potent therapeutics. Seaweed has been shown to kill bacteria, boost the immune system, heal ulcers, stop the

outside

seaweed/salt bath

salt body scrub

*seaweed hair & body
  pack*

inside

seaweed medicine food

167

growth of cancer in animals, reduce cholesterol, lower blood pressure, prevent strokes, and thin the blood. It has been proposed that the high consumption of seaweed in Japan is one of the factors in the low incidence of breast cancer among Japanese women. A sheet of seaweed a day...

For better health, seaweed should be a part of the daily diet. The refreshing, invigorating sensation we get from the sea air, a brisk ocean swim, or a warm sea-salt bath at home indicates that the benefits of the sea can also come from the outside in.

seaweed

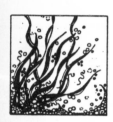

outside

funori *seaweed shampoo*

wakame *seaweed shampoo/hair pack*

kombu & wakame *seaweed shampoo/ hair pack*

There would not be virtually thousands of shampoos and conditioners on the market if consumers were satisfied with available products. The evidence shows that there's not a lot of fidelity to hair products. A look at what women used traditionally to cleanse the hair sheds some light on the problem.

In past eras in most parts of the world, there was no such thing as the daily shampoo. The hair was washed comparatively infrequently, and the presence of oil in the hair was seen as a desirable and natural condition. Many of the traditional shampoos thus cleansed and nourished the hair without removing the natural oils. Further, oils were used in dressing the hair and to protect it from damage from cold and sun. The goal: oily, lustrous hair!

This method of cleansing and caring for the hair must have created healthier tresses, but would the same approach work in the modern world? The problem with current customs and products is that the hair is washed too often and too thoroughly, causing eventual dryness and damage, which condition necessitates ever more treatments and conditioners. The difficulty is, none of the conditioners work quite as well as the scalp's natural oils.

In Japan, one very early traditional shampoo was made from clay—while this cleanser obviously acted to pull oil and dirt from the hair and scalp with the powerful "vacuum" action that is clay's property, it also had a drying effect. Women who used clay began to exhibit reddish or brownish locks—a color change that in black hair is a common sign of damage. Only those who could not afford the more expensive shampoo made from seaweed used the clay shampoo.

The seaweed shampoo was a hair beautifier used in Japan for centuries. At first only the wives of samurai could avail themselves of it, and it was believed in early Japan that the seaweed gave those upper-class women their sleek, black, thick hair. Of all the traditional Japanese shampoos, it is perhaps the only one that might find favor among modern women. A true mineral-rich beauty treatment, it leaves the hair in sublime condition, though still not with the squeaky cleanness one gets from a commercial shampoo.

There are two seaweed techniques to try. The first is the *funori* shampoo. This purple-red seaweed is used as a starch and appears in some Japanese dishes. It is available in supermarkets in Japan. To prepare the shampoo, place a couple of handfuls of *funori* in a nonmetal pot with water in a 1:3 seaweed-to-water ratio. Simmer for 20–30 minutes or until the liquid grows thick and mucilaginous. Remove from the heat and let stand until cool, then drain the solids and save the thick pink-purple liquid. To shampoo, pour the seaweed liquid onto dry hair and massage. Allow to remain on the hair for 10 or 15 minutes, then rinse very thoroughly. (Finish with a vinegar-in-water rinse to erase any marine fragrance!)

Another cleansing seaweed treatment is a hair pack or shampoo consisting of powdered *wakame* or a mixture of *wakame* and *kombu*.. One may buy the commercially prepared powder (buy organic to avoid additives) or make it oneself by grinding dried seaweed in a food-grinder. Stir about 4 tablespoons of the substance into a cup of very hot water, then allow to sit for 30 minutes. When the mixture thickens, apply to the hair as above. Both seaweed recipes can also be used in conjunction with a small amount of commercial shampoo—women who like a stronger removal of the natural oils of the hair will prefer that method. For a hair pack, no shampoo should be added. A little *tsubaki abura* —camellia oil—added to the rinse water will put some moisture back in, the old-fashioned way.

One of the above shampoos will be about as traditional as most contemporary women will want to get. Two other Japanese shampoos are oil-based—one an *azuki*-bean-and-olive-oil recipe, the other a camellia nut technique employing the raw oil … for those who want to achieve that heavy, lank, dense-curtain Heian look for the hair.

sesame

Sesame oil is one of several oils used in traditional Japanese beauty care, and it is invaluable as a treatment for skin and hair.

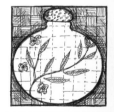

Any sesame oil that you use externally must be pure (no red pepper!) and of the highest quality. There are many grades available, so buy carefully. Those with normal or oily skin may use sesame instead of heavier oils, but those with dry skin, who require a great deal of moisture, may have to look for something richer in emollients. Sesame oil nourishes and protects the hair, and it is said that a daily sesame oil scalp massage will help slow hair loss. Just a few drops are necessary; apply daily going to sleep and do this over an extended period of time.

Another scalp/hair treatment is the ginger juice-sesame oil massage. To prepare, grate a piece of ginger and squeeze through cheesecloth to obtain juice. Combine the juice with the oil in a 1:1 ratio and beat with a whisk until blended. Massage well into the scalp to treat dandruff or falling hair. Ginger is a potent stimulant and will certainly benefit the circulation of the scalp, giving life and vigor to the hair. Use daily. (Lower the amount of ginger if you feel a stinging sensation.)

The oil is an effective, nongreasy skin softener. Massage a little of it into the skin after cleansing (after a bath is a good time), or rub it all over before a sauna session.

And finally, many believe that the daily consumption of roasted black sesame seeds will prevent the graying of hair and even restore natural color to hair that has begun to whiten.

I can't vouch for this, but it won't hurt to try! Sesame seeds are tasty and high in calcium, whether or not they give you a whole new head of glorious hair.

silk

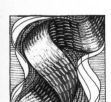

During beauty-sensitive Heian times in Japan, on the Ninth Day of the Ninth Month a Chrysanthemum Festival was held, upon which occasion those present at the Imperial party drank chrysanthemum-infused wine, composed poetry, ate small white trouts, and viewed with wonder the Imperial chrysanthemums. The chrysanthemums were wrapped in silk on the eve of the festival, and this silk could later be used to rub one's face with, to prevent the wrinkles and lines of age.

Japanese beauties have washed their skin with silk since ancient times. The soft caress of the fabric against skin or hair is said to impart a luscious softness and sheen. The silk washing-square or mitt is easily made: use the finest white silk you can find and hem it, layering the fabric several times to give it substance. A raw silk version will supply gentle exfoliating powers. Make small silk herb-bags to set afloat in the bath or to encase flower sachets for your drawers.

Sleep on silk sheets, or at least lay your precious head upon silken pillows. Wear silk in all its guises: red silk when you're in need of talismanic protection, white silk when it's cleansing and purification you desire. There's nothing wrong with a little magic … and nothing like silk for weaving a very feminine spell.

spirits

Do you know what to do with leftover champagne? Used as a rinse on fair hair, it's said to encourage gleaming golden highlights. It is also a nice, silly, luxurious feeling to pour a bottle of bubbly over your head—never mind the benefits to beauty!

A beer dousing is the plebeian answer and will provide similar conditioning, leaving hair soft, silky, and shiny.

For a more tropical adventure in hair beauty, try rum as a potent and aromatic rinse. With any of these beverages, apply after shampooing, leave on the hair for a few minutes, then rinse. You'll be rewarded with a happy head of hair, full of shine and vigor. As a shampoo rum can be used with egg yolk in a traditional European recipe. Froth up an egg yolk or two in a cup, add 100 ml/^{1}/$_2$ C of rum and a little warm water, then apply the mixture to the hair, proceeding as for a standard shampoo. This is a wonderful shampoo, leaving the hair somewhat moist and naturally oiled.

Another way to use alcohol is in a *sake* bath, a popular Japanese technique for achieving satin-smooth skin. You can buy special bath *sake*, but any big bottle will do. Simply add one full bottle to your hot bath, and plunge in. Relax as the *sake* works to beautify your skin and remove toxins.

I have some Swedish friends who splash Aquavit on the hot rocks in their sauna, then sit and "drink" in the vapors … they claim this gives them an effervescent tingle. I don't recommend this one to the uninitiated! The combination of extreme heat and alcohol can be dangerously heady.

If you have anything left in your bar after these experiments, here's a toast to a beautiful you!

strawberry

In early summer, both city and country are abloom with color: fresh strawberries have arrived in the shops, blossoms of vivid hues are bursting forth in gardens, and the world is refreshingly green again. To harmonize with nature in this festive mood, and to renew your beauty in the most gentle and natural fashion, use fruits and flowers in season for your beauty rituals.

The succulent strawberry is so decorative and sweet that one is almost surprised to learn it has medicinal qualities. Strawberries evidently possess the ability to block the formation of carcinogenic nitrosamines, and are antioxidant and rich in anticancer polyphenols. In lab tests, strawberries have been found to destroy viruses cultivated in test tubes.

Strawberries contain lots of pectin, which is said to be very effective in reducing blood cholesterol. Pectin apparently can also reduce the number of calories absorbed by the body. The high level of potassium in the berries helps blood pressure into the bargain. All this, and one cup of strawberries has only about 45 calories!

Folk medicine traditions all over the world have long respected the strawberry as an efficient but gentle diuretic, laxa-

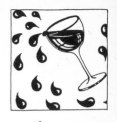

outside

champagne rinse for
* fair hair*

beer rinse for hair

rum rinse for hair

egg yolk & rum
* shampoo*

sake *bath*

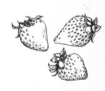

outside

strawberry facial tonic

strawberry face pack

inside

strawberry medicine
* food*

tive, and astringent. In essence, it would seem that the sugary red berry is a purifier, helping the body to cleanse and protect itself against disease.

Externally the strawberry has been used in both east and West as a protector of skin beauty. It will help to calm and heal acne, eliminate certain fungi, and heal simple skin inflammations. The Japanese grandmother has long known of the strawberry's ability to whiten the complexion and soothe skin burnt by the sun.

The simplest way to use the strawberry is to rub a cut berry over the skin after washing, like a tonic. A pack may be made by mashing the ripest fruits you can find, then lying down for 20 minutes with fragrant strawberry purée on your face. As an astringent, the pack will benefit oily skins, sensitive skins, or skin that has received too much sun.

tea

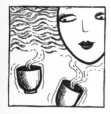

outside

green tea skin lotion & facial rinse

black-tea-bag eye compress

black tea infusion/bath

inside

tea medicine food

"Better to be three days deprived of food than a single day without tea." The ancient Chinese were right. As usual. Once again, modern science has found that the old folk wisdom about tea is accurate, and suddenly everyone wants to drink it. Why? Well, here are some of the reasons.

Japanese research shows tea to be a powerful enemy of the hated "free radicals," which cause degeneration of all sorts; America's National Cancer Institute lists tea as an anticarcinogenic food.

Green tea is taken to prevent tooth decay and to reduce the risk of cancer—recent studies have shown it to be one of the most effective plants in cancer prevention. The Japanese recommend not only drinking it but eating the leaves as a medicine food. Applied topically, the liquid will reduce itching and swelling caused by insect bites and reduce bleeding from minor wounds. Green tea reinforces the immune system.

Oolong tea, especially the type known as *puerh* or *polei*, is taken internally immediately after eating a rich meal in order to reduce blood cholesterol. Japanese scientists have found evidence that it lowers hypertension and improves the health of the arteries. Retiring sumo wrestlers and others who wish to lose weight report great success with *puerh* or *polei* tea.

Black tea is a good antidiarrhea remedy. The Chinese use it for hangovers. A steeped tea bag will refresh tired eyes. To cure a sunburn or soothe inflammation caused by insect bites, make an infusion and apply locally, or take a tea bath.

A well-known French cosmetics company includes green tea in its skin beauty capsules along with seaweed, vitamin E, and beta carotene. As a diuretic, tea is useful against water retention. The theophylline in tea is a fat-gobbling agent, one of the xanthine family to which caffeine also belongs. Tea is now being included in slimming creams, and if one follows the inside/outside beauty dictum, applying the creams would seem to be a happy complement to drinking the beverage.

Green tea makes a wonderful facial rinse. Steep as for drinking, cool, then apply to the skin after washing. It will tighten the pores, calm sensitivity, and ostensibly provide anti-aging benefits if used with regularity.

I suppose it seems obvious that one must simply apply tea in all its forms, internally as well as externally, to take advantage of the extraordinary *Camellia sinensis Kuntze*, which is the source for all the types we've mentioned here. (The various teas are obtained via different drying methods.)

ume

In June the plum rains (*tsuyu* in Japanese) may coax your *Prunus mume*—a type of apricot, to be precise—to fall green and hard from your plum tree. In kitchens all over Japan, plum-related activity begins. The summer plums are set to pickle or steep, to soak in salt or syrup—captured and preserved for round-the-year use. The sour *ume* is made into *umeboshi*, or pickled *ume*, into *ume* liquor, *ume* wine, and *ume* extract—all beloved elements of the Japanese diet.

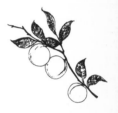

outside

green plum skin tonic

The *ume* is prized for its antibacterial properties; used internally as well as externally, it is said to be a potent eliminator of toxins. Green plum tonic, a traditional lotion for beautiful skin, has the *ume* as its primary ingredient. On one of those long gray days of summer rain, try concocting this Japanese beauty elixir.

Markets in Japan abound with green plums at this time of year (early June), so if you don't have a plum tree, don't despair. Outside Japan you will find *ume* in season wherever Japanese are living. The plums, a bottle of good *shōchū*—tasteless and colorless distilled spirits with a 20–45% alcohol content—and a wide-necked glass bottle or canning jar are all you will need for this recipe. (Very close to the plums in the market you are likely to find the bottles and jars used for making plum wine and plum liquor. One of those will be perfect.)

Wash 150 g/5 ¼ oz of unripe *ume*—they must be green, not yellow—and remove the hulls. Dry the fruits gently with a cloth. Place the *ume* in a sterilized bottle, add 240 ml/1 C of *shōchū*, and seal tightly. Store the bottle away from sunlight for a period of two months. When ready, rebottle in smaller glass jars and store in the refrigerator or a cool place.

When your green plum tonic is well steeped and ready for use, employ it as you would any tonic lotion. Apply with gauze, or splash onto freshly washed skin morning and night; do not rinse.

The *ume* lotion will tone, refresh, and purify the skin, destroying surface bacteria and refining pores. Just right for August, when the tonic will be ready to use. Green plum tonic is appropriate for all skin types (though very dry or sensitive skin may not appreciate the alcohol), and it may be used daily if desired.

umeboshi

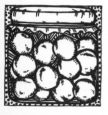

outside

umeboshi *skin tonic*

inside

umeboshi *medicine food*

I have always felt a particular affection for the *umeboshi*, that talismanic, salty, sour, wrinkled red ball that is the faithful consort of Japanese white rice. To my surprise and delight, I recently discovered that there is a use for the *umeboshi* in beauty care! Perhaps that should not be so entirely surprising—the *umeboshi* plays a starring role in Japanese folk medicine. During the course of my research, I have gathered at least 50 different *umeboshi* health remedies, for everything from ulcers to headaches.

In beauty care, the *umeboshi* is used to concoct a skin lotion or tonic. Prepare as follows:

1. Remove the salt from several *umeboshi* by soaking them in warm water for 2 days. The water should be periodically renewed.
2. In a clean, sealed glass bottle, soak the salt-free *umeboshi* in 180 ml/ $^3/_4$ C of good-quality *sake* for a week or 10 days.
3. At the end of this time, strain the liquid through cheesecloth and discard the *umeboshi* solids. Store in the refrigerator.
4. The resulting *umeboshi* lotion may be used daily as a skin tonic. It is said to beautify and stimulate the complexion, purifying it of toxins and acting to destroy surface bacteria.

For those who wish to explore other of the *umeboshi*'s many talents, some things to try:

—*Umeboshi* with *okayu* (rice porridge), the medicinal meal for one who is sick.

—An *umeboshi* with meals, to prevent food poisoning.

—At the very beginning of a cold, a cup of *ban-cha* tea with *umeboshi* in it may ward off the illness.

—Take one *umeboshi* as a quick remedy for indigestion.

—Eat an *umeboshi* daily to keep you looking and feeling young.

—For strength and stamina, *umeboshi*.

—To purify your blood, a daily *umeboshi*.

—Take an *umeboshi* for sluggish digestion.

—When you have a headache, stick a big soft pitted *umeboshi* to your forehead.

—For a splinter, apply an *umeboshi*.

—For a sore throat, gargle with *umeboshi* decoction.

—For a cough, drink a cup of water with charred *umeboshi* in it.

—Also for a cough: wrap some pitted *umeboshi* in cheesecloth and apply to the chest.

—Before an exam or an important interview, tuck an *umeboshi* into your *obi* sash for good luck.

vanilla

It's not hard to understand the special allure of the vanilla bean—it was the essence of all those lovely childhood aromas: ice cream, cookies, the archetypal mother baking away in the kitchen…. Although vanilla may not immediately come to mind as a star ingredient in women's perfumes, it is indeed one of the classic elements in some of the world's most popular fragrances.

I will confess here that back in my impoverished-student-in-a-Paris-garret days, I used to dab humble vanilla extract onto my pulse points. It was one of my favorite do-it-yourself scent discoveries. (Another was the clove necklace—I made that by soaking cloves until they became soft, then stringing them with needle and thread into a necklace.) Some years later I learned about a scientific scent study in which male subjects had been exposed to hundreds of different aromas, including foods, expensive perfumes, and assorted other scented things, like tobacco and cut grass. The big winner in allure? Vanilla.

The scientists conjectured that it was due to unconscious associations with mother and the warm hearth—but I personally feel it could just as likely have been unconscious associations with cookies and ice cream! Well, then again, perhaps that amounts to the same thing—food being the equivalent of mother in the lexicon of symbols.

Happily, for those who are already vanilla aficionados, vanilla-redolent perfumes are more prevalent than one might think. If you have yet to discover it, have a whiff of the vanilla-fragrant scents before making your next perfume choice. Vanilla may unexpectedly seduce you.

Many vanilla perfumes are not constructed from the vanilla bean itself but from its chemical substitute, vanillin. It appears that the strength of the natural essence makes it difficult to work with, while the vanillin blends well with other aromas.

Grown in Polynesia and other tropical paradises, vanilla releases its scent only when the bean is dried under the burning sun. A complex ritual of successive sessions of drying, aerating, reheating, wrapping, soaking, and storing is carried out until the bean is finally ready to release its sweet and sensual odor.

And vanilla extract? The common cheap sort is fake vanilla in

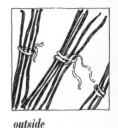

outside

vanilla fragrance

vanilla & egg yolk & camellia oil & rum hair treatment

vanilla bath

vanilla hair fragrance

lots and lots of alcohol, but still, it's serviceable for certain purposes. In a pinch—say if I were stranded on a desert island without my "Habanita"—I might even apply some to a wrist. The more expensive extract of pure vanilla, available in gourmet shops, carries a headier punch.

For a hair treat, add a little of the real extract to an egg yolk-camellia oil-rum hair treatment. Wrap the head in a warm towel or relax in a sauna for an hour, then shampoo and rinse. You'll emerge with gorgeous, vanilla-scented tresses! (Don't tell anyone your secret.)

To experiment at home with vanilla, try grinding the bean to a fine powder, then adding it to the bath or brushing it through your hair for a subtle scent.

---

some vanilla-redolent fragrances

Lagerfeld: "KL"
Brosseau: "Ombre Rose"
Laura Ashley: "No. 1"
Armani: "Gio"
Thierry Mugler: "Angel"
Comptoir du Sud Pacifique: "Vanille," "Vanille Abricot," "Vanille Café"
L'Artisan Parfumeur: "Vanilia"
Herbiers du Provence: "Vanille Florale"
Guerlain: "Shalimar," "Jicky"
Molinard: "Habanita," "Miss Habanita"
Yves St. Laurent: "Opium"
Dior: "Poison"
Cacharel: "Loulou"
Guerlain: "Samsara"
Lancôme: "Trésor"

---

vinegar

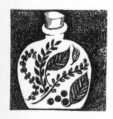

When winter lingers, the last weeks of snow and icy winds and cold drafts make of us dedicated bath aficionados. A steaming Japanese-style bath, and with it an abrasive skin scrub, combine to produce a relaxation and warmth that effectively banish the winter chill. Add to the bath ritual an old French tradition—the friction rubdown—updated with aromatherapy, and bathtime will become truly sublime.

The friction rub is a method of stimulating the circulation of the skin by the brisk application of a very light eau de cologne, eau de toilette, herbal vinegar, or diluted mixture of essential oils to every part of the body. In Europe one may buy enormous one-liter bottles of friction water or cologne for this purpose. Commercially made waters for such a skin-softening, toning, energizing rubdown often contain a mixture of fragrant essential oils in alcohol and water. Such ingredients as ylang ylang, neroli, sandalwood, lavender, mandarin orange, and other aromatic plants contribute the virtues that give skin vitality and freshness.

One may create one's own homemade *vinaigre de toilette*—beauty vinegar—with a mixture of 25–30 drops of essential oils, 2 1/2 teaspoons of vodka or rubbing alcohol, 120 ml/4 oz of vinegar, and 240 ml/2 C of spring water. To make, mix the essential oils together, add to the alcohol, and shake well. Leave to sit before adding vinegar. Wait a day, then add water and shake. Strain.

Witch hazel is a good old-fashioned product that is perfect for the friction rub; dilute it with 50% rosewater for a lighter effect. Japanese *hechimasui* (loofah-vine water) might make a lovely rubdown water—the *hechima* is skin softening, lightening, and protective.

First, how-to. After the bath, which by all means should be accompanied by a good scrubbing with a loofah, a bath brush, or a *tawashi*, lightly towel-dry. In the Japanese manner, the skin should be just slightly moist when applying the product. Using the bare hands, apply the aromatic water, oil, or vinegar to every square inch of the body. Beginning at the extremities (don't omit the soles of the feet!) work in brisk strokes moving toward the heart. The entire operation should take just a minute or two. When you're done, wrap yourself up nice and warm.

What are the benefits of the friction rub? The old European wisdom held that a good daily rubdown with lavender water or cologne strengthened and stimulated the skin, and the strong, well-functioning skin would in turn strengthen and invigorate the entire being. The rubdown action itself is effective, of course, but the addition of a product with soothing, softening, stimulating, and healing properties compounds the rub's benefits.

The skin acts as one of the body's defense systems as well as a primary means of toxin-and-waste-elimination. The Asian techniques of *shiatsu* and acupuncture stimulate the *tsubo*, or pressure points upon the skin, as a means of balancing the energy flow and health of the entire organism. The daily stimulation of the entire surface of the body is thought in both Eastern and Western traditions to help prevent illness and promote a healthy longevity.

The local stimulation of the circulation sets up a beneficial process in the body: cells receive more oxgen, wastes are eliminated more efficiently, and water retention is ameliorated. Such conditions as cellulite and sluggish circulation can benefit enor-

outside

*essential oil friction rub
for the skin*

*beauty vinegar tonic
for the skin*

mously from this type of daily skin stimulation. And it feels wonderful into the bargain!

For a homemade tonic water try the following recipe: fill a wide-necked glass bottle $2/3$ full with red wine vinegar, apple cider vinegar, brown rice vinegar, or soybean vinegar. Add enough dried herbs so that the liquid reaches the top of the bottle. Let the mixture sit for 10 days, then strain, discarding the plants. Reserve the vinegar and apply as directed above.

While the traditional plant to use is lavender (calming, stimulating), other possibilities are geranium leaf (refreshing, stimulating), sage, rosemary, or pine (antifatigue, stimulating), cinnamon or clove (stimulating, refreshing, antibacterial), oregano, thyme, cinnamon or eucalyptus (cold remedy), mint (stimulating, sore muscle soother), or a mixture of your own. For a Japanese touch, try green tea (stimulating, astringent), *shiso* (stimulating, antibacterial), or field horsetail (*sugina*) (soothing, moisturizing).

water

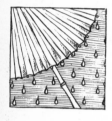

One fundamental beauty secret is so obvious that it is very easy to overlook: WATER. It's a natural resource that is present in delightful abundance, in the form of humidity, ocean, streams, lakes, rain, mist, snow, sea, and hot springs.

Not only is water a natural richness in Japan, but the cultural reverence for the element has resulted in various refined ways of appreciating it. The tea ceremony, the ritual of rinsing the hands and mouth at a Shinto shrine, the hot-spring bath, the bath at an inn, and the elegant carp pool in a quiet garden are some of the many ways to enjoy the "art of water" in Japan.

When one considers that water is the most important element (second to air!) in maintaining health, all this water-appreciation does not seem odd. For beauty, too, one must begin with water and build from there.

The wet air of Japan is good for the skin, and a relaxed walk in the misty plum rains will work magic for your complexion. Taking lots of baths, soaking in *onsen*, and drinking liters of pure water are the very basics of a good beauty regimen. Externally, water not only cleanses, moisturizes, and refreshes, but it relaxes and soothes the soul.

Internally, water is "responsible for and involved in nearly every body process, including digestion, absorption, circulation, and excretion, is the primary transporter of nutrients throughout the body and is necessary for all building functions in the body." (*Nutrition Almanac*)

If you are not drinking enough water (and many people do not) it will show in your complexion. A recommended amount is a liter/4 C per day, and more in hot weather. For pure drinking water, spring or bottled water (taken from sources far from industrial pollution) are your best bets.

Water in its various forms has been adversely affected by the excesses of modern man, so that special care must be taken to avoid pollutants and chemicals. An innocent walk in the rain can subject you to acid rain, so use an umbrella. (Your complexion will still benefit from the moisture in the air.)

Drink untested tap water, and you may be ingesting not only the usual antibacterial chemicals but also a variety of pollutants and wastes. Boiling water will destroy bacteria, but heavy metals and nitrates in the water will become more concentrated. So be informed about your water sources. Get the best water you can for drinking, and drink a lot! Take lots of baths, go swimming, walk in the rains and the dewy mists … indulge in the wonders of water.

yarrow

Visiting Colorado—the wide sunburnt desert land at the foot of the Rocky Mountains—I've been inspired to write about yarrow. On a recent hike through pine-fragrant hills, I came across the medicinal plant with its pale delicate flower clusters, and felt moved to pay my respects in writing to this ancient oracle-herb. Yarrow is a noble plant that figures in the oldest of international folk medicine traditions: archaeologists have found evidence of yarrow with several other healing plants at a 60,000-year-old Neanderthal burial ground in Iraq.

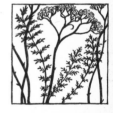

outside

yarrow-tea skin lotion

yarrow healing poultice

inside

yarrow tea

Yarrow—*Achillea millefolium* in Latin, *nokogirisō* in Japanese—is a beautiful pale green plant with a downy delicate stem, feathery fernlike leaves, and neat clusters of yellow-centered, pink- or cream-colored flowers. The plant grows to between 8 inches and 3 feet in height. A perennial herb, yarrow is found growing wild in open, sunny fields and pastures in temperate areas of the world. It is native to Europe and Western Asia and is a member of the daisy family (the Compositae).

As with other extremely powerful medicine-plants, yarrow has been regarded as a magical agent in many cultures. Those who are familiar with the ancient Chinese system of divination (presented in book form in the *I Ching*) will know that another name for the system is The Yarrow Stalk Oracle, for the dried stalks were traditionally thrown to determine the hexagrams. The Druids and Anglo-Saxons also employed yarrow in divination and in fashioning talismans. In many of the places where yarrow was used as a medicine, it was regarded both as a protector against evil and as a tool of black magic. Yarrow, like mugwort, was known to be a favorite herb of witches.

In the English herbal tradition, yarrow is one of a small group of plants known as allheal. The native Americans of the Navajo tribe consider yarrow a "life medicine," a general tonic and panacea. The genus name *Achillea* refers to the hero Achilles of Homer's *Iliad*, who prescribed yarrow to stop the bleeding from his soldiers' wounds. In all cultures, yarrow has been used to heal wounds, stop bleeding, soothe burns, and alleviate bruises. The plant has also been utilized as an astringent and a pain-reliever, as a treatment for earaches, as a fever reducer, appetite stimulant, and anti-inflammatory agent. The entire plant is official. Of particular importance in the treatment of the digestive and circulatory systems, yarrow is diaphoretic, astringent, hemostatic, antibacterial, stimulating, and carminative. Yarrow is a major curative in both the Chinese and European medical traditions. As a Bach Flower Remedy, yarrow brings protection from harm by inspiring reliance on inner strength.

In beauty, yarrow has great value as both a healing and a cleansing astringent. This combination of attributes makes it a treasured treatment for oily or problem skin. Applied externally in infused tea form (see appendix for directions), yarrow will heal rashes and blemishes. For a more intensive treatment, fresh macerated or mashed leaves or the dried and powdered herb may be applied directly to problem areas for quick healing. Yarrow infusion may be used every day on oily and normal skins as a gentle astringent rinse after washing; it will supply additional healing and toning benefits at the same time.

Very dry skins will not tolerate that daily astringent action but can make use of yarrow occasionally to treat inflammations or blemishes. Every skin type will benefit from the ingestion of yarrow tea, which improves the circulation and acts as a general tonic, strengthening the body's own healing processes.

A look at the literature on yarrow reveals that not only has this plant been used just about everywhere and for just about everything, but it had a particularly interesting function in old England as a love-divination. It is said that in bygone days one might discern the trueness of one's love by placing a yarrow leaf in one nostril and twitching it while intoning, "Yarroway, Yarroway, bear a white blow; if my love love me, my nose will bleed now." Given yarrow's reputation as a cure-all, doesn't it seem more likely that it would alleviate a nosebleed than cause one? One wonders how many romances came to an abrupt end when that so-desired nosebleed didn't materialize.

the

spirit-magic

of

scent

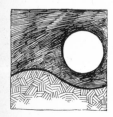

A male friend, describing his reaction to the presence of a perfumed woman, says, "It is as if a fairy tale happens, a sort of floaty magic feeling; the moment she enters the room there is a transformation of the atmosphere into something wonderful." I love this description. Although many might say merely that they find perfume seductive or feminine, its diffusion through space actually does something very close to an act of magic: reality is changed on a chemical, molecular level, by means of a substance both potent and unseen.

In most cultures where scent in some form is used, it is seen as a power in itself—something that penetrates the boundaries of matter in the same way that spirit can, or that *ki* (the vital energy), is able to do. Of great interest too is the fact that scent and medicine are one and the same: the essences that are the origin of fragrance are also curative substances, with the power to effect healing. Further, the mind and emotions may be influenced by aroma; the power of scent to trigger memories or to alter mood is well documented.

Incense accompanies religious rituals in many parts of the world, and its use is always regarded as both transformative and purifying. It is looked upon as a mover between worlds, between the seen and the unseen. Scent is present at rites of passage, at the boundary between life and death. As a symbol of the threshold and the crossing of the threshold, scent both precipitates transformation and protects against its dangers. Scent is used in the beauty ritual as an attractor, in medicine as a mind/body transformer, in magic and religion as invocation and blessing.

"The moon smells like flowers," say the Batek Negrito people of Malaysia, whose entire world is defined by aroma. Hindus employ sandalwood to cleanse the third eye, to induce concentration, and to raise the spirits. Among the Swahili people of the East African coast, where I lived for a time, night-blooming jasmine is used in great quantity for its aphrodisiac perfume: women wear bundles of the blossoms in their hair and strew the sweet-smelling fresh petals in the bed before a night of love. In modern

Japan, mood-altering scent is used in office buildings: lemon, lavender, or rose currents are piped in with the air to make workers relaxed, cheerful, or more alert.

In Japan the ancient tradition of incense as an aromatic, both to perfume one's clothing and to softly sweeten the atmosphere of the house, continues to this day. The incenses of Japan are subtle and light—very different from the incenses of India, which tend to be bright, dense, and rather dominating.

Incense in Japan is also employed for religious purposes: *kenkō* is the burning of incense for Buddha and the gods, and *shokō*, the burning of incense for the souls of the deceased. But even incense used as an aromatic is believed to function as a charm against evil.

Incense for aromatic uses appears in two forms: the *nioibukuro*, or scent bag, and *soradakimono*, incense for burning. Both types are traditionally available in the following fragrances: clove, musk, sandalwood, daphne, pine, borneol, and Japanese yew.

The *nioibukuro* (also sometimes referred to as *kakekō*) is a bag of silk containing kneaded incense or chopped aromatic barks and grasses. The bag may be hung in a room to impart a delicate fragrance to the air, or worn tucked inside the clothing. Traditionally, two scent bags tied to either end of a cord would be hung around the neck, with each bag concealed within the sleeves of the kimono. Alternatively, a bag might be tucked into the *obi* or the bodice. This use of scent creates an enchantingly vague aroma, a whispering waft of fragrance that fascinates by its very subtlety.

Nioibukuro are also tucked between the folds of stored kimono. Before the kimono is worn, it is hung to air on a kimono hanger. Kimono can be scented by another method: underneath a basket containing the kimono one is to wear, *soradakimono* is placed and lit, thus permeating the kimono with fragrance; the effect is smokier and heavier.

For perfuming a room, incense is always burned in an inconspicuous place, usually in another, nearby room; in this way the aroma has no visible origin and is mysteriously light; there is just the suggestion of something pleasant in the air.

An exploration of scent properly begins with the primary materials in their original forms: scented barks and fragrant woods. From there, a look at the essences drawn from these, the oils of aromatherapy. Finally, a glance at perfumes, themselves elixirs created by elegant interweavings of the fragrant essences, to arrive at scent in its most refined state.

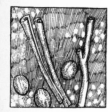

Fragrant woods, barks, roots, and nuts have a special place in the panoply of health and beauty botanicals. While blossoms, leaves, fruits, and vegetables are often fragile, in need of drying or other means of preservation, the hardier parts of plants may hold their fragrance and efficacy for longer without manipulation.

Earlier in history, those parts provided the simplest, easiest ways of perfuming the body, clothes, and home. Each fragrant wood has unique therapeutic benefits, making this natural form of perfume a healing indulgence.

Cinnamon (*Cinnamomum zeylanicum Ness.* and *C. cassia Blume.*), in Chinese *rou gui* (bark) and *gui zhi* (wood), is an astringent aromatic. Added to hair rinses, cinnamon imparts a fresh, spicy perfume to the hair and brings out chestnut tones. Made into an infusion, cinnamon can be used as a disinfectant skin wash. In Chinese medicine cinnamon wood is employed as a stimulant for the circulation, while the internal bark commonly known to us as cinnamon is used as a *ki* stimulant, an energizer, and a kidney tonic. A warming treatment, cinnamon is prescribed in cases of asthma and for difficulties in menopause. Western uses focus on digestive benefits. Precautions for both internal and external use: due to warming properties, avoid use during fever; because it is a strong uterine stimulant, it must also be avoided during pregnancy. Used as fragrance, cinnamon will promote a sensation of warmth, happiness, and energy. Traditional Japanese fragrance often included a subtle dash of cinnamon.

Fennel, *uikyō* in Japanese and *Foeniculum vulgare* in Latin, is an aromatic of particular interest in beauty for its usefulness in slimming (the Greek name for fennel is *marathron*, from a verb that means "to become slender"). Another warming herb used in traditional fragrance, fennel in seed and root form stimulates the circulation, improves lactation, and has anti-inflammatory, expectorant, and diuretic properties. Fennel taken internally is beneficial to the eyes. Chinese medicine employs fennel to cure stomach troubles, babies' colic, and digestive colds. A fennel-tea facial rinse is a calming, strengthening astringent for the complexion. As fragrance, fennel produces a piquant, warm, refreshing note.

Sandalwood is *Santalum album* in Latin and *byakudan* in Japanese. With its wonderful scent and its power as a relaxant and sedative, sandalwood would seem magical even without its many other medicinal properties. A remedy for acne, catarrh, skin infections, menstrual problems, and depression, sandalwood has been used as a rejuvenative antiseptic and perfume for over 4,000 years. In India sandalwood constitutes a delightfully simple night-time beauty treatment, especially recommended for oily or blemished skins. Take a small piece of sandalwood and rub with a little water against a stone. Spread the light paste thus obtained upon the face, and leave there all night. In the morning, remove the dry sandalwood pack by rinsing with rosewater. A little powdered sandalwood brushed through the hair will impart a lovely fragrance and cleanse and beautify the hair.

Known as *kanzō* in Japanese, *Glycyrrhiza glabra* and *Glycyrrhiza uralensis Fisch.* in Latin, and *gan cao* in Chinese, licorice root is another traditional aromatic that is also a potent medicine. In external beauty uses, licorice root acts as an emollient. The Chinese give it the appellation "the great detoxifier" and use it as an overall tonic. Licorice stimulates the production of hormones, acts as an anti-inflammatory and expectorant, and lowers the blood cholesterol. A refreshing herb, licorice root has 50 times as much sugar as does glucose. A mixture of licorice root and ginseng, made into a tea, is a beneficial daily tonic, but those with hypertension or problems of the arteries must abstain.

Nutmeg, *Myristica fragrans* in Latin and *rou dou kou* in Chinese (*nikuzuku* in Japanese), is a common ingredient in perfumes. Used externally, nutmeg stimulates circulation and soothes aching joints. Said to possess aphrodisiac properties, nutmeg will exercise a hypnotic effect on the mind if it's taken in large quantities. While an overdose (more than 7 g/$\frac{1}{4}$ oz at a time) can be dangerous and even cause hallucinations or convulsions, in small amounts this nut is beneficial. Nutmeg is useful for stomach problems; in Chinese medicine it is employed as a regulator of *ki*. The French add nutmeg oil to honey to treat bad breath, and it's a standard ingredient in cakes and other baked sweets. Witches find the spice to be indispensable in any love potion, with the nutmeg-redolent cake casting a particularly potent enchantment over a desired one.

Play with the scented barks and fragrant woods by mixing them in arrangements of your own devising, then enclose them in silk bags to wear or hide in nooks and crannies of your home.

What is aromatherapy? The principle underlying aromatherapy is this: fragrant essential oils derived from plants can effect changes in body and mind, and thus they may be used in the cure or treatment of a variety of conditions. (The concept is ancient, dating to at least 2,000 years B.C.) It is thought that essential botanical oils function as the hormones of plants, that they are indeed the source of the life force in plants, and that by introducing them into the human organism either internally or externally we can stimulate healing.

While the therapy was practiced in various ways in ancient Egypt and China, then in Greece and Rome, it wasn't until the thirteenth century that the practice appears to have arrived in England. It was noted during the Middle Ages that perfume makers seemed immune to cholera and the epidemics that swept through Europe in that period. Essential oils have been shown in recent studies to possess antiviral, antibacterial, and antiseptic properties.

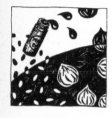

For centuries in China and Japan, fragrant plants have been culled for healing; the use of incense, hair oils, and skin oils redolent of sandalwood, musk, and camphor dates to very early times. Both women and men appropriated a personal fragrance as much for its healing and talismanic properties as for its more obvious power to attract the opposite sex and evoke an aura of beauty.

While cheaper chemical versions of essential oils were developed in the nineteenth century and found uses in fragrance and medicine, the side-effects associated with those man-made substances gradually led in the twentieth century to a renewal of interest in the natural essential oils. In the 1920s, the French chemist Gattefosse presented new modern evidence that essential oils were therapeutic and could penetrate the skin to circulate within the blood and lymph systems and ultimately reach the organs of the body. (If you wish to test this theory yourself, try rubbing fresh garlic on the soles of your feet—within a short time evidence of garlic will be found on your breath!)

Dr. Jean Valnet was a French physician who applied aromatherapy for healing, particularly in the form of essential oil compresses. Also in France a biochemist, Madame Maury, developed her own massage system for aromatherapy—her application of this technique to beauty therapy led to the popular aromatherapy massage that is today so widespread.

Essential oils are taken internally, and can be introduced into the bloodstream through other means such as massage (including *shiatsu*), baths, inhalations, and compresses. While a serious aromatherapy treatment program would best be placed in the hands of a specialist, it is simple enough to experiment with oils on one's own.

The therapeutic use of fragrance can include burnable or non-burnable incense, potpourri, scented candles, and personal or ambiance perfumes and scents, but true aromatherapy calls for the essential oil itself in some form. The materials available for aromatherapy use are base oils, macerated oils, essential oils, base creams, and oil burners. The techniques include massage, room-scenting, inhalation, baths, compresses, and internal use, usually in the form of teas.

Essential oils for aromatherapy are not usually made in the same way as oils for perfume, or as those for the food-flavoring industry. Aromatherapy requires oils of the utmost purity, distilled from fresh, usually organic, plant sources. Different parts of a plant may be utilized in distillation, and this can have a great effect on the quality and efficacy of the resulting oil. Roots, barks, seeds, berries, fruits, leaves, wood, flowers, and gums or resins may be the primary material from which a volatile oil is extracted. Distillation is done with water or steam, or a combination of the two, depending on the particular plant as well as on local tradition. Occasionally flower oils are extracted with solvents, and citrus rind oils by cold pressing. An aromatherapist will insist on oils that have been produced under the purest conditions and that consist of the appropriate parts of the plant.

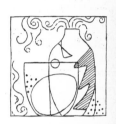

To prepare massage oils, one dilutes essential oils in a base or carrier oil. The lightest and most easily absorbed of these is grapeseed; sweet almond oil and apricot kernel oil are light but oily; all three are lacking in fragrance. Olive oil, wheat germ oil, and avocado oil are richer—any of these are beneficial to dry skin but possess their own fragrance. All three are good for the prevention of stretch marks and increasing the resilience of the skin. Evening primrose oil is another healing oil. Soybean oil is nourishing. Hazelnut oil is rich and fragrant. Jojoba oil is good for oily skin. Generally, one chooses a mixture of base oils to ensure the appropriate combination of qualities, but for the novice a simple grapeseed or soybean oil can be fine.

Macerated oils, also used as base or carrier oils, are oils in which plant materials have been steeped and then removed, leaving the oil with the properties and fragrance of the botanical ingredient.

A massage oil consists of approximately 2% essential oil to 98% base oil. It can be mixed in small amounts for each massage or in 100 ml/3 1/2 oz quantities. For 100 ml/3 1/2 oz, add about 40 drops of essential oil.

Base creams are simply less oily carriers for the essential oils. For the beginner in aromatherapy, using base oils and creams is safer than using essential oils in more concentrated ways.

An oil burner is a water-filled vessel in which essential oils are diluted for scenting a room. A candle burning underneath helps to impart scent into the room for purification or for a therapeutic adjustment of the atmosphere. For inhalations, a few drops of oil are added to a bowl of very hot water, then a towel is placed over the head for inhalation of the steam. For baths, 7 or 8 drops of essential oil are enough for benefits, and for teas, a drop or two is enough, but only a specialist should prescribe internal use. The unskilled should avoid compresses.

Never apply oils directly to the skin, and avoid black pepper, cinnamon, and clove, along with citrus oils. Don't experiment at all during pregnancy, but see a specialist. Don't use oils on

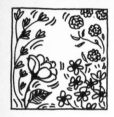

babies or children, and don't use them on anyone for more than a couple of weeks at a stretch, once per day.

Let's look at a few oils that are safe for the beginner who wants to experiment. Remember, always, that these benign-seeming fragrant oils are intensely concentrated and are absorbed into the skin to real effect.

The entire efficacy of the system depends on this ability of the essential oil to reach all parts of the organism. Handle with care.

ROSE: This is the least toxic of all the essential oils, and a good place to start. Good for all skin types, rose is antiseptic, with benefits for dry or irritated skin as well as aging or sensitive complexions. The oil is said to improve blood circulation, and combat depression, insomnia, tension, and stress; ameliorate menstrual problems and other reproductive system ailments; treat conjunctivitis, earache, and headache; and offer relief for a variety of digestive problems. Rose oil is one of the most expensive oils; its fragrance is of course delightful. Very tiny amounts will have powerful effects, but as this is fundamentally a relaxing and soothing oil, there is not much danger in employing it. Rose is acquired from either *Rosa centifolia* or *Rosa damascena*.

CHAMOMILE: A lovely oil low in toxicity and high in healing power, chamomile is employed for all manner of skin troubles: acne, skin allergies, burns, dermatitis, sensitivity, irritations, blemishes, wounds, and wherever an antiseptic is warranted. Chamomile is calming, refreshing, and relaxing, and therefore assuages anxiety, depression, insomnia, and children's tantrums. It acts as a tonic to the nervous system. Chamomile will soothe muscle aches and other pains, normalize menstrual irregularity, and assuage earaches, headaches, and teething pain, as well as various digestive problems. Chamomile is distilled from *Anthemis nobilis*, *Osmanis mixta*, or *Matricaria chamomilla* and contains a substance called azulene. Chamomile will lighten hair. Chamomile oil should be avoided during pregnancy.

LAVENDER: Lavender is one of the most popular oils due to its versatility. It has applications for skin problems, all sorts of bites and burns, sunburn, eczema, dermatitis, and inflammations. Lavender benefits the circulation, and the digestive system and fights, respiratory problems, headache, menstrual problems, muscle aches, anxiety, depression, fluid retention, and female hair loss. While not quite as all-around safe as rose or chamomile, when used very sparingly it is generously therapeutic, refreshing, and relaxing. The oil is distilled from *Lavendula vera*.

JASMINE: A relaxing, soothing, uplifting oil, jasmine promotes emotional well-being and body/mind harmony. It is antidepressive and is said to improve self-confidence! An aphrodisiac, jasmine is beneficial to both men and women in the realm of love. Jasmine is good for all skin types, especially sensitive, dry, or irritated skin, and it ameliorates respiratory and menstrual complaints. Jasmine oil is obtained by enfleurage or with solvents from the flowers of *Jasminum grandiflorum*.

NEROLI: Also known as NEROLI-BIGARADE or simply OIL OF ORANGE BLOSSOM, neroli is the ultra-relaxing oil. Calming and uplifting, neroli will fight depression, hysteria, exhaustion, confusion, and all illnesses resulting from nervousness or anxiety. It is an antidepressant and is used for treating shock. Its low toxicity makes it useful in treating skin inflammations and in healing scar tissue and skin problems caused by sensitivity or inflammation. It is beneficial for dry, damaged skin. This very fragrant oil is used for digestive disorders caused by stress, and nervous system disorders. Neroli-Bigarade is distilled from the blossoms of bitter orange, or *Citrus aurantium L./Citrus Bigaradia Riss.* (The oil of sweet orange, or Neroli Portugal, made from the zest of the *Citrus sinensis Osbeck*, is less useful.)

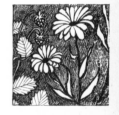

Begin with the lovely scents described above and discover the delights of using natural fragrances therapeutically—all five of them are classics in the realm of body/mind healing, working on the emotions and spirit as much as on the physical being. But remember that quantities are always minute, and while the information presented here is meant to guide you safely through a confusing domain, I would always advise consultation with a specialist if you have a tendency to sensitivity, allergies, or have any health problem or condition that might require special consideration. True aromatherapy is a serious system for health and beauty care; it is advisable to consult with a physician regarding all treatment options and any possible contraindications.

Perfume is perhaps the most ephemeral form of scent, used entirely for its magical promise of beauty and love (or at least attraction). Perfume is talismanic, and the bottles that hold it are designed to convey this. Perfume is all about the power of suggestion.

Perfume can express a hidden aspect of the self. Women often choose a perfume for themselves that conveys an unrealized aspect of the identity. The shy wallflower who wears some passionate, aggressive fragrance, or the dynamic career woman who wears something innocent or flowery are behaving out of character, but at the same time providing an intriguing counterpoint to the presence. Perfume can offer the subtle suggestion of something hidden.

Perfume *is* atmosphere, and as such it is mysterious. How to find one's way through this world of the ephemeral? What follows are a few fundamentals to serve as a guide in the art of choosing perfume.

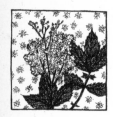

First, become familiar with the gamut of scents. You need not initially know the classifications—woody, green, spicy, floral, and so forth—but merely have a sniff of as many different fragrances as possible. You will find that your nose becomes confused quickly, so it's best not to overdo it. Have a brief encounter with several perfume bottles just to break the ice.

Now that I've advised you to smell the bottled perfume, let me tell you why this method is not too useful beyond the roughest scent-acquaintance stage. A perfume is composed of top note, middle note, and base note. What you smell first in a perfume is the top note, the most volatile aspect of the fragrance. The top note is palpable for less than 30 minutes, during which time it gives way to the slower-developing middle note.

The middle note takes over where the top note leaves off. The middle note adds its own character to the top note, establishes itself while the base note develops, and lasts for two or three hours. The middle note is the perfume's central fragrance. The base note takes longest to develop and forms the foundation of the perfume. This note lingers longest. Thus, a perfume might start out fresh and green, then become deeper and warmer when the scent has developed.

To really know a perfume, then, you must spend time with it. Apply a small amount and wear it for a day. In choosing a fragrance gift for someone else, one can approximate the time test by asking for smelling strips—small pieces of stiff paper that have been sprayed with a small amount of the fragrance. Smell the strip right away for the top note, an hour or two later for the middle, and four hours later for the base note, which is the perfume's "true" nature. It won't help much in this case to dab or spray a perfume on your own skin, as every skin reacts slightly differently to scent ingredients.

Have a whiff of a lot of fragrances. Right away, there will be some you dislike. Follow your impulses. If you like a perfume, ask for a smelling strip and write the name on it. Carry it and any other appealing scents around for a few hours or a day. Give your nose a rest and sniff again later. By the way, don't hold the strip right up to your nose. Instead, wave it in the air slightly so that you can easily "catch" the scent.

What you're looking for is a strong positive response, a visceral reaction to the fragrance—something as simple as "I like it!" If it's a scent you feel drawn to, if it's a scent that enchants you, that's the one to buy.

Once having chosen the scent, you must decide among its forms. You will find that the most expensive is *parfum* or *extrait*, usually 15–20% perfume and 80–85% alcohol. Next is *parfum de toilette*, 12–15% perfume, with the rest alcohol and water. *Eau de toilette* is 5–12% perfume, with more water than alcohol, and *eau de cologne* is 2–6% perfume, mostly water and a bit of alcohol. The *parfum* lasts longest and is most expensive, while the *eau de cologne* is very light, lasts only an hour or two, and is the least expensive. The *parfum*, of course, is the most precious, and often its bottle will be a work of art.

The essential rule in the use of any type of scent is moderation. Subtlety is best. Learn to hint, to suggest, to create an aura of imperceptible magic. This is the realm of emanation, and the art of emanation is fundamental to beauty.

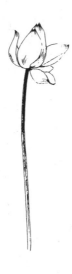

the beauty that is unfinished

The Japanese liking for the unfinished, whether in a sentence, a woodblock print, a tea bowl, or the face of a woman, results in a type of vague beauty that suggests rather than displays itself to the viewer. Such beauty leaves room for the imagination, invites the eye to engage with it, explore it, invent what is missing. Imperfection; a detail roughed over; a small uncertainty; an understated element; simplicity.

In an ink painting, we see the single branch of a cherry tree in the act of disappearing, with a few delicately evoked blossoms hesitating on the limb; surrounding this we see a generously rich, serenely satisfying expanse of pristine, pure, empty space. In woman's beauty, too, we see the face sketched in lightly, quietly, with no attempt made to illuminate it fully. The sensation that something remains innate, unrealized, lost—this reticence draws the observer close, searching. An intimation of potential, secrets hidden, facts unknown, is more disturbing, more moving than the face that holds back nothing, complete, richly colored, fully blossomed into elaborate perfection, self-contained and self-sufficient, without the depth of mystery.

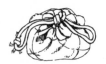

the

black,

the

white,

&

the

red

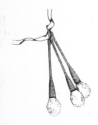

M ake-up. It's a universal feminine practice, this applying of color to the face as a means to perfect it, or to provide illumination to some nascent quality or feature that might otherwise remain unseen. The Japanese have evolved a way of feminine "face design" that—like their other forms of design—comes pretty close to ideal. Stylized yet understated, the make-up that depicts the design can be carried out on any face with splendid results.

brushes, powder, & the red of flower petals

Making up the face is an ancient feminine ritual. The Japanese approach to face design, while entirely modern, is strongly influenced by the traditional aesthetic in feminine beauty. What's interesting about it is that this Japanese way of make-up operates upon a foundation of timeless and universal elegance that can be enhancing to the woman of any culture.

Like any design approach that is based on classic principles, the Japanese face make-up always looks right. We'll start our exploration in make-up by discovering ways to borrow from that approach and adapt it to our own needs. We'll be using the ultimate in beauty tools: the Japanese brush.

The classic Japanese writing tool is the brush. Used for ink painting and calligraphy, the brush offers stunning grace of line and sensitive precision of application, producing the full range of possible shadings, textures, and densities, with subtle variations in rhythm, width, and softness, crispness, or boldness of line. The brush, so responsive to the hand wielding the utensil, requires a certain finesse from the artist.

Brushes, like other practical Japanese tools, exist in a breathtaking variety of forms, sizes, shapes, and weights. They are all beautiful. Each astutely fills its precise function.

The brushes used in beauty are very like those used in painting and writing. The modern Japanese cosmetics brushes basically conform to the traditional standards of shape, size, and texture, standards evolved over the centuries.

Like the beauty of ancient Japan, the modern woman delights in these efficient and elegant brushes, brushes to be used in applying a generous dusting of white powder, a gentle fog of rouge around the eyes, a fine black mist for the eyebrows, to paint perfect scarlet lips and, finally, to polish and smooth the whole sublime composition.

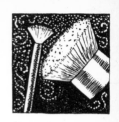

Because of the precision and range possible with the brush, many professional make-up artists prefer to work with this tool. Brushes may be used wet or dry; brushes may be used to apply powders, liquids, or creams. Brushes can draw and define, give a faint suggestion of color, build color up to a smooth, soft-edged density, refine and unify a surface. Using brushes—supplemented by fingers and sponges and an occasional fine-tipped cotton swab—one can create a make-up that is a delicate work of art.

Nine basic brushes are required for the accomplishment of all the steps in the make-up ritual. Among contemporary brushes, those by Shu Uemura are among the best.

The traditional brushes are still manufactured and sold in Japan, available in great array at the small shop called Hyaku-suke, in Asakusa. (See the appendix for further information.) Art stores carry a wide selection of brushes, of course, among which are some that are virtually identical to traditional make-up brushes and may be used for that purpose.

A complete collection of brushes will include the following:

A POWDER BRUSH: This brush has a thick, medium-length handle and a round "collar"; the bristles are long, thick, and soft, ideal for puffing on powder. This is the fattest of the brushes. It is known in Japanese as the *botanbake*.

A ROUGE BRUSH: This brush is similar to the powder brush but is smaller and has a flattened collar, giving the bristles a semiround shape. Bristles are medium-soft and rounded, with the slight stiffness offering greater precision of application but still a softness of edge. The traditional equivalent is the *hōbeni no hake*.

A FINISHING BRUSH: A flat, wide, short-handled brush that resembles a crumb-broom. It has soft but short bristles that are used to remove rather than apply powder. This brush is used to dust off excess powder and unify the surface of the face. The *itabake* in Japanese.

AN EYE-COLOR BRUSH: This long-handled, flat, short-bristled brush resembles an oil-painting brush. The bristles are medium-stiff for precise application of soft-edged color. This brush is used to apply a suggestion of color to the eyelids, sometimes to eyebrows as well. A sponge-tipped applicator with a flat round end may be substituted. Traditional brushes were not made for this modern purpose, but either the *sumihatsushi* or the *mayu-hatsushi*, originally for the hairline or eyebrows, will do nicely.

AN EYELINER BRUSH: This is a very fine-tipped brush with short, pointed, flexible bristles of medium stiffness and, usually, a handle of medium length. This brush is used to apply color close to the lashes; a fine-pointed sponge-tipped applicator may be substituted. Among traditional brushes, a *benifude* may be adapted for this purpose.

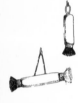

AN EYEBROW-COLOR BRUSH: This is a long- or medium-handled brush with very stiff short bristles, tightly packed and blunt-ended, that emerge from a small round collar. This brush is designed to deposit a dense mist of color to the eyebrows; a semiround version of the eye-color brush or a sponge-tipped applicator with a tapered round tip may be substituted.
Sumihatsushi or mayuhatsushi.

AN EYEBROW/EYELASH COMB AND BRUSH—This tool is usually designed to contain both brush and comb. The comb is the size of the lashes, and is meant to separate and align lashes or brow hairs. The brush is similar in size, and may be used to groom the brows or to apply color to brows and lashes. The traditional counterpart is the *hakurofude*, made from three bound pheasant feathers.

A LIP BRUSH—A short-handled, flat-collared, narrow, medium-stiff-bristled, flat-ended brush, used to apply lip color with precision. *Benifude*.

A CONCEALER BRUSH—Similar to the lip brush but smaller, this is used to apply cream or liquid concealer to imperfections and shadows. The *benifude* may be used.

a rice-cake complexion

The first important step in the ritual of applying make-up is the preparation of the face with foundation and powder. The face is readied for color in much the same way that a painter prepares a canvas.

The purpose of foundation is not only to supply a surface onto which colors will slide smoothly and adhere well, but also to render the face uniform in color and texture. Once the face is thus unified, with all slight imperfections erased and the natural unevenness in pigmentation rectified, then and only then is the face ready for color and line. The oval of the face is illuminated by this first step. And of course, properly applied foundation and powder create the delightful illusion of flawless skin.

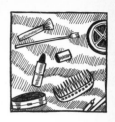

In the Japanese tradition: *a beauty has skin so translucent, so delicate, so white, that when she drinks tea one should see it flowing down her throat.... A beautiful complexion conceals seven defects.... A beauty has the complexion of a lily.... A beauty has rice-cake skin.* The sayings may be old, but the aesthetic stills holds true. The fact that Japanese women have kept their skin from the sun for centuries certainly plays a part in the visibly fine, seemingly ageless complexions one often sees in Japan.

The woman of times past employed every possible means at her disposal to further perfect her complexion. To achieve skin that was luminous, smooth, soft, fine, and very white, she masked her face with heavy powder.

Before the adoption in 692 A.D. of Chinese-style face powder, which, ironically, contained poisonous, skin-darkening lead, Japanese women used a mixture of rice flour and earth to whiten their faces. Other substances later used in varying proportions— and often mixed with the lead-based powder—were powders of mercury and alum, titanium powder, the powder of *kuzu* root, wheat flour, rice flour, and chestnut flour.

Used almost continuously from the 7th century to the beginning of the 20th, white powder (*oshiroi*) was produced in several forms: as a hardened, pressed brick; as a softer, creamy block; as a paste, suspended in solution with water; and as loose powder. After the skin was prepared with an oil or pomade, the powder, first softened or dissolved in water, would be applied to the neck, the back, the chest, and finally to the face. The powder was applied so thickly that the natural complexion was entirely concealed under a mask of luminous snowy white.

Because lead powder adhered well to the face and gave a superior finish, even after the Japanese government warned of its dangers in the late 1800s women continued to use it faithfully. The substance was finally prohibited in 1934. Japanese manufacturers had begun to market lead-free powders at the turn of the century; at about the same time European flesh-tinted face powder began to arrive in Japan. Gradually the fashion of white-face met its demise.

Still, in modern Japan pale is preferred, and this is a preference that benefits the skin, which is hidden from the sun behind sunscreens, hats, and parasols. Some of the world's most exciting breakthrough-products in skin lightening and sun protection have been developed in Japan, in response to the demands of the sun-wary female population.

So in modern times, what can be done to create the lily-like complexion of myth? We are lucky to be living at a time when powders and foundations not only make us beautiful in the most subtle fashion but actually act as treatments for the skin at the same time! Almost every company now offers superior products in both powder and foundation categories, and these are often designed to suit particular skin types; some guard against the sun or moisturize, others keep an oily complexion matte for hours.

Once you've invested in the appropriate products, here's what you do to achieve a diaphanous complexion:

—First prepare the skin by applying an emollient or moisturizing lotion, unless the foundation contains moisturizer.

—Use a neutral foundation that is either exactly your skin tone or ever so slightly paler. Dark or golden skins should not go paler, at the risk of looking chalky or ashy—instead aim for a warmer look. Apply the foundation with sponge or fingertips by massaging it into the skin. A white base, primer, or complexion-perfecter may be mixed with the foundation or applied alone or as a concealer, to give a luminous radiance to the face.

—With a fine brush apply a concealer to the sides of the nose, the eye area, and any areas of shadow or imperfections. Blend well with sponge or fingertips.

—Apply a generous, extravagant dusting of loose, pale or translucent powder to face and neck. The tool for this step is a big, fluffy, puffy brush.

—Next, using a flat wide finishing brush, dust the face briskly to remove excess powder and to refine the surface.

—Touch up through the day with pressed powder.

red lips

In the Japanese tradition as in others, the woman has limited the use of color in make-up to black, white, and red. These three colors accentuate and stylize the natural drama of the woman's face, especially so when she has Asian coloring—pale skin, dark eyes, and dark hair. Practically all that's needed is that vital touch of red! But even in many European cultures, the potent trinity of black, white, and red has been the basis of women's make-up throughout history.

Whereas in the doll-like mask of the geisha we find the black-white-red concept carried to its ultimate, exalted expression, in the modern woman's make-up these colors are used so subtly that they are almost not there at all. In the Japanese aesthetic, the made-up feminine face is meant to be restful, not exciting, to the viewer, and this approach differs strongly from the Western goal of heightened vivacity. The Japanese end result is subtle, but the work that goes into the masterpiece is studied and intricate.

If a woman were to paint only one feature of her face, the choice would most certainly be the lips. So, proceeding from the pale, matte, powdered face, let's look at the mouth. Japanese tradition dictates that it should be a small, elegant, sensual red flower in an expanse of lily-white.

Old-style Japanese lip color is reminiscent of the red of autumn maple leaves, the rich warm red of a lacquer bowl, the flame red of the rising sun over a snowy dawn landscape. The color of the safflower has historically been the source of this magical, feminine red.

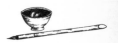

Coating the inner surface of a clamshell or a porcelain *sake* cup, safflower red lip-paint, *kyōbeni*, is silvery green, iridescent. Applied in successive layers, the color turns mysteriously from red to otherworldly elfin green. Between the 7th century, when safflower *kyōbeni* first reached Japan from China and Korea, and the turn of the 20th century, when the use of the lip-paint began to wane in favor of Western-style lipstick, there was one period—in the early 19th century—when the strange glowing green was fashionable. And because *kyōbeni* was so expensive, those women who could not afford to apply it in thick layers would simply paint an undercoat of black *sumi* ink to darken the red to greenish black. But the mid-19th century, Japanese lips were once again a more seemly red. Safflower lip-paint is still available for sale in Japan but is now worn only by geisha and some traditional performers.

To apply the color, which goes on after foundation and powder, a fine-pointed lip brush is first moistened in water, then brushed over the dry lip-paint to pick up color, which is then applied to the lips. A look at the history of Japanese make-up reveals a variety of lip color designs, with lip-paint applied to lower lips only, to only the center areas of both lips, or in a natural lip shape but smaller than life. The preference for small lips persists, but the highly stylized bud of earlier times may now be seen only on geisha or the actors of the kabuki.

The traditional Japanese aesthetic, in feminine face design as in much else, being based on a keen understanding of principles of line, color, and composition, may be applied to the modern woman's face, whether of East or West, with stunning results. Adjustments are necessary only in the degree of stylization: away from the artificial and toward the natural. A face that presents vivid lips in a matte, neutral, monochrome setting possesses a purity of design that is universal and timeless.

To try the Japanese approach to lips:
—The color chosen is less important than its texture—it should be rich, whether matte or brilliant, and not a gloss or a stain. As this color will supply the only discernible color on the face, it must be in harmony with hair and skin, and must not overpower

the face. Choose a color that has both subtlety and vitality.

—Once you've got your own special color, apply it with a lip brush. This has always been the tool of choice for those purists who are serious about make-up. The natural lipline may be very delicately perfected with this tool—if any lip redesigning is done, it should aim to lift just minutely the center bow of the lips or to accentuate the curve, and to give the tiniest touch of extra color to the midpoint of the lower lipline, creating a mouth that is plump, rounded, and full, but with corners refined and tapering. A small elegant pout.

the mysterious glance

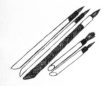

So far we've created a face that is pearly-pale but for the surprise of poppy-red lips. It looks interesting in a kind of underdone, blank-eyed way, but if you want a classic face, you're not there yet. Of course, you say, the eyes need something!

Yes, the eyes need something. In traditional Japan, that something was rouge, a relative of the safflower-red used on the lips. And while pure red for the eye area is still seen pretty often on Japanese faces, it's just as likely to be a blush of yellow or mauve or pink these days. Color choice aside, there is still a traditionally informed approach to the application of eye color.

In the old way, the very faintest of reds, in the same tone as the red of the lips, is swept delicately over the lids and the outer corners of the eyes, creating a soft warm glow.

Though in earlier times red was sometimes also brushed or painted along the sides of the bridge of the nose or painted quite vividly at the eyelid edges, the color was never used to create a healthy-cheeked outdoorsy bloom or a rosy girlish blush as it has been in the West. Cheeks, when given any color at all, even in modern Japan, have never veered toward the noticeably red. In Japan, the apple-cheeked girl has connotations of the inelegant broad-faced farmgirls of the oh-so-unrefined *inaka*, or country regions.

From the point of view of design, the choice—to gently color the eye area with a red that echoes the red of the lips, and to neutralize the cheeks—is brilliant. Bright cheeks in a face vie for attention, competing with eyes, eyebrows, lips, complexion. Without blank space, the beauty of the face gets lost, buried in detail. The composition is crowded, inelegant; there is no balance. The decision to accentuate the natural interplay between the most important facial features—the eyes and the mouth—while reducing the rest, results in a countenance that is both striking and simple.

Emphasizing the already important eye area with a mist of warm color rather than shadows or lines—when these are present they are of an infinite delicacy—makes two things happen: softness and life appear in a face that might otherwise seem too strict, too stark; and by echoing the red of the lips in the eye area, relationship is brought to the two features.

The original Japanese rouge, way back in the beginning, was red earth or natural cinnabar—a poisonous substance also known as red mercuric sulphide—with subsequent compositions based most commonly on safflower red mixed with white powder.

At various times in history, rouge was used in liquid, powder, paste, or solid dried forms and applied with the fingertips or special rouge brushes, sometimes made from a rabbit's foot with the claws removed. Most often, rouge was applied with the aid of water in a series of sheer, translucent layers. After first neutralizing any natural red color in the face by the application of white powder, rouge was applied to the outer eye area and the uppermost edges of the cheeks, to be followed by another layer of powder, over which yet another layer of rouge would be applied. The aim was then as it is today: the faintest shading of color, like the pale hue of pink at the center of a white flower.

To experiment with eyelid rouge:

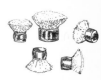

—Choose a color that is translucent and soft. It is essential that this color be identical in hue to the lip shade, in a fainter, "diluted" version. Choose a color that leaves only a hint of its presence when applied in a single layer.

—The best tool is a soft, puffy brush, similar to a face-powder brush but smaller. The brush should allow the powder rouge to float onto the skin without demarcations or concentrations of color.

—Experiment with application techniques. Color may be applied to the entire eyelid and up to the eyebrow, ever so faintly; or infinitesimally, only to the outer eyelid; or just to the upper and outer edges of the cheeks; or to the outer eye area, as a whispered suggestion of a glow extending from the outer eye corner toward the hairline, either as is or with a slightly more intense shade of color at the top of the outer eyelid, applied with a stiffer, smaller eyebrow brush.

—Don't make the mistake of thinking the color must be noticeable to be effective. The opposite is true. Aim for secret red. And stay away from the cheeks.

the eloquent eyebrow

We are now in mid-make-up, having mastered the white and the red but still lacking the black. On, then, to the eyebrows.

A French friend—a connoisseur of feminine beauty—once told me that there is no detail in a woman's face as important as the eyebrow. It was his view that too many women understimate

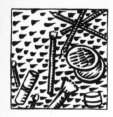

its power—they leave this feature pretty much to its own devices rather than enhance its role. Not so in Japan—Japanese interest has been obsessive for centuries, and the eyebrow still gets plenty of attention today.

The Japanese passion for perfection of design, when applied to the human face, resulted in an interesting phenomenon. During almost a millennium, the Japanese redesigned the basic proportions of the face by shaving forehead hairlines and eyebrows, redrawing new hairlines higher on the forehead, and inventing entirely new eyebrows. Eyebrows were not only given the precise curve, thickness, and shape considered desirable, but placed in entirely new locations.

Consider the face for a moment. An engineer or a designer, presented with the human face and asked to manipulate it, would quickly realize that only two elements were moveable: the eyebrows and the hair. From the point of view of volume, only the coiffure offers a range of possibilities. Considering the aspects of color, line, plane, and angle, the designer sees that only color and line offer the opportunity to create illusions of relief, plane, and angle.

Working within the natural limitations but pushing them as far as possible stylistically—not unlike the work of a Japanese master gardener—the face designer chooses to limit color to the original trinity of red, white, and black. These colors are intensified and purified, carried to their ultimate states, perfected. Thus is the skin rendered whiter, the lips more red, the hair and the eyebrows a deeper black. The balance and harmony of the composition is altered in striking ways with the help of the moveable eyebrow's linear energy, and by the use of the hair as a sculptural frame.

The traditional high-on-the-forehead eyebrow placement was generally considered to have a softening effect on the face, giving what was described as a mild, feminine, aristocratic expression. And while the eyebrows are no longer moved around the face like the features in the traditional *fuku warai* (funny face) game, they continue to play a very important role in the overall harmony of the face. The eyebrow is subtly shaped—from above, most often—by tweezing and trimming, darkened and defined with black or brown, and brushed to linear perfection.

While Western eyebrows are usually brushed upward and outward, winglike, the Japanese eyebrow-brushing tends to be straight across or even downward, suggested by the natural pattern of brow growth. Because the area underneath the brows is not rendered hairless, the effect is a "misty" one. Too-long hairs are trimmed, so the overall effect is neat and refined.

In a face that is pale and matte, the graphic verve of the brow supplies important punctuation. The look is elegant and even natural, in a pristine and classical way. Because color is used so unobtrusively, the dark eyebrows give a necessary spark, a quiet bit of spirit and a very personal, expressive look to the face. With the eyes understated and the lips bright, the total effect is serenely, simply beautiful.

To try the Japanese approach to eyebrows:

—While the old-fashioned beauty might have employed charred cork, carbonized egg yolk, *sumi* ink, lamp soot, lamp soot with gold leaf and sesame oil, a charred stick of paulownia wood, or even a burnt matchstick, the modern woman may prefer to use a commercial product, whether powder, pencil, or eyebrow mascara. The most subtle effect is achieved with a powder in a neutral shade, slightly darker than the natural eyebrow. Eyeshadow powders may be applied with a pointed sponge-tipped applicator or a small, slightly stiff brush. To achieve a natural effect with pencils or liquid colors, greater expertise is required.

—Eyebrows are groomed by tweezing only the obvious strays, and by trimming the ends of any long hairs. Before applying color, comb or brush the eyebrow in the direction of natural growth, not upward unless that is their original tendency.

—It is traditionally correct to draw the left eyebrow before attending to the right one. Brush color onto the brows with subtlety, leaving no obvious lines or demarcations. The brows may be brushed or combed a final time.

—At night, apply camellia oil to the eyebrows to keep them glossy and thick.

a note on color & the seasons

Beauty from nature. Even as we borrow the botanical elixirs, the aromatic flower oils, the mineral-rich muds of the earth in our pursuit of beauty, we can also be inspired by the changing colors and tints of the natural world in our use of color for make-up and clothes. In the season of autumn, when trees become a rich brocade of red, gold, and scarlet, it is fitting that these are the tones we want to drape ourselves in, the same warm colors we want for lips, even for hair. Winter brings the blue-reds and the smoky grays, the violets and the icy pinks. And true red in winter is a surprise and a challenge to the chill in the air! In spring and summer our seasonal sense of color brings us to translucent, airy tones, a move from young springy pastels and pale hues into blues and greens for summer coolness, brights that echo the berries and fruits of August. Make-up may be thought of as a personal, painterly way to harmonize with the changing look of the landscape.

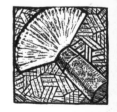

the ceremonial object

One of my most treasured possessions is an antique Japanese face powder compact presented to me by a friend. The large round compact is satisfyingly heavy in the hand, and a delight to the eye, with its black-lacquered lid inlaid with silver and green in a stylized bamboo-leaf design. It is an early Shiseido creation, and it is still possible to buy pressed powder that fits inside.

Certainly, one of the pleasures of the beauty ritual is the handling of the beautiful objects that accompany it. Or was, for the world—Japan included—seems to have transferred its allegiance from the enduring treasure to that which can be used briefly and discarded.

As might be expected of a culture so long enamored of tools, utensils, and implements, and the boxes, chests, purses, bags, and wrappings used to contain them, the traditional Japanese toiletries kit existed in a wondrous array of forms, each designed to perfectly suit the contents and their methods of use.

The smallest portable compact often contained face powder, rouge, lip-paint, a tiny lip brush, and an eyebrow pencil, each item fitted into the container as in an intricate puzzle box. Medicines and one's personal seal were carried tucked in an *inrō,* the portable masculine kimono accessory. A woman on an outing might carry a *shingenbukuro,* the small drawstring bag still in use today, containing needle and thread, a handkerchief or sheaf of rice paper, a small mirror, face powder, rouge, lip-paint, eyebrow pencil, and a brush or two for applying make-up.

In the days when well-bred women formulated their own fragrances and participated in incense games and ceremonies, there were handbags designed to hold complete fragrance-making kits in their own special compartments. A portable toiletries kit for travelling was sure to contain all the basic necessities: a small sewing kit, a make-up kit with powder, rouge, lip-paint, and brushes, and a hairdressing and grooming kit holding combs, scissors, tweezers, razor, pomade or oil, a file, a mirror, and a container for incense. A stationary kit containing rice paper, inkstone, brush, and water dropper might also be included.

In her home, a woman would keep an extensive collection of chests and containers designed to hold the objects used in the beauty ritual and in other exclusively feminine activities. She would own two large round mirrors—or a single, artfully jointed one—and their folding mirror-stand. From the rungs of a brush stand would dangle a full array of make-up brushes. A woman would possess as well a silk square for wrapping, a *tenugui* towel hanger, a small tub, basin, and pitcher for water, and arranged within a special toiletries chest of drawers, a tiered porcelain powder box, a small basin for mixing face powder with water, a rouge container, a small basin for mixing rouge with water, a lip-paint container, an oil or pomade container, eyebrow black, *ohaguro* (tooth-blackener), several lidded containers, lip brushes and eyebrow-color brushes, a tray for cosmetics items, a razor in its own box, tweezers, scissors, a comb-shaped basin for hairdressing liquid, combs of various types, and an incense container and burner. A woman would own further small chests, each of distinct specialized design, each made to hold her personal items of a particular category: writing, sweets, sewing. These containers were finely crafted possessions in themselves, objects of great beauty and value, often made of elegantly lacquered wood, inlaid with mother-of-pearl, gold, or silver, and tied with sumptuous tasselled cords of silk. It is not difficult to imagine with what a reverential, quiet sense of ceremony—and pleasure!—such articles were used.

beauty

games

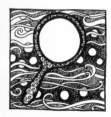

I n the presentation of yourself to the world, a certain degree of realism and self-knowledge is required. The old adage about being true to oneself is apt; although undeniably any outward self is by definition partial. But what must take place for one's external image to correspond as closely as possible to the true self is that a kind of self-definition must transpire. To clarify: to cultivate and project what is a true reflection of oneself, to present oneself at one's best, is an achievement of power, an assumption of self. It requires independent thinking; it requires courage; it requires a certain amount of presence and the ability to project; it requires a little bit of theatre. In this aspect of beauty, it is perhaps not the Japanese but the French who are the true teachers. When we've mastered the basics of inner beauty and inside/outside beauty, which we learn from the East as holistic techniques for spiritual, emotional, and physical health, which are shown outwardly as beauty of being as well as beauty of physical form, then we can turn to the West for lessons in the arts of style, adornment, individual beauty, chic, and élan. (Perhaps that's another book!) In the meantime, on the following pages you are provided with a few games, exercises to inspire you in your exploration.

a short course in discovering your true beauty

How can a woman discover her own unique beauty? I have known so many women who think of themselves as unbeautiful, when all they lack are the tools with which to see what they possess and learn to illuminate it. The process may be likened to the transformation of a diamond, as it is taken from its raw state embedded in ordinary granite to its eventual incarnation as a polished, facetted, scintillating gem. The beauty may be natural, but to be seen and brought into its own a little attention is necessary. Are you a diamond in the rough? I offer the following beauty-making exercises to you, and invite you to discover yourself. I assure you that you will enjoy the process.

It is my sincere belief that absolutely everyone has beauty.

There are basically two common barriers that can impede the realization of one's own unique beauty. The first is the need for accurate self-assessment: you need to be able to look in the mirror and see what is really there in an objective way. The second is knowing what to do with what you've got.

Most people have some difficulty with these two things, and quite a few people can't cope with them at all. The situation is thus: the woman looks in the mirror hoping to see a reflection of whatever fits her (culturally imposed) ideal of beauty. She then sees only her "shortcomings" and magnifies them in her mind into enormous flaws. She sets about trying to hide these things from view in order to come as close as possible to her imagined standard.

What often happens in the process is that the entire woman goes into hiding. Whatever is unique about her is eliminated. Further, there is an atmosphere about her that hints at her low self-esteem. If she does not think herself attractive, it is unlikely that anyone else will. For beyond the actual physical presentation, what is perceived as beauty should often more properly be termed confidence, aided by grace and self-awareness.

I am assuming, however, that the raw materials have not been outright abused. If one is either underweight or overweight as the result of unhealthy eating, if the body is out of condition due to lack of exercise, or if the hair, skin, and nails look terrible due to neglect, then to realize one's unique beauty is an impossible dream. First attend to those fundamental aspects of diet, exercise, and external grooming!

To become beautiful requires a simple training—or re-training, as the case may be. One thing to try immediately is to study yourself in the mirror with an objective eye. Remove your clothing and look at yourself. (Don't try this under a fluorescent light—those antibeauty light sources will discourage you immediately! Try low natural light, curtains drawn, or any indirect soft lighting.)

Have a pen and notebook at hand. Study yourself without applying judgment to what you see, but if a "pro" or a "con" comes to mind, jot it down. Jot down neutral observations as well. Finally, you should have a very detailed list of observations. Group your observations under these headings: Things I Dislike About My Appearance/Things I Like/Unique Things. (Write "pros" and "cons" under this last heading.)

On a separate piece of paper, describe in detail how you envision yourself looking after one of those magazine makeovers. It would be a daring and successful makeover that corresponds to your secret self-image. You can change hair color and cut (don't forget about wigs and hairpieces), make-up, and most importantly, your overall image.

Put that makeover description aside for the moment and take

a look at your first list—the disliked things. Now, you will first explore in writing whatever it is that you currently do to disguise each of those things, and then you will consider them as potential *attributes*! As perverse as it may seem, think of how you might accentuate those "flaws." (If the flaws exist due to some physical disability or impairment, the proper course will depend on the nature of the condition. A battered sense of self-esteem combined with social ostracism or other forms of discrimination increases the difficulties, so it's advisable to seek the help of a counselor specializing in such matters.)

Examples from real life: A woman I'll call Ann has spent her life walking hunched over in order to conceal her 40-inch bust. She indeed conceals it, but in the process she has lost all presence, grace, and harmony. When she can bring herself not only to stand up straight but to carry herself with pride, she instantly becomes stunning! The simple act of straightening up is almost all she needs to do! She reclaims her body as it really is, and discovers she is beautiful.

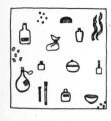

Another woman has a nose that she describes as witchlike and beaky. In order to hide it, she wears her hair down around her face. What happens? The total effect is actually distressingly witchlike, thereby reinforcing her insecurity. What should she do? Start by getting a different haircut, perhaps something short and swept off the face, with height at the back to balance the nose and present the profile proudly. A chignon would also work. Add to this a good make-up that accentuates lips or eyes with drama, and she achieves the kind of haute, exotic beauty that the button-nosed woman can't dream of.

The idea here is what the French call turning your flaws into assets, and this is so important a lesson to learn, but such a difficult one, that I'm placing it first in our beauty-making program. Perhaps you have realized by now that it is necessary that you transform your ideas about what exactly is beautiful. It may take some time, but eventually you may become fond of your flaws!

Let's assume there is a young woman who considers herself overweight by about 5 kilos/10 pounds. In this ubiquitous scenario, it is the woman's self-image—she sees herself as downright fat!—that really gets in her way, not the 5 kilos. She is undoubtedly using stick-thin role models as her ideal standard, and since she doesn't match up, she considers herself a hopeless case. The result? She carries herself badly and practices camouflage dressing, and she ends up looking both self-negating and shapeless.

What can she do? This is indeed a hard one. One useful tactic—useful in the case of any type of perceived flaw: big nose, short legs, small eyes, crooked teeth, whatever—is to locate a role model that resembles her. Are there women in the public eye who are considered beautiful in spite of or even because of their more rounded forms? What about Isabella Rossellini, Beatrice Dalle, Juliette Binoche?

Once a few role models are located, the woman in question can set about to alter her perceptions, her ideas about what is beautiful. She must begin to consider the possibility that her slight plumpness might be becoming. (She might even take a trip to Italy, where a couple of extra kilos are thought to lend a lovely soft voluptuousness to the form and so are much appreciated.) Only when she has truly accepted this premise, by whatever means, can she begin to use it to her advantage.

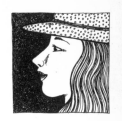

The same approach may be used in the case of age. Are there older beauties around to reinforce the idea that "older" and "beautiful" might not be mutually exclusive conditions? Certainly: Jacqueline Bisset. Catherine Deneuve. Jeanne Moreau. Sophia Loren. Lauren Hutton. I'm sure you can think of many more.

Once you have truly begun to identify your flaws and turn them into assets, you will not only appear outwardly to be more beautiful but you will actually begin to like yourself, which in turn will positively affect your appearance. This may sound like a truism, but it is so common for women to dislike their own appearances (even when they are seen by others as beautiful!) that one can almost assume this to be the norm. A photographer-friend, a man who has taken pictures of many famous beauties, told me he has yet to encounter someone who is completely secure about his or her appearance. Women in particular seem to lack both confidence and objectivity in regard to how they look.

Using this information as a guide, it is safe to assume that you probably look better than you think you do. It is also safe to assume that you do not project utter confidence in your carriage and your way of dressing and your entire demeanor! So do me a favor. Try this experiment for a week. Choose your worst flaws. Decide they are beautiful and stop disguising them. Be proud: walk tall; believe in yourself! Pin up photos in your house of beauties who resemble you.

Now, back to those lists. You have identified your flaws and made them assets; you have wherever possible presented them proudly, accentuated them where appropriate, or at the very least stopped hiding them. Hiding is the worst thing to do because it communicates on the important nonverbal level that you are ashamed of something.

Now what about those lovely "Things I Like"? This should be fun! These assets are what you can run with. Beautiful red hair? Take extra care of it, get a great cut, dress to accentuate the color. Amazing legs? Don't let anyone talk you into long skirts. Let your legs contribute grace to the landscape! Wear short skirts, heels, interesting hose. You get the idea.

Unique things? These elements are probably present on both of the other lists. As you probably realize by now, what you are identifying is what is special about you; get it into your head that to be oneself and unique is the way to be beautiful. The other route—conformity—leads nowhere, to nonentity-dom.

Perhaps as you go through the process outlined here, you will begin to see that a certain amount of courage is required in the pursuit of beauty. It's true. You've got to be willing to go against the herd a little bit, to stand out, to be you. If nobody else is wearing man-tailored clothes and that's what you look good in, you've got to be able to resist the urge to fit in. If you've got dark skin and the fashion is porcelain, you've got to hold on to your inner sense that you are beautiful in a different way from what is touted all around you.

(And by the way, another nice thing will be happening as you pursue this process of becoming yourself, blossoming in all your unique beauty. You will be developing *style*.)

Go back to the imaginary makeover I asked you to describe, and look at it again. It represents how you would like to look. Is it realistic? Is it based on you, your particular attributes? Or is it an idealized image that doesn't come close to what you are?

If the image portrays a woman that you could not possibly become without major surgery, the task is to refashion the picture in your mind. What are the nonphysical qualities in the image? Elegance? Romantic softness? Urban chic? Traditional reserve? Sportiness? Mystery? Purity? Think about retaining those qualities you admire without necessarily being limited by the physique, which is—admit it!—not you. The nonphysical qualities are the key to what will become your own unique style; hold onto them.

If your makeover image is merely a more-so interpretation of yourself, you are already on the right track. Now, in both cases, the next step is to take the plunge and actually realize this most beautiful version of yourself. Your tools? Haircut and color, make-up, fashion. There are also those more ephemeral tools of voice, gesture, movement, posture, facial expression, and gaze, but let's assume for the moment that you are already cultivated in those areas. (No? Well, simply put, it's a matter of standing beautifully tall, placing conscious awareness into gestures and movement, keeping a softly relaxed face with a light in the eyes, and speaking with a timbre and intonation that is comfortable and makes the best of your natural voice. Practice grace in everything!)

For the act of redesign that you are about to undertake, remember that underlying its success is realism. If you have, for

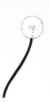

example, fine, thin hair, you must say, "I have fine, thin hair." You must stop saying, "I want my hair to be a big and wild mane!" You will fight a losing battle, neither respecting the nature of your hair nor allowing it to suggest its own particular tendencies in matters of style. You must not only accept your hair as it is, but you must begin to search for the way in which it can be its most naturally beautiful. In the case of the hair type in question, this is likely to mean a sleek, close-to-the-head look—the hair will not be very long, probably blunt-cut into a bob or other geometric shape.

What you will need, then, is a very good haircutter. Have your hair cut and colored according to its true nature. Choose a shape that accentuates and flatters your features and facial outline. Resist the urge to go against nature—by this I mean forcing your hair by chemical or other means to do what it is not inclined to do. Not only is this a high-maintenance and often damaging strategy, but you will almost always do better by following your hair's own dictates. But when it comes to choosing one style from several suitable ones, be daring. Try the one that comes closest to your personal vision of yourself, as revealed in your makeover description. Aim for the fantasy you.

With make-up, again, start with what you've got. Work with your natural skintones; a session with a make-up artist can be very helpful in educating oneself in the art of choosing colors. Once you are working with the correct tones and hues, begin to play. Choose a feature—your best? your worst?—to accentuate. Try smoky *khōl*-rimmed eyes; try scarlet '40s lips; try pale '60s lips; try a pale powdered face; try a sunny sporty dewy face; try arched eyebrows; try everything. You are looking for the one little touch that makes everything else come to life!

If you are doing a sincere redesign, by now you will have begun to evolve a unique look. You will have your own hair look, and your own face look; from these plus clothing you will fashion a totally new you that is gorgeous. With fashion, fantasy and imagination can really come into play. Although a distinct personal style will already be emerging with the revamped hair and the face, it is the clothes that will complete the look.

When you're evolving into a more fully beautiful you, it may be useful to begin to think of clothing as a form of communication, as a way of expressing and providing outward definition of how you see yourself. While make-up, hair, and attitude certainly form the foundation, the clothes you wear will either make or break what you have. Not only does fashion convey an instant impression of who you are, but clothing entrains the physical self and in turn affects the "atmosphere" of the image to an extraordinary degree. Try donning a kimono or a sari or a pair of cowboy boots and watch what happens to your movement and stance, then in turn to your way of speaking, your facial expressions, and finally to your sense of self. Clothing is theatrical; make use of its power.

Personal style is essential to individual beauty. How is a total presence created? The field of image counseling has become an important one in recent years; sometimes a trained and objective eye can identify a person's nascent style-tendencies and yearnings more clearly than she herself can. Sometimes it's a matter of knowing what questions to ask of oneself—for true personal style obviously is derived from one's unique history, personality, and aesthetic sense. With or without the help of an image consultant, the process is detective work.

Personal style is not about fitting into a mold. It is about, simply, knowing what we look like, how we want to look, and how to employ the colors, textures, and forms that please us in the service of that image.

Shall we do a little style searching? In my experience assisting women in this pursuit, I've found the following self-survey to prove illuminating. Answer rapidly, without giving too much thought to the responses.

1. List 20 items of clothing or accessories from childhood that you cherished.
2. Next to each item, list one-word reasons for its appeal.
3. Repeat 1, but for adulthood.
4. Repeat 2 (for items listed in 3).
5. If you had 10 minutes to pack for a trip to your favorite city, what items would you reach for first?
6. What women of past or present do you admire for their style?
7. If you could spend time in another period of history (past or future), which periods would be your first 3 choices? Describe the things you would wear and the reasons for their appeal.
8. What would you love to wear or look like, but do not have the courage to try?
9. Are you following other people's dictates in the area of your appearance? If so, those people and describe the images they expect you to conform to.
10. Read back over what you have written. When an interesting observation regarding any of your answers comes to you, jot it down.
11. Writing quickly, cover 4 sheets of paper with your thoughts on what you have written and any related

ideas or emotions. Try to uncover the thread that runs through all your responses.

12. Write 10 sentences beginning "I love" (fill in with article of clothing or related object). Write 10 sentences beginning "I want to look" (fill in with the first thing that comes to mind).

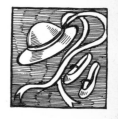

What you are trying to uncover in this exercise is the real you underneath the habits, the urge to conform, the limited self-image. You will find that your sense of style was already formed in childhood, and that you can return to those early cues for illumination. Not that you want to resemble a child now, but what was magical for you back then? Which items held a personal meaning for you, and why? Did you cherish a pair of green shoes? Full skirts? A certain white blouse? How can you rediscover that sense of magic in what you now wear?

Reading over all your answers, you will begin to see an image emerge, one that combines what you knew as a child, what you are within, and how you would like to be. Honor this revelation! Begin to plan your wardrobe with it in mind. At first, buy small items that seem to belong to what you see emerging as your own style. Be playful, for true style always has a playful spirit. This is a game, and its goal is to make you happy.

Did I forget something? Yes. Go through your closet with an iron hand. Remove everything you don't adore, and certainly everything you haven't worn in a long time. Get rid of it, or if you daren't do that, pack it all in boxes, with careful labels so you know what's there in case you want it. (You never will!) It's best to embark unencumbered on a voyage of self-discovery.

appendix

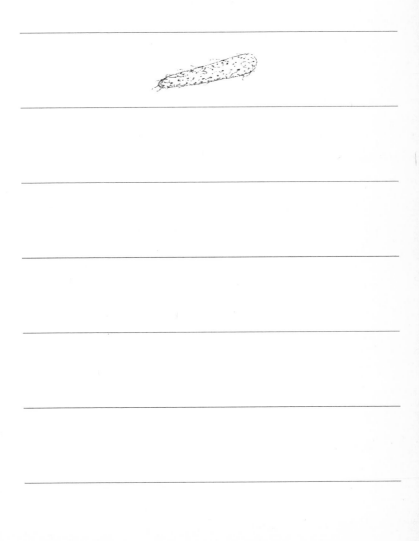

I

Glossary

This glossary offers the English equivalent of all Japanese words included in the text. Words and phrases from other languages are generally employed only once and are defined upon introduction in the text. For further information on ingredients, please refer to the ingredient guide that follows.

abura:	oil
arame:	sea plant, in Latin *Eisenia bicyclis, E. arborea*
azuki:	*azuki* bean
azuki no kona:	*azuki* bean powder
bainiku ekisu:	extract of *umeboshi*
ban-cha:	the lowest grade of green tea; mature tea leaves with twigs and stems
banira:	vanilla
bara:	rose
benibana:	safflower
benifude:	lip-color brush
biiru:	beer
biwa:	loquat
biwa no ha:	loquat leaf
botanbake:	large, full cosmetics brush used for powder
budō:	martial arts
budō:	grape
byakudan:	sandalwood
cha; -cha (suffix):	tea
chōsen ninjin:	ginseng; specifically, Korean ginseng
daikan:	the season of "the greater cold"
daikon:	giant radish
daizu:	soybean
dō, -dō (suffix):	path, or way
dō-in:	Japanese system of breathing and movement training
dokudami:	*Houttuynia cordata*, a wild medicinal plant
fuku warai:	funny face game; blindfolded players pin features on a blank face
funori:	sea plant; in Latin *Gloiopeltis furcata*
futon:	foldable bedding used traditionally in Japan
genmai:	brown rice
genmai-cha:	*ban-cha* tea mixed with puffed brown rice kernels
gobō:	burdock
goma:	sesame
goma abura:	sesame oil
gyokuro:	high-grade green tea
gyūnyū:	milk
hachimitsu:	honey
hakobe:	chickweed
hakurofude:	cosmetics brush
happa:	green leaf (or leaves)
hara:	stomach
hatomugi:	pearl barley, or Job's Tears
hatomugi-cha:	tea that contains pearl barley
hechima:	loofah
hechimasui:	loofah-vine water
hijiki:	sea plant, in Latin *Hizikia fusiformis*
hinoki:	Japanese cypress
hōbeni no hake:	brush for applying cheek rouge
hōji-cha:	roasted *ban-cha* tea
ichigo:	strawberry
ichō no mi:	ginkgo nut
ikebana:	Japanese tradition of flower arrangement
inaka:	back country
itabake:	cosmetics brush
jinenjo:	mountain yam
kabocha:	Hokkaido pumpkin
kaisō:	seaweed

kakekō:	fragrance bag (see *nioibukuro*)
kaki:	persimmon
kaki no ha-cha:	persimmon leaf tea
kaki no ha:	persimmon leaf
kampōyaku:	botanical medicine of the Asian tradition
kanten:	agar-agar
kanzō:	licorice root
karuishi:	pumice stone
keichitsu:	the season of "the end of insect hibernation"
kendō:	the way of the sword
kenkō:	burning of incense for Buddha and gods
ki:	vital energy
kikō:	the practice of harnessing and directing the flow of *ki*
kiku:	chrysanthemum
kiku-yu:	chrysanthemum bath
kinako:	roasted soybean flour
kinu:	silk
kō:	incense or fragrance
kombu:	kelp
kombu-cha:	kelp tea
komenuka:	rice bran
konnyaku:	devil's tongue root
koto:	Japanese traditional stringed instrument
kudamono:	fruit .
kuki-cha:	tea consisting of twigs and stems of the tea plant
kuko (kuko no mi):	Chinese wolfberry (the berry)
kumazasa:	bamboo grass
kurogoma:	roasted black sesame seed(s)
kuromame:	black soybean
kurorera:	chlorella
kurozatō:	black sugar; unrefined sugar
kurumi:	walnut
kuwa (kuwa no ha):	*Morus alba*, mulberry (the leaf)
kuzu:	*Pueraria Thunbergiana Benth.* (*Leguminosae*); so-called Japanese arrowroot
kyōbeni:	traditional safflower lip-paint
kyūdō:	the way of the bow; Japanese traditional archery
kyūri:	cucumber
matcha:	powdered *gyokuro* green tea
matsu:	pine

matsuba-yu:	pine bath
mayuhatsushi:	brush for painting eyebrows
mekabu:	root of *wakame* seaweed
mikan:	type of tangerine
miso:	fermented soybean paste
mitsuba:	trefoil
mizu:	water
mochi:	rice cake; glutinous rice that is steamed, pounded, and dried
mogusa:	material used in moxabustion, usually a small cone of dried and powdered mugwort
momo:	peach
momo no ha:	peach leaf
mugi:	barley
mugi-cha:	roasted barley tea
myōga:	a root used in *miso* soup
nasu:	eggplant
nattō:	fermented soybeans
negi:	onion
nikuzuku	nutmeg
ninjin:	carrot
ninniku:	garlic
nioibukuro:	fragrance bag (see *kakekō*)
nokogirisō:	yarrow
nori:	laver seaweed
nuka:	rice bran
nukabukuro:	cotton or silk drawstring bag used for washing face and body; may be filled with rice bran, *azuki* bean powder, pearl barley powder, or other substances
ōbako:	plantain
ocha:	green tea
ofuro:	Japanese bath
okara:	tofu lees
okayu:	rice porridge
omamori:	protective talisman; good luck amulet or charm
ōmugi:	barley
ōmugi no wakaba:	young shoot of barley
onsen:	hot spring
oroshigane:	grater

oshiroi:	white powder
oyu:	hot water
polei:	a form of oolong tea, also known as *puerh*
puerh:	a form of oolong tea, also known as *polei*
renkon:	lotus root
rokai (aroe):	aloe vera
ryokan:	Japanese traditional inn
sake:	rice wine or alcohol in general
sakura:	cherry tree
sekken:	soap
sen-cha:	medium-grade green tea
seri:	double dropwort
shakuhachi:	traditional Japanese flute
shiatsu:	pressure-point massage
shiitake:	Black Forest mushroom or *Cortinellis shiitake*
shinju:	pearl
shinju no kona:	pearl powder
shiso:	perilla or beefsteak plant
shōbu:	iris
shōchū:	distilled spirits; colorless, odorless; 20–45% alcohol
shōga:	ginger
shōji:	rice-paper latticed screens for doors and windows
shōjin-ryōri:	Zen temple cuisine
shōkō:	burning of incense for souls of deceased
shungiku:	edible chrysanthemum
shungiku-yu:	chrysanthemum bath
soba:	buckwheat
soradakimono:	incense for "empty burning" (no religious purpose)
su:	vinegar
sugina:	field horsetail
-sui (suffix):	water
suikazura:	Japanese honeysuckle
sumi:	black ink
sumi-e:	Japanese ink painting
sumihatsushi:	cosmetics brush
suribachi:	mortar
surikogi:	pestle
tai chi chuan:	Chinese system of breathing and movement
taikyoku-ken:	stick-breathing practice
take:	bamboo
takenoko:	bamboo shoot
tamago:	egg
tamagozake:	egg-*sake* drink
tampopo:	dandelion
tatami:	thick woven rice-straw matting used on floors of traditional rooms
tawashi:	turtle-shaped scrubbing brush
tengusa:	sea plant, in Latin *Gelidium amansii*
tenugui:	fine-textured cotton towel
tōki:	*Angelica sinensis*
tsubaki:	camellia
tsubaki abura:	camellia oil
tsubo:	pressure points
tsuyu:	plum rains; misty rains of early summer/late spring
uguisu no fun:	bush warbler droppings
uikyō:	fennel
ume:	a variety of apricot that falls green from the tree and is used in making *umeboshi* and other items; *Prunus mume Sieb. et Zucc (Rosaceae)*; so-called Japanese plum
umeboshi:	so-called pickled plum made from *ume*, salt, and perilla
wakame:	sea plant, in Latin *Undaria pinnatifida*
wasabi:	bitingly hot green root grated and used as a condiment for sushi
yakinasu no hamigakiko:	eggplant toothpaste
yakusō:	Japanese herbs used in folk medicine
yomogi:	mugwort
yu, -yu (suffix):	bath; hot water
yunohana:	flowers of sulfur
yuzu:	citron
zaru:	basket
zazen:	sitting meditation in Zen Buddhism

preparation guide

utensils & materials

When working with botanical ingredients, metal should be avoided. Instead, use glass, enamel, or ceramic bowls and pans. Utensils should likewise be nonmetal. The following utensils and materials will be useful in preparing the recipes in this book:

mortar (*suribachi*) and pestle (*surikogi*)
The Japanese version is a heavy ceramic bowl, textured on its interior, used with a large wooden pestle. This duo is very efficient for grinding, crushing, and puréeing ingredients. The technique requires only gentle pressure in a rotating and pressing motion. The mortar should be set on a damp cloth to prevent slipping. A blender or food processor may substitute.

bamboo draining baskets (*zaru*)
These are ideal for the draining, rinsing, and sorting of ingredients. They must be washed in plain water—no soap, no soaking—and stored in the open air.

graters (*oroshigane*)
The Japanese graters for ginger and *daikon* are wonderful tools. The ginger grater is extremely fine, made with tightly set bumps or spikes, while the *daikon* grater is similar but less fine, with bumps, spikes, or spiked holes. The traditional graters are ceramic. To grate, a circular motion is used. The graters must be washed with salted, vinegared water. A food processor may substitute.

glass or enamel cooking pans

glass, enamel, or ceramic bowls

mill
A coffee bean grinder or grain or spice mill is very useful for making such things as bean powder and pearl barley powder.

utensils
High-quality knives, wooden chopsticks, wooden spoons, and a whisk are useful tools. A small bamboo tea whisk for whipping powdered green tea may be enjoyed for its beauty as well as for its functionality.

cloth
Many recipes call for cloth, for wrapping ingredients to add to a bath, for scrubbing, or for filtering. Cheesecloth, muslin, gauze, or silk may be used, but whatever the material, it should be all-natural, undyed, and unbleached.

measuring utensils
A scale, measuring cup, measuring spoons.

wide-necked dark glass bottles and jars
Like all the utensils used in preparing beauty treatments or internal teas, these should be absolutely clean, sterilized if possible (simply achieved by immersing in alcohol, or in boiling water if the glass is heatproof).

pure spring water
The purest water available should be on hand for use in the recipes.

plant gathering

The first rule of plant gathering is proper identification. If you're unfamiliar with the plant, consult a botanical guide with photographs to avoid making a mistake. The second rule is to know the proper harvesting times:

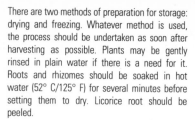

leaves

Pick them just before flowering time, on a warm dry day when the sun is well up but not yet hot, and after the dew has dried. Cut only 1/3 of a plant's foliage, using sharp scissors. Avoid crushing or bruising the leaves.

flowers

Pluck them gently just as they have fully opened, at midday in dry weather.

fruits and seeds

Gather fruits on a warm dry day when fully ripe. Seeds should look dry and hard but not yet be dispersing.

bark

Peel from young branches in damp weather; don't take too much at one time—never peel a complete ring around a branch. Best gathered in the summer when the sap has risen.

roots and rhizomes

Harvest in autumn when the above-ground plant is withering. Annuals should be harvested at the end of the year's growth cycle; perennials every 2 or 3 years. Unearth the whole root structure without damaging it, separate the portion desired, then replace the remaining root carefully in the ground (to replant perennial plants).

whole plant

Harvest just before the flowers bloom.

stems

Gather when the flowers bloom or when the fruits are first born.

preparation for storage

If plants will be used within a few days of harvesting, they will keep in the refrigerator tightly sealed in air-filled plastic bags. (They may be lightly rinsed before refrigeration if they seem dirty.)

There are two methods of preparation for storage: drying and freezing. Whatever method is used, the process should be undertaken as soon after harvesting as possible. Plants may be gently rinsed in plain water if there is a need for it. Roots and rhizomes should be soaked in hot water (52° C/125° F) for several minutes before setting them to dry. Licorice root should be peeled.

drying

There is divided opinion over whether plants should be dried in the sun or in the shade. The Japanese approach is generally to choose sun-drying, perhaps because the climate is so moist, and mold or mildew are likely to develop with shade-drying. Sun-drying is quick, but exposure to the sun may remove some of the plant's active properties. Fragrant or aromatic herbs and colorful flowers or fruits should dry in the shade.

In dry climates, a warm, arid, dark location that receives good ventilation is the optimum drying situation. For the first 24 hours, temperatures should be around 32° C/90° F, with slightly lower temperatures preferable thereafter. Drying may take anywhere from 3 days to 3 weeks, with 10 days being average.

Plants may be tied and suspended from an eave or a ceiling for drying. Whole plants should be tied together at the stems in small bunches, while whole fruits or sections of bark should be tied so that they hang separately from one another. If drying seeds in this manner, place a box beneath the plants to catch seeds as they fall.

Another method is to spread muslin over a wire rack or a wooden frame, upon which plants may be placed in a single layer. Large items such as fruits, roots, or bark pieces must be turned periodically.

storage

Plants are ready to be stored when leaves are dry, brittle, and fragile, but still green. It should be ascertained that no moisture remains in any portion of the plant.

Leaves should be removed from their stems, while flowers should be removed whole, not petal by petal. Don't crumble or cut the plant parts.

In Japan's wet climate herbs are stored in paper, as glass can seal in even tiny amounts of moisture that may cause mold or mildew. In drier climates, dark glass jars may be used. Whether of paper or glass, the container must be tightly sealed. Do not use metal or plastic.

Each container should be clearly labeled with the contents and the date of storage. Green plants generally stay good for 6 months to a year, while roots, seeds, and bark will last for 2 to 3 years.

Containers are best placed in a dark location away from moisture and high temperatures. A slightly cool temperature is preferable. The traditional Japanese method was to suspend paper-wrapped herbs from the ceiling.

freezing

This method of plant storage requires no drying process. Plants are merely rinsed and dried well, then immediately packed in small quantities in polyethylene bags, which are in turn placed loosely in freezer boxes to avoid damage to the contents.

processing methods

charring

The plant is washed and left moist, then wrapped tightly in aluminum foil, placed in a cast-iron pan over high heat, covered, and left to roast until it is charred.

powdering

The dried plant is chopped, then crushed with a mortar and pestle or ground in a mill.

salting

Leaves and sea salt are placed in alternating layers in a wide-necked jar, and oil is poured over the lot. The jar is sealed tightly and stored in the refrigerator. This keeps for several weeks.

juice extraction

Plants may be cut with scissors, then crushed in a small amount of water with a mortar and pestle; ground with a grater; pulverised in a blender; rubbed with sea salt to induce the emergence of juice. The substance obtained by these methods may be filtered through cloth to obtain juice.

cold extraction

A good method for fragile flowers, 15 ml/1 T of the plant is added to 300 ml/1 1/4 C of tepid water in a covered nonmetal container, which is set in the sun for a whole day, after which time the water is filtered and the solids discarded. Stored in the refrigerator, the water will last 3 days or so.

maceration

A glass jar is packed tightly with crushed fresh herbs, topped up with vegetable oil, vinegar, or alcohol, then sealed to steep for 2 weeks in a dark location. The jar is shaken daily. The herbs may be filtered out and the process repeated if desired. The solids are finally removed by filtering. The liquid will keep indefinitely.

tincture

A tincture may be prepared by adding herbs to *shōchū* or vodka in a 1:3 ratio, or less or more as desired. These ingredients are placed in a sterilized wide-necked bottle, which is then tightly sealed and stored in a cool, dark location. The minimum length of time for steeping is 2 weeks, during which time the jar is shaken daily. Some tinctures or spirits are steeped for much longer, up to a year, depending on the ingredient. When the jar is opened, the contents are filtered to remove solids, then the liquid is returned to the container. Keeps indefinitely.

infusion

The basic method of infusion consists of pouring boiling water over the herbs in a nonmetal bowl, covering to steep—anywhere from 10 minutes to overnight—then filtering to remove solids. Another method involves adding the herb to the water in a nonmetal pot, covering to bring just barely to a boil, then removing from heat to steep, covered, until cool. The ratio of fresh herbs to water is 15 ml/1 T – 50 ml/3 T of plant to 300 ml/ 1 1/4 C of water; of dried herbs, 5 ml/1 tsp – 15 ml/ 1 T to 300 ml/1 1/4 C of water. An infusion lasts for a few days in the refrigerator, or may have tincture of benzoin added as a preservative.

decoction

While an infusion is generally preferred for tender and fragile plants, a decoction is used for roots, wood, bark, and seeds. The plant substance is first crushed, chopped, scraped, or grated, then added to a nonmetal pan with water, to be brought to a boil and then simmered, covered, for anywhere from 3 to 40 minutes. The mixture is steeped, covered, for a few minutes or until cool, at which time it is filtered to remove solids. Some recipes call for the addition of enough water to bring the volume to half the original volume. Proportions are the same as for the infusion method.

II

appendix

For the reader living in the West who wishes to delve further into any of the areas presented in this book—Japanese health foods, the Japanese bath, *tsubo* and traditional Asian medicine, inner beauty—a list of suggested books is offered. For more active exploration, one may consult the local telephone directory for resources. In most cities in the Western world, it is possible now not only to buy a variety of Japanese foods and household items—including futon, *tatami*, and wooden hot tubs—but it is possible as well to study Zen meditation, *shiatsu*, calligraphy, flower arrangement, or *kendō*. Expert practitioners of *shiatsu* and acupuncture and doctors of traditional Chinese medicine are readily accessible for those who would try such treatments.

In the section on resources outside Japan, a list of mail-order companies is provided. It is possible to obtain nearly all of the ingredients listed in this book from these companies. By mail one can get natural foods, macrobiotic and other traditional Japanese health foods, highest-quality seaweeds, organic produce (including exotic Japanese vegetables), brushes, rice paper, seeds, live plants, dried herbs, Chinese herbs, Japanese kitchen utensils, grain mills, even Japanese music.

For those who wish to do their shopping in person, a list of retail sources is provided. This is in no way an exhaustive list! For more resources in your area, check the telephone directory under headings such as these:

Art Supplies	Imports
Bath	Japanese
Beauty	Macrobiotic
Botanical	Natural Foods
Chinese	Oils, Essential
Cosmetics	Oriental
Gourmet	Pharmacies, Chinese
Health Foods	Pharmacies, Natural
Herbs	

The ingredient guide section supplies suggestions for locating each ingredient. The first place to check is a well-stocked natural foods store—the macrobiotic way of eating is based on traditional Japanese foods, and the items in such stores are likely to be as pure and natural as will be found anywhere. Natural foods stores often carry good Japanese kitchen utensils and natural-fiber bath brushes, sponges, loofahs, even wooden combs.

Oriental or Japanese markets not only carry the staple food items and condiments but often stock fresh produce in season—things like *daikon*, green plums, lotus root, burdock, *shiitake*, and ginger. Korean greengrocers, now prevalent in many parts of the U.S., may also carry such produce. A supermarket in an Asian or cosmopolitan neighborhood will carry a selection of Asian foods. Gourmet food stores often stock Japanese foods and supplies.

The best herb stores carry Asian herbs along with the Western ones. (In many cases, the same herbs are used in both traditions.) For such ingredients as cherry tree bark, licorice root, safflower petals, pure oils, benzoin, camphor, and sandalwood, check an herb store. If a Chinese traditional medicine store is available, it will likely offer a huge bounty of roots, barks, leaves, and berries. (Any urban Chinatown will have a Chinese medicine store.)

Ordinary drugstores, bath shops, and beauty goods stores may be explored for bath brushes, sponges, combs, and pumice stones. Art stores for Japanese brushes and rice paper. Import stores for kitchen goods and incense. Finally, for a few items, search the natural world: forests, gardens, vacant lots. Carry a well-illustrated botanical reference for certainty of identification.

The section on resources in Japan is intended for the resident or visitor on a health-and-beauty quest. The best sources for ingredients and supplies are listed, along with some information on a few companies offering natural or traditional beauty products. Also listed are beauty and health-care resources: Tokyo hot-spring bathhouses, herbal skin care, *shiatsu* practitioners; a list of learning resources for those who would strengthen their spirits through the way of tea, archery, or calligraphy; Tokyo restaurants whose menus nourish both health and beauty. (Part of the appeal of the multicultural way of beauty is the adventure of seeking it out!)

ingredient guide

The following guide includes all the ingredients mentioned in the book. It is not a field guide for identifying plants in the wild, but rather serves to specify each substance's purported properties and to provide tips on where to find the items: in food stores (F), specialized food stores such as Asian or gourmet (S), herbalists (H), Chinese apothecaries (C), or natural foods stores (N), and where commonly found there, in gardens (G). (*Never attempt to harvest a plant growing wild without expert assistance in identification.*) For readers living in Japan or China, many Asian items will be widely available, so the where-to-find indications are included largely for the benefit of readers in the West. Very important ingredients for inside/outside beauty are indicated with a * next to the entry. Each entry is set up as follows:

English term: *Japanese term: Chinese term where applicable: Latin term:* part of plant used: (O) properties attributed to the substance used outside/externally; (I) properties attributed to the substance used inside/internally: F/S/H/C/ N/G recommended sources as explained above: F known contraindications

alfalfa: *arufarufa: Medicago sativa:* leaf: (O) exfoliates; heals; high in chlorophyll and iron, vitamins and minerals; beautifies hair; (I) nourishing; stimulates hair growth and health; increases lactation; contains estrogenic properties: H/N/G: ✦ external use may provoke allergic reaction in those susceptible

almond (sweet almond): *arumondo: Prunus amygdalus Batsch; Amygdalus communis L.* (*Rosaceae*): nut, oil from the nut: (O) nourishes; tones dry skins; calms irritations; heals; lightens complexion; cleanses; (I) antianemia; antispasmodic; laxative; remineralises; nourishes: widely available: ✦ toxic in internal overdose

aloe: *aroe/rokai: lu hui: Aloe vera; Aloe arborescens; Aloe barbadensis* (*Liliaceae*): leaf gel, dried leaf: (O) antiseptic; heals; soothes inflammation; heals burns; reduces scarring; moisturizes; cools; useful for sunburn; chapped skin; dermatitis; eczema; blemishes; oily skins; (I) purgative; laxative; detoxifies; tonic: C/N/G: ✦ dangerous in pregnancy; avoid during lactation; dangerous in overdose (powerful emetic)

angelica: *tōki* (=Angelica sinensis): *dang gui* (=Angelica sinensis), *bai zhi* (=Angelica anomala): *Angelica species* (*Umbelliferae*): root, dried seed, fresh leaf, and stem: (O) (A. archangelica, leaf) soothes skin irritations; (root) soothes joint pains; all varieties are warming; (I) (A. archangelica) anti-inflammatory; antispasmodic; diaphoretic; expectorant; diuretic; used to treat a broad variety of minor illnesses; tonic; uterine stimulant; (A. sinensis) blood tonic; circulatory stimulant; laxative: H/C/N: ✦ dangerous in pregnancy and for diabetics; increases photosensitivity when used externally

anise: *anisu: bajiao: Pimpinella anisum* (*Umbelliferae*): seed, oil: (O) cleanses; antibacterial; fragrant; beautifies hair; revives hair color, (I) calms; antiseptic; soothes coughs and colds; sedative: F/H/N: ✦ may be toxic in overdose

apricot: *anzu: xing ren: Prunus armeniaca L.* (*Rosaceae*): fruit, fruit kernel, oil from kernel: (O) (oil) softens; heals; anti-aging benefits; (I) (fruit) antianemic; astringent; laxative: widely available: ✦ the fruit can provoke allergic reactions; the kernel is highly toxic

***arame* see seaweed**

avocado: *Persea gratissima Gaertn.* (*Lauraceae*): fruit flesh, oil from nut: (O) (flesh) nourishes; rich in vitamins A, B, & E; beneficial to fragile skins; (oil) used as nourishing carrier oil in aromatherapy; (I) antibiotic properties; nourishing: widely available

***azuki* bean:** *azuki: hong tou: Phaseolus species:* seed: (O) tones, smoothes, exfoliates; cleanses;

lightens; stimulates local metabolism; contains saponins; (I) detoxifies; nourishes: F/S/N: ✦ raw bean is toxic in internal overdose

baking soda: *jūsō/itansan suiso natoryūmu. sodium bicarbonate:* powdered mineral: (O) removes residues from hair and skin; cleanses: draws out toxins; soothes; relieves tension; warms; beautifies skin: widely available

balm, lemon balm, melissa: *Melissa officinalis* (*Labiatae*): fresh leaf: (O) lemony fragrance; stimulates hair growth; heals skin blemishes; (I) lifts spirits; relieves colds, headaches: H

*bamboo: *take* (**bamboo shoot:** *takenoko*): *zhu ye. Phyllostachys nigra:* root, leaf, shoot, stem, *tabaschir.* (O) calms; astringent; (I) (root) astringent; antipyretic; styptic; (leaf) antipyretic; diuretic; astringent; (shoot) sedative; anti-emetic; (stem) sedative; antipyretic; (*tabaschir*) antipyretic; antispasmodic; strengthens skin, hair, nails; rich in silica; tonic; reinforces cartilage, tissues, bones; anti-aging tonic: S/C. See also **Mylitta lapidescens Horan**.

bamboo grass: *kumazasa. Sasa veitchii:* dried leaf: (O) calms; astringent; (I) astringent; styptic; antipyretic; diuretic; sedative: C

ban-cha see **tea**

*barley: (*o*)*mugi* (**barley sprout:** (*o*)*mugi no wakaba*): *mai ya. Hordeum vulgare* (*Graminae*): grain, germ, dried germinated sprout: (O) (grain) emollient; soothes; calms; cleanses; heals; (I) (germ) contains an adrenalin-like substance; nutrients; enzymes; amino acids; chlorophyll; abortifacient; (grain) antidiarrhea; soothes; sedative; nourishing; cleansing; diuretic; elimination of fats; laxative; stomachic; digestive: grain widely available; sprouts and sprout powder at N/C: ✦ germ and germinated sprout may be toxic in overdose, absolutely not to be taken during lactation and pregnancy

basil: *bajiriko: Ocimum basilicum* (*Labiatae*): leaf: (O) fragrant; relaxes; in magic, invites love (!); anti-acne; promotes hair growth; conditions hair; (I) relieves nausea; sedative; fights colds and flus; tonic; digestive: F/H/G

bean curd see **soybean**

bean sprouts see **soybean**

beer: *biiru:* (O) conditions hair; gives shine: widely available

bitter orange: *Citrus aurantium* L., *Citrus Bigaradia Riss* (*Rutaceae*): flower, **neroli**, *neroli-Bigarade* (essential oil from the flower), fruit: (O) (**neroli**) antidepressant; aromatic; sedative; softens skin; (I) (fruit) mobilizes *ki*; stimulates digestion; nervous system sedative: H/C/N: ✦ abstain during pregnancy

black pepper: *koshō: Piper nigrum* L. (*Piperaceae*): fruit: (I) warming; aromatic; stimulates digestion: widely available

black soybean: *kuromame: dou chi. Glycine max* (*Leguminosae*): seed: (I) (fermented beans) sedative; antipyretic; soothing to coughs and colds: S/C/N. See also **soybean**.

black sugar/ molasses: *kurozatō: Saccharum officinarum:* sugar-cane-stem extract: (O) nourishes; cleanses; heals; stimulates: soothes itching; heals blemishes; calms rashes; (I) nourishes; beautifies skin and hair; rich in calcium and iron; eases stress; antianemia; F/S/N

borage: *Borago officinalis* L. (*Boraginaceae*): flower, leaf, seed: (O) (leaf) soothes dry skin; heals infection; anti-eczema; good for sensitive or dry skins; (seed oil) anti-eczema; astringent; (I) (leaf) aphrodisiac; rich in minerals; stimulates adrenal gland; stimulates heart; beautifies skin; (flower) invites happiness or elevates mood; calms coughs: H/G: ✦ overdose of fresh leaves may be dangerous

borneol: *ryōnō: long nao xiang: Dryobalanops aromatica (Dypterocarpa):* aromatic resinous fissures of the Borneo camphor tree: (O) aromatic; antiphlogistic; (I) sedative; antispasmodic: H/C

brewer's yeast: natural fungus used in brewing beer: (O) stimulates local circulation; nourishes; not for sensitive skins; antibacterial properties; (I) nourishes: beautifies skin and hair; rich in vitamin B, minerals, and amino acids; strengthens; revives: N: ✦ used externally, may cause allergic reactions in those susceptible

broom, butcher's broom: *Cytisus scoparius* (L.) Link (*Papilionaceae*): top of flowering plant just prior to blooming: (O) brightens hair; soothes sore muscles; anticellulite; relieves congestion; (I) diuretic; laxative; detoxifies; vasoconstrictor; heart tonic: H: ✦ bears a resemblance to other wild plants that are highly toxic; overdose may be toxic

buckwheat: *soba: Fagopyrum esculentum* (*Polygonaceae*): seed, flour from seed: (O) soothes; nourishes; calms; detoxifies; beautifies hair: acid astringent; cleanses; strengthens tissues; purifies; (I) detoxifies; nourishes; blood-purifier; strengthening tonic; stimulates; beautifies skin; rich in amino acids, potassium, rutin, and sulphur; improves lactation: F/S/N: ✦ causes allergies in those susceptible

*burdock: *gobō: niu bang zi. Arctium lappa* (*Compositae*): root, leaf, seed: (O) varicose vein remedy; heals acne; soothes inflammations, rashes, and eczema; diaphoretic; antifungal; antibacterial; soothes sore muscles; (I) stimulates digestion; detoxifies; strengthens: beautifies skin; aids in slimming; diuretic; diaphoretic; high in iron; increases vitality; normalizes body functions; beneficial to kidneys: F/S/H/C/N/G

bush warbler droppings: *uguisu no fun:* from birds of the *Sylvidae* species: the dried, powdered droppings: (O) smoothes; lightens; exfoliates: available from birds: ✦ may cause irritation in sensitive skins

cabbage, Chinese cabbage: *kyabetsu, hakusai. pe tsai. Brassica oleracea L/B. campestris (Cruciferae)*: leaf: (O) diuretic; aids in slimming; heals; detoxifies; soothes; beautifies skin; high in vitamin C: widely available

calendula see **marigold**

camellia oil: *tsubaki abura. Camellia linne Japonicus (Theaceae)*: oil pressed from the fruit kernel/nut: (O) moisturizes; conditions hair and skin; nondrying; stable; softens; nourishes: H/N

camphor: *shōnō. Cinnamomum camphora T. Nees et Ebem. (Lauraceae)*: leaf extract, wood: (O) aromatic; warming; stimulates; soothes sore muscles; (I) cardiac stimulant: H

*carrot: *ninjin. Daucus sativus Hayek, Daucus carota L. (Umbelliferae)*: root, seed, green: (O) (root) antiseptic; rich in vitamin A; heals sores; prevents scarring; cleanses; (I) antidiarrhea and anticonstipation properties; diuretic; sedative; stimulant; increases lactation; beautifies skin; anti-aging benefits: widely available

cayenne pepper see **red chili**

cedar: *sugi. Cedrus, Thuja, and Juniperus species (Cupressaceae)*: bark, needle, oil made from wood: (O) stimulates hair growth; tonic; stimulates; aromatic; relaxes; astringent; (I) astringent; diuretic; sedative: H; ✦ dangerous abortifacient; not to be used during pregnancy; overdose is toxic

chamomile, camomile: *kamitsure. Hungarian/German. Matricaria recutita, Matricaria chamomilla; Roman: Chamaemelum nobile, Anthemis nobilis (Compositae)*: petal: (O) brightens fair hair; cleanses; draws out impurities; soothes; diaphoretic; reduces swelling; calms inflammations; (I) calms; sedative; eases stomachache: H/N ✦ some possibility of allergic reaction; avoid essential oil during pregnancy

champagne: the alcoholic drink made from grapes; a sparkling wine: (O) brightens fair hair; conditions hair: widely available

cherry: *sakura. Prunus nipponica (Rosaceae)*: bark, blossom, fruit, fruit stem, leaf: (O) (bark) beautifies hair and gives dark red tones; soothes and heals scalp and skin; (fruit) tonifies skin; good for oily skin; (leaf) stimulates circulation; cools; soothes inflammations, rashes, heat rash; refreshes; (I) (fruit) rich in vitamins A and B; detoxifies; diuretic; refreshes; laxative; (blossom) lifts spirits; (oil) antidepressant; (fruit stem) diuretic; cleanses: H ✦ pit is toxic

chickpea: *Cicer arietinum L.*: legume: (O) cleansing; toning; smoothes skin; (I) lowers cholesterol in blood; low in fat; high in protein, iron, potassium, B vitamins: widely available

chickweed: *hakobe. Stellaria media (Caryophyllaceae)*: leaf: (O) demulcent; benefits skin problems, blemishes: (I) diuretic; tonic; benefits skin; rich in vitamin C and phosphorus; nourishing: H/N/G

Chinese wolfberry: *kuko no mi. gou qi zi (berry); di gu pi (root skin): Lycium Chinense Mill. (Solanaceae)*: berry, skin of root: (I) (berry) liver & kidney tonic; nourishes semen; beautifies hair and skin; (fresh root) lowers blood pressure and blood sugar: C

chlorella: *kurorera. Chlorella*: microscopic green algae, powdered: (I) high in nutrients; antipollution; detoxifies: N

chrysanthemum: *kiku/shungiku. ju hua. Chrysanthemum species (Compositae)*: edible green and blossom: (O) stimulates circulation; antiseptic; heals wounds and soothes irritations; antibacterial; astringent; (I) sedative; astringent: S/G

cinnamon: *gui zhi* (twig): *rou gui* (bark): *Cinnamomum cassia Blume, C. zeylanicum Ness. (Lauraceae)*: interior bark of the young shoots, dried as is or powdered: (O) aromatic; antiseptic; tints hair; promotes happiness; (I) warming; diaphoretic; stimulates circulation; stimulates *ki*, kidney and liver tonic; carminative; antiseptic; benefits colds, flu, and digestive disorders; astringent: widely available; ✦ avoid use during fever and abstain during pregnancy as it is a uterine stimulant

citron, cedrat: *yuzu. Citrus medica (Rutaceae)*: fruit, rind:(O) purifies; lightens complexion; aromatic; astringent; stimulates circulation; beautifies skin; fights sun damage; anti-aging; (I) stomachic; regulates *ki*: S/C

citrus see individual listings: **bitter orange, citron, lemon, orange, tangerine**

clay/mud/earth. doro: (O) refines; stimulates; detoxifies; absorbs oil: H/N

clove: *chōji. ding xiang. Syzygium aromaticum, Eugenia caryophyllus, Carophyllus aromaticus (Myrtaceae)*: dried floral bud: (O) darkens and reddens hair; aromatic; local anesthetic; breath-freshener; astringent; antiseptic; relieves melancholy; calms; (I) stimulates circulation; warms; anti-emetic; facilitates labor in childbirth: F/S/H/C

coconut: *Cocos nucifera*: oil, fruit: (O) nourishes; moisturizes; cleanses; beautifies skin and hair;(I) nourishes: widely available

*comfrey: *Symphytum officinale (Boraginaceae)*: root, leaf: (O) heals; soothes sore muscles; revives aging skin, tissues; relieves dry skin, heat rash; cell regenerative; cell proliferant; emollient; astringent; (I) stimulates; tonic; relaxes; heals ulcers: H/N/G ✦ *Warning.* whether or not there is danger in ingesting comfrey in root or leaf form is controversial; the high levels of pyrrolizidine alkaloid substances in the plant can conceivably lead to serious medical problems if the root or leaf is consumed without a specialist's supervision

corn: *tōmorokoshi. Zea mays L. (Graminae)*: kernel, corn silk: (O) (kernel) remedies constipation; reduces risk of cardiac disease; diuretic; emollient; tonic; (silk) healing to urinary tract; diuretic; widely available

cucumber: *kyūri. Cucumis sativus (Cucurbitaceae)*: vegetable flesh, juice: (O) cleanses; lightens skin; cools; smoothes; good aftershave; heals; bleaches freckles; softens wrinkles; good for sunburn; corrects excess oiliness; astringent; (I) refreshes; diuretic: widely available: ✦ may cause allergic reactions in some; taken internally is difficult to digest

daikon: Raphanus sativus L. (Crucifereae): root, seed, leaf: (O) (leaf) removes toxins; clears skin; anti-acne; stimulates metabolism; warms; affects female reproductive system; stimulates circulation; cleanses; deodorizes; (root) anti-acne; draws out toxins; antibacterial; (I) (root) cleanses; beautifies skin; helps eliminate fats; detoxifies: S/N: ✦ avoid overuse of greens in bathing for their effect on the reproductive system

***dandelion:** tampopo: pu gong ying. Taraxacum officinale Weber (Compositae)*: rhizome, root, leaf, stem sap: (O) (stem sap) removes warts; (leaf) beautifies skin; anti-eczema; (I) (leaf) skin beautifier; tonic; liver tonic; high in vitamin A; diuretic rich in potassium; improves lactation; (root) liver tonic; lowers cholesterol; treats female hormone imbalances; digestive; detoxifies; anti-candida agent; beautifies skin: H/C/N/G: ✦ the stem sap can cause skin irritation, so should be applied directly to warts or eczema patches only; a strong diuretic, should be avoided by children for internal use

daphne: *jinchōge: Daphne genkwa Sieb. et Zucc. (Thymelaeaceae)*: flower, root: (O) (root) vesicant; aromatic; (I) (flower) diuretic; stomachic; soothes coughs: C: ✦ poisonous; to be taken only under medical supervision

devil's tongue root: *konnyaku. Amorphalus konjac:* root processed into gel form: (O) cleanses; (I) useful in weight control; cuts appetite; reduces assimilation of fats; lowers blood cholesterol; aids in constipation: S/N

dill: *Anethum graveolens (Umbelliferae)*: leaf, oil: (O) antibacterial; aromatic; cleanses; (I) calms; sedative; digestive: H/G

***dokudami:** Houttuynia cordata (Saururaceae):* whole plant: (O) (fresh leaf) benefits skin problems; good for dry skin, liver spots; antirheumatism; helps eczema, prickly heat; stimulates circulation; soothes muscle aches; strengthens resistance; beautifies hair; (I) diuretic; cleanses;

beautifies skin; detoxifies: C: ✦ observe caution in dosage

double dropwort see **meadowsweet**
dulse see **seaweed**

egg: *tamago:* (O) nourishes; conditions hair; the **white** refines skin; tightens skin; stimulates skin; (I) beautifies skin and hair: widely available

eggplant: *nasu. Solanum melongena, Solanum esculentum (Solanaceae)*: vegetable flesh, calyx: (O) (calyx) cleanses; contains alkaloids; (I) diuretic; emollient; laxative: widely available: ✦ calyx is toxic

elderflower: *Sambucus canadensis, S. nigra (Caprifoliaceae)*: leaf, berry, flower: (O) (berry) darkens hair; (flower) astringent; cools; refreshes; heals; good for dry/normal skin; fragrant; cleanses; bleaches freckles; soothes sunburn; calms; (leaf) softens; cools; (I) diaphoretic; diuretic; laxative; emollient: H

eucalyptus: *Eucalyptus Globulus Labill. (Myrtaceae)*: leaf: (O) antiseptic; aromatic; astringent; disinfectant; (I) stimulates; tonic; reduces fever: H/G

evening primrose: *Oenothera biennis (Onagraceae)*: leaf, stem, seed, oil from seed: (O) beautifies skin; anti-aging benefits; (I) (seed, oil) relieves premenstrual tension; reduces menopausal discomfort; aids psoriasis, thrombosis, multiple sclerosis; (leaf, stem) soothes coughs: H

fennel: *uikyō. hui xiang. Foeniculum vulgare Mill. (Umbelliferae)*: fruit, seed, leaf, stem: (O) fragrant; soothes eyes; antiseptic; analgesic; warms; stimulates; cleanses; soothes skin; relaxes; (I) aids in slimming; calms; stomachic; increases lactation; regulates *ki*. S/H/C/N/G: ✦ in pregnancy, no more than a couple of fennel seeds daily; at all times avoid overdosage; misuse of essential oil may cause convulsions

field horsetail: *sugina. Equisetum arvense (Equisetaceae)*: stem: (O) heals; reduces scarring; astringent; helps prevent stretch marks; stimulates hair growth; eliminates dandruff; tones aging skin; restores moisture balance; cleanses; (I) antifat retention; diuretic; remineraliser; regenerator; antifatigue; strengthens bones, tissues, cartilage, tendons: H/C: ✦ taken internally, may reduce menstrual bleeding; consult herbal practitioner before ingesting

fruit: *kudamono:* see individual listings
funori see **seaweed**
***garlic:** ninniku. da suan. Allium sativum (Liliaceae)*: fresh bulb: (O) antiseptic; antibacterial; heals acne; antiviral; stimulates hair growth; (I)

diaphoretic; vermifuge; lowers arterial tension and cholesterol levels; anticoagulant; beautifies skin; antidote; tonic; stomachic; said to be anticancer agent; stimulates immune system; antibiotic and antifungal properties: widely available

genmai-cha see **tea**

geranium: *Pelargonium species* (*Geraniaceae*): leaf, flower, oil: (O) antifat; astringent; aromatic (not only the flowers but the leaves are fragrant, with apple, orange, incense, rose-peppermint, rose-lemon, and rose among the various geranium aromas); stimulates; (oil) treats lice, ringworm, shingles; beneficial to all complexions; anti-aging; antidepressant; anti-insomnia; repels mosquitos; (I) (flower, leaf) edible; astringent; antidiarrhea: H/G

ginger: *shōga: gan jiang. Zingiber officinale Rosc.* (*Zingiberaceae*): rhizome: (O) stimulates scalp; battles hair loss; stimulates circulation; heals; warms; anticellulite; purifies; cleanses; (I) tonic; hot stimulant; anticold; antinausea; helps prevent seafood poisoning; stimulates delayed menstruation; vermifuge; prevents motion sickness; diaphoretic; may ease morning sickness: widely available: ✦ not for sensitive skin; may irritate skin used externally; avoid large dosages or concentrated direct application; avoid when stomach ulcers are present and during pregnancy

ginkgo: *ichō: Ginkgo biloba* (*Ginkoaceae*): nut, leaf: (O) benefits varicose veins; soothes skin; purifies; protects; (I) (leaf) increases blood flow; combats free radicals; brain tonic; regulates neurotransmitters; stimulates metabolism; supplies oxygen to brain; improves memory; stimulates circulation; anti-aging benefits; (nut) antituberculosis; astringent; sedative; antitussive; antiasthma: S/H/C: ✦ outer layer of nuts can cause dermatitis; overdosage of nuts or leaves can be highly toxic; avoid prolonged use or large quantities

ginseng: *chosen ninjin: ren shen: Panax ginseng* (*Araliaceae*): root: (O) benefits dry skin; conditions skin; cleanses; restorative; (I) tonic; rejuvenative; regulates blood pressure and blood sugar; promotes sex hormone secretion; tonifies *ki*; aphrodisiac: H/C/N: ✦ avoid all tea and turnips when taking ginseng; overdosage may lead to high blood pressure, depression, insomnia; exercise caution during pregnancy or where there is hypertension

gold thread: *Coptis trifolia*: whole plant: (O) brightens hair; astringent; heals blemishes; (I) benefits liver: H/N: ✦ may cause allergic reaction in those susceptible

golden seal: *Hydrastis canadensis* (*Ranunculaceae*): root: (O) brightens hair; astringent; heals skin conditions; (I) antiviral; antibacterial; lowers blood pressure; restorative: H/N: ✦ use for short periods only, even externally, as cumulative overdose is toxic; overdosage can cause oversecretion of mucus; avoid during pregnancy due to uterine stimulation; fresh plant can cause dermatitis

Gotu Kola: *Hydrocotyl asiatica, Centella asiatica* (*Umbelliferae*): root, leaf: (O) (root juice) heals cutaneous wounds; prevents scarring; benefits varicose veins; stimulates circulation; anticellulite; stimulates tissue repair; tonifies veins; reduces swelling; (I) (leaf) digestive; tonic; purifies blood: balancing tonic; calms; energizes; sedative; rich in vitamin B; tranquilizing action; nerve tonic; restorative; diuretic: H/C/N: ✦ narcotic in overdose

grape: *budō: Vitus species:* fruit, oil from the seed, leaf: (O) (grapeseed oil) used as carrier oil in aromatherapy; astringent; (fruit) cools; demulcent; tonic; soothes; moisturizes; benefits all skin types; (leaf) astringent; restorative; (I) (fruit) purifies; nourishes: widely available

gyokuro see **tea**

hazelnut: *hashibami: Corylus Avellana L.* (*Betulaceae*): nut, oil from nut, leaf, stem, branch: (O) (nut, oil) encourages hair growth; nourishes skin; heals; benefits circulation; (I) stimulates circulation; nourishes; reduces fever; counters obesity, edema, and varicose veins: encourages weight loss; astringent: widely available

henna: *henna: Lawsonia alba, L. inermis*: leaf, flower: (O) (leaf) dyes hair and skin red or other colors; gives volume to hair; slightly drying; antiseptic; stimulating; (flower) aromatic: H/N: ✦ may cause allergic reaction in those susceptible

hijiki see **seaweed**

hōji-cha see **tea**

Hokkaido pumpkin, *kabocha*: (seeds) *nan qua zi. Cucurbita moschata* (*Cucurbitaceae*): vegetable flesh, seed: (I) (seed) anthelmintic: F/S/N

*honey: *hachimitsu. feng mi: Apis mellifers* (*Apidae*): (O) stimulates circulation; nourishes; moisturizes; heals; humectant; good for aging, sensitive, or dry skins; exfoliates; clears blemishes; eliminates blackheads; antibacterial; (I) laxative; soothes internal areas; sedative; longevity tonic: widely available

honeysuckle/Japanese honeysuckle: *suikazura. jin yin hua: Lonicera Japonica Thunb.* (*Caprifoliaceae*): whole plant: (O) (flower) soothes delicate skin; removes freckles and sunburn; stimulates circulation; regenerates; benefits heat rash and other irritations; tones; nourishes; (bark oil) wrinkle-softener; (I) antibiotic; diuretic; laxative; diaphoretic: C/G: ✦ may cause allergic reaction in those susceptible; berries poisonous

hops: *Humulus lupulus* (*Cannabaceae*): strobiles:

(0) brown hair dye; contains estrogen-like compounds; softens skin; soporific; aromatic; (I) calms; sedative; diuretic; analgesic; antibacterial; aphrodisiac in men; regulates menstrual cycle: H/N: ✦ may cause allergic reactions in those susceptible; external contact causes dermatitis in some

horse chestnut, Indian chestnut: *Aesculus hippocastanum* (*Hippocastanaceae*): seed skin, seed: (0) anticellulite; astringent; aids in slimming; benefits varicose veins; beautifies skin; cleanses; (I) astringent; vasoconstrictor; soothes: H

hyssop: *huo xiang. Agastache rugosa, Hyssopus officinalis* (*Labiatae*): leaf, stem: (0) diaphoretic; cleanses; aromatic; (I) relaxes; stomachic; diaphoretic; prevents colds; tonic; antiviral: H/C/N: ✦ avoid large doses; abstain during pregnancy or in the case of high blood pressure or epilepsy

incense: *kō*. made from powdered or chipped aromatic woods, leaves, seeds, etc.: (0) supplies fragrance; relaxes; depending on type, can influence mind and body in various ways: H/N and specialty stores

iris: *shōbu. Iris florentina, Iris germanica, Iris versicolor, others of Iridaceae species*; note that while this type of blue, lavender or white-flowering iris may sometimes be referred to as **sweet flag** (or **blue flag**), it should not be confused with the A*corus Americanus, A. calamus* (*Araceae*) which is also known as **sweet flag**: leaf, root, flower: (0) (leaf) diaphoretic; purifies; cleanses; stimulates circulation; (I) (root) violent purgative; expectorant; diuretic; G: ✦ all parts of the plant can be dangerously toxic taken internally

Irish moss see **seaweed**

ivy: *tsuta. Hedera helix L.* (*Araliaceae*): leaf: (0) tones; firms; soothes; relaxes tissues; eliminates fluids; anticellulite; soothes sunburn; helps prevent and remedy stretch marks; beautifies hair; (I) analgesic: H: ✦ berries poisonous

Japanese cypress: *hinoki. Chamaecyparis obtusa*: aromatic wood: (0) aromatic; antibacterial; refreshes; soothes; relaxes; available from lumberyards

Japanese yew: *ichinoki. Taxus cuspidata* (*Taxaceae*): aromatic wood, resin, seed, leaf: (0) (wood, resin) aromatic; (I) (seed) vermifuge: C: ✦ the bark, leaves, seeds, and fruit are highly poisonous; the seed and the seed oil can be fatal

jasmine: *Jasminum officinale* (*Oleaceae*): blossom, leaf, root: (0) aromatic; heals; softens skin; soothes sensitive dry skins; cleanses; (I) soporific; calms; sedative; soothes coughs; purifies blood; aphrodisiac; (root) relieves headaches and insomnia: H/N: ✦ may cause allergic reactions in those susceptible

jojoba: *Simmondsia chimemsis* (*Buxaceae*): bean, oil from bean: (0) (bean oil) soothes inflamed skin; fights psoriasis, acne, eczema; nourishes hair;

cleanses; strengthens hair and skin; protects against elements: H

kabocha see **Hokkaido pumpkin**

kelp see **seaweed**

kombu see **seaweed**

kuki-cha see **tea**

kuzu: *ge gan. Pueraria thunbergiana Benth.* (*Leguminosae*): processed powdered roots (white starch): (I) nourishing; tonic; treats digestive problems; detoxifies; calms: S/C/N

*lavender: *Lavandula vera, L. officinalis* (*Labiatae*): flower, leaf, oil: (0) anticellulite; anti-acne; astringent; aromatic; stimulates sore muscles; soothes aches; cools; refreshes; stimulates hair growth; eases fatigue; local anesthetic; good for oily hair; normalizes oil secretion in skin; antiseptic; cleanses; antifungal; antibacterial; helps varicose veins; (I) calms; soporific; stimulates; relieves headache and fatigue; tonic; nerve tonic; carminative; eases headache: H/N: ✦ pregnant women should abstain

laver see **seaweed**

lemon: *remon. Citrus limon* (*Rutacae*): fruit, rind, oil: (0) (fruit) lightens skin and hair; astringent; deodorizes; heals; exfoliates; antioxidant; preservative; (rind, oil) benefits oily skin; aromatic; brightens hair; antibacterial; (I) relaxes; soothes; cools; antibacterial; antihistamine: widely available: ✦ used externally, oil may cause allergic reaction in some

lemon balm see **balm**

lemon grass: *Cymbopogon citratus* (*Graminae*): leaf, oil: (0) benefits oily skin; normalizes oil secretion; rich in vitamin A; aromatic; repels insects; eases sore muscles; deodorizes; treats ringworm; (I) treats irregular menstruation, diarrhea, digestive problems; destroys bacteria: S/H

licorice root: *kanzō. gan cao. Glycyrrhiza uralensis Fisch.; Glycyrrhiza glabra L.* (*Leguminosae*): root: (0) soothes; emollient; (I) benefits all organs; tonic; antidote; analgesic: H/C/N: ✦ dangerous in overdosage; abstain during pregnancy or if suffering from high blood pressure or kidney disease

lime: *Citrus aurantifolia, C. limetta* (*Rutacae*): blossom: (0I) soporific: H/N

linden: *Tilia Europaea*: flower: (0) relaxes; sedative; antiseptic; cools; (I) calms; diaphoretic; sedative: H/N

loofah: *hechima* (**loofah-vine water:** *hechima-sui*): *si gua luo. Luffa cylindrica Roem.; Luffa aegyptiaca* (*Cucurbitaceae*): fruit, fruit fibers, vine sap: (0) cools; soothes; smoothes; moisturizes; lightens; softens wrinkles; lightens freckles; refreshes; (I) (fruit) cools: not widely available unless cultivated

loquat: *biwa. pi pa ye. Eriobotrya Japonica Lindl.* (*Rosaceae*): leaf: (0) antiseptic; heals; purifies; soothes inflammations; stimulates circulation; anti-cellulite; tones skin; warms; (I) expectorant;

anti-emetic; treats skin problems; antifatigue; improves appetite: C

lotus: *hasu /renkon: he ye: Nelumbo nucifera, Nelumbium nelumbo Druce.* (*Nymphaeaceae*): whole plant, esp. roots: (O) cleanses; beautifies skin; (I) beautifies skin; aids in weight control; astringent; poisoning antidote: S/C/N

marigold: *Calendula officinalis* (*Compositae*): petal: (O) gives red/gold tones to hair; heals; conditions skin and hair; stimulates skin; soothes skin; helps varicose veins; antibacterial; antifungal; prevents scarring; (I) stimulating; tonic; diaphoretic; used in cancer treatments; purported antitumor properties: H/G

marjoram: *Origanum majorana* (*Labiatae*): leaf: (O) calms; mild antiseptic; aromatic; antioxidant; soothes muscle cramps; soporific; antidepressant; (I) digestive; diaphoretic; antiviral: H

matcha see **tea**

meadowsweet, double dropwort: *seri: Filipendula ulmaria, F. vulgaris, Spiraea ulmaria* (*Rosaceae*): flower: (O) aromatic; astringent; diaphoretic; heals blemishes; (I) calms; sedative; contains salicylic acid and was the origin of the first aspirin drug; eases pain; digestive; antiseptic; diuretic: H
mekabu

melissa see **balm**

melon: *meron/makuwauri: Cucurbitaceae* family. flesh, seed: (O) cleanses; refines skin texture; most melons are good for all skin types, although the honeydew has particular benefits for dry skins, and the Persian melon for oily; (I) cleanses; nourishes; diuretic: widely available

milk: *gyūnyū: niunai:* (O) nourishes; smoothes; moisturizes; softens wrinkles; relaxes; (I) soporific: widely available. See also **yogurt**.

mint: *minto: bo he* (*Mentha arvensis*)(*Labiatae*): leaf: (O) refreshes; soothes; smoothes; stimulates; (I) relaxes; digestive; soothes inflammation; eases headache; antibacterial; antifungal: H/C: ✦ avoid overdosage; pregnant or lactating women and children and babies should abstain. See also entries for **peppermint**, **spearmint**.

miso see **soybean**

mistletoe: *Viscum album:* leaf, flower, twig, bark-sap (birdlime): (O) heals skin problems; (I) calms; sedative; nerve tonic: H: ✦ berries poisonous

mugwort: *yomogi: ai ye: Artemisia vulgaris L.* (*Compositae*): leaf: (O) used in moxabustion; analgesic; astringent; soothes sore muscles; exfoliates; softens skin; calms inflammations; soothes heat rash; (I) benefits female reproductive system; warming; analgesic; tonic; stomachic; hemostatic; improves lactation: H/C/N: ✦ may cause allergic reactions in those susceptible; avoid overdosage or continued use; pregnant women abstain

mulberry: *kuwa:* **white mulberry:** *sang shen:* **white mulberry leaf:** *sang ye:* **white mulberry:**

Morus alba (*Moraceae*);. **black mulberry:** *Morus nigra* (*Moraceae*): branch, twig, leaf, root, fruit: (O) (leaf) cools; strengthens hair; prevents hair loss; (I) (white mulberry branches and twigs) rheumatism aid; analgesic; soothes; (black mulberry root skin) relieves toothache; (white mulberry root skin) cough remedy; aids in bronchitis and asthma cases; expectorant; sedative; diuretic; (black mulberry) anti-inflammatory; (white mulberry) yin tonic; anti-insomnia; remedies hypertension; nourishes blood and *ki*; laxative; relieves pain; (black mulberry leaf) tonic; laxative; relieves pain; antibacterial; expectorant; fever remedy; astringent; antidiabetic agent; (white mulberry leaf) antipyretic; liver sedative, antibacterial; expectorant; cold remedy; antidiabetic agent: H/C/N: ✦ may cause allergic reaction in those susceptible

musk: *jyakō: she xiang: Moschus moschiferus* (*Cervidae*): secretion from the preputial follicles of the musk deer: (O) aromatic; (I) cardiotonic; stimulant: H/C

Mylitta lapidescens Horan.: (*Polyporaceae*): fungus that grows in association with the roots of bamboo: (I) vermifuge: C: ✦ mildly toxic; to be taken only by prescription and with specialist supervision

nattō see **soybean**

neroli see **bitter orange**

nettle: *irakusa: Urtica dioica* (*Urticaceae*): leaf: (O) encourages hair growth; stimulates; activates circulation; (I) purifies blood; encourages hair growth; blood tonic; stimulates circulation; contains iron with vitamin C; increases lactation; lowers blood sugar; mild laxative and diuretic; astringent: H/N/G: ✦ may cause allergic reaction in those susceptible; wear gloves and protective clothing when harvesting

nori see **seaweed**

nuka see **rice**

nutmeg: *nikuzuku: Myristica fragrans* (*Myristicaceae*): seed: (O) analgesic; stimulates circulation; aromatic; (I) aphrodisiac; digestive; regulates *ki*; in magic, brings love; stimulates appetite; carminative; eases nausea; anti-inflammatory: widely available: ✦ dangerous taken in amounts greater than 7 g / 1/4 oz; may cause convulsions or palpitations

***oats:** karasu-mugi: Avena sativa L.* (*Graminae*): grain, bran: (O) clears skin; heals; anti-infection; soothes irritated skin; exfoliates; stimulates; (I) anti-insomnia; antidepressant; tonic to the nervous system: widely available

ocha see **tea**

okara see **soybean**

olive: *oriibu.* (**olive oil:** *oriibu oiru*): *Olea Europaea* (*Oleaceae*): oil from the fruit, fruit, leaf: (O) (oil) soothes; mild tonic; moisturizes; anti-aging; (I) diuretic; beautifies hair and skin; laxative: widely available

onion, **green onion:** *negi. Allium cepa L.* (*Liliaceae*): bulb, stem: (O) promotes healing and scarring process; emollient; (I) antiseptic; warming; affects lungs and stomach; cough remedy; cardiotonic; diuretic; expectorant; laxative; stimulant to whole system: widely available

oolong tea see **tea**

orange, **trifoliate orange:** *orenji. zhi shi. Citrus sinensis Osbeck, Poncirus trifoliata* (*Rutaceae*): fruit—ripe and unripe, flower, rind: (O) (fruit) whitens skin; soothes; anti-aging; (flower) aromatic; deodorizes; calms; relaxes; uplifts spirits; heals skin problems; (rind) aromatic; mobilizes *ki*, (I) (fruit) digestive; sedative; tonic: widely available: ✦ essential oil or rind may cause allergic reactions in some, used externally; skin of nonorganic oranges may contain pesticide residues so do not use in recipes calling for orange peel

pansy: *Viola tricolor* (*Violaceae*): leaf, flower: (O) contains salicylic acid; astringent; heals; cools; emollient; reduces scarring; an inside/outside regime of long duration beautifies skin; tonic; (I) relaxes; laxative; diuretic; beautifies skin; sedative; emetic; tonic: H/G: ✦ may cause allergic reactions in those susceptible

papaya: *papaya. Carica papaya* (*Cucurbitaceae*): fruit, fresh leaf: (O) eliminates dead skin cells; heals; good for oily skin; cleanses; (I) vermifuge; stimulates digestion: widely available: ✦ may cause allergic reactions in those susceptible

parsley: *Petroselinum sativum Hoffm.* (*Umbellifereae*): leaf: (O) nourishes; tones; cleanses; heals skin problems; (I) cleanses; beautifies skin; tonic; antianemia; diuretic; sedative: widely available

passionflower: *Passiflora incarnata* (*Passifloraceae*): flower, leaf: (O) calms; (I) calms; sedative; benefits the nervous system: H/N: ✦ may cause allergic reactions in those susceptible; overdosage may cause nausea and vomiting

patchouli: *Pogostemon cablin, P. patchouli.* oil, powder: (O) aids in slimming; fragrant; stimulates; tonic; good for dry skin; repels insects; rejuvenates skin: H/N

peach: *momo* (**peach leaf:** *momo no ha*): *tao ren: Prunus persica Batsch* (*Rosaceae*): fruit, leaf, fruit kernel, blossom: (O) (leaf) soothes skin inflammation; cools; heals; relieves itching, heat rash; emollient; (fruit) soothes irritated skin; tonic; refines skin; good for oily and normal skins; (I) (leaf, flower) calms; sedative; laxative: widely available: ✦ the fruit pit, flower, and leaf contain toxins, so must be consumed only by prescription and under the supervision of a specialist

pearl: *shinju* (**oyster shell:** *kaki no kai*): *mu li. Ptera margaritiferia* (**oyster:** *Ostrea rivularis* [*Ostreidae*]): pearl powder, shell powder: (O) calms; smoothes; softens; activates cell regeneration; lightens freckles and age spots; (I) sedative; relaxes; supplies calcium; astringent; benefits eyes; restorative; blood purifier; detoxifies; eliminates saturated fats: C

*pearl barley, **Job's Tears:** *hatomugi. yi yi ren. Coix lacrymae Jobi L.* (*Graminae*): seed: (OI) clears skin; eliminates warts, blemishes, freckles; diuretic: H/C/N: ✦ as an effective diuretic, overdosage of more than 2-3 cups or portions per day is to be avoided

pennyroyal: *Mentha pulegium, Hedeoma pulegoides* (*Labiatae*): leaf, oil, vinegar: (O) (leaf) diaphoretic; soothes itching; deodorizes; repels insects; (vinegar) heals burns, bruises, skin blemishes; (I) diaphoretic; eases headache, cold congestion, menstrual pain: H/N: ✦ may cause allergic reaction in those susceptible; can cause contact dermatitis; must be avoided by pregnant women or by those with kidney problems

peppermint: *Mentha piperita* (*Labiatae*): leaf, oil: (O) cools; antiseptic; heals; good for oily skin; (I) analgesic; relieves insomnia; calms; relieves abdominal pain, nausea, colds, headaches, fever, and flu; stimulates; tonic: H: ✦ avoid overdosage; children, babies, and lactating women abstain

*perilla: *shiso. zi su zi. Perilla frutescens Britt.* (*Labiatae*): seed, stem, leaf: (O) antiseptic; fragrant; preservative; diaphoretic; antibacterial; deodorizes; moisturizes; beautifies skin and hair; stimulates local metabolism; (I) calms; antitussive; warming; laxative; diaphoretic; stomachic; antiseptic; antiasthma; brain food; stimulates circulation; improves metabolism; prevents colds; retards hair loss; beautifies skin and hair: S/C: ✦ not to be consumed in large doses or taken by children

persimmon: *kaki* (**persimmon leaf:** *kaki no ha*): *shi di. Diospyros kaki L.* (*Ebenaceae*): fruit—fresh and dried, leaf, calyx: (O) (leaf) warms; beautifies skin; eases sore muscles; improves circulation; lightens skin; nourishes skin; (I) (leaf) beautifies skin; cold remedy; (ripe dried fruit) stomachic; astringent; (fresh fruit) lowers blood pressure; improves blood circulation; reduces arterial tension; (calyx) soothes coughs: F/S/C

pickled plum see **ume**

pine: *matsu. Pinus* family: needle, resin: (O) fragrant; cools; refreshes; stimulates; tones; antiseptic; soothes; stimulates cell regeneration; anti-acne; good for aging skin or irritated skin; (I) tonic; stimulates circulation and metabolism; anti-aging; rich in vitamin C: H/G

pineapple: *painappuru. Ananassa sativa L. (Bromeliaceae)*: fruit: (O) astringent; good for oily skins; exfoliant; contains the enzyme bromeline; lightens skin; stimulates cell regeneration; (I) rich in vitamins and minerals; accelerates digestion of proteins; nourishing; detoxifies; diuretic; aids in slimming; beautifies skin; anti-arteriosclerosis: widely available

plantain: *ōbako. che qian zi. Plantago major L., P. asiatica (Plantaginaceae)*: leaf: (O) stimulates; cleanses; heals; reduces inflammations; diuretic; detoxifies; (I) antiallergy; useful in respiratory treatment; lowers high blood pressure; helps eyes; beautifies skin; diuretic; aphrodisiac; tonifies kidneys: C/H/G: ✦ may cause allergic reactions in those susceptible

plum, plum extract, plum vinegar, plum liquor see *ume*

polei, puerh see **tea**

quassia: *Picrasma amara, P. excelsa, Quassia amora (Simarubaceae)*: bark: (O) brightens hair; cleanses; antidandruff; (I) benefits liver and eyes: H: ✦ may cause allergic reactions in those susceptible

red chili, cayenne pepper: *tōgarashi. Capsicum frutescens L. (Solanaceae)*: fruit: (O) aids lumbago, arthritis, rheumatism; activates blood circulation; warming; (I) tonic; stimulates circulation; cold remedy; digestive; carminative; antiseptic; nerve tonic; antibacterial: widely available: ✦ seeds are toxic; overdose may damage liver or cause gastroenteritis; abstain during pregnancy and lactation; may blister the skin if contact is too direct or prolonged; avoid contact with eyes or broken skin

rhubarb, medicinal rhubarb: *daiō. da huang. Rheum officinale Baill. (Polygonaceae)*: root, rhizome: (O) brightens hair; relieves pain and swelling; (I) astringent; purgative; laxative: stomachic: C/H: ✦ avoid tea and turnips when taking medicinal rhubarb; may cause allergic reactions in those susceptible

rice: *kome* (**brown rice:** *genmai. rice flour: jōshinko/mochiko/shiratamako*): *Oryza sativa L. (Graminae)*: grain, flour, oil from germ, bran, wine: (O) (flour) soothes; nourishes; calms: anticellulite; softens skin; relaxes; (I) (whole grain) beautifies skin; aids in slimming: widely available

> **rice bran:** *nuka, komenuka.* (O) soothes skin inflammation; cleanses; moisturizes; balances any skin type; heals; nourishes; (I) nourishes: S/N
> **rice vinegar:** *komezu.* (OI) cleanses; heals: S/N
> **rice wine:** *sake.* (O) detoxifies; smoothes; exfoliates; (I) diaphoretic; stimulates: S

rose: *bara.* (*mei gui hua*. flowers of *Rosa rugosa* Thunb.; *jin ying zi*. rose hips of *Rosa laerigata* Michx) *Rosa damascena, Rosa gallica, Rosa Chinensis, Rosa multiflora (Rosaceae)*: petal, hips, seed, oil, vinegar: most rose species share similar traits; where the properties are specific this is indicated: (O) (petal, oil) astringent; deodorizes; fragrant; good for dry skin; lightens complexion; tonic; soothes; stimulates circulation; antidepressant; aids digestive system; eases headache; anti-insomnia; regulates menstruation; (I) (petal) calms; sedative; aids headache, sore throat; (rose hips) tonic; ki tonic; diuretic; rich in vitamin C; cold remedy; (*Rosa Chinensis, Rosa rugosa*, petal) tonic; circulation stimulant; *ki* tonic; benefits digestion; blood tonic; (*Rosa multiflora*, seed) diuretic; laxative: widely available

rosemary: *Rosmarinus officinalis (Labiatae)*: leaf: (O) astringent; conditions hair; anticellulite; stimulates hair growth; diaphoretic; (I) stimulates; tonic; relaxes; stimulates circulation and digestion; soporific: H

rum: (O) conditions and nourishes hair; gives shine: widely available

safflower: *benibana. hong hua. Carthamus tinctorius. L. (Compositae)*: seed oil, petal, seed: (O) (petal) heals; soothes skin problems; red dye; (I) (petal) stimulates circulation; blood purifier; eliminates age spots, stress, and liver complaints; general tonic; calms; astringent; regulates menstruation; eases bruises and joint pain; powerful effect on female reproductive system: C/H: ✦ the herb is never to be taken during pregnancy

saffron: *safuran. Crocus sativas (Iridaceae)*: stamen: (O) brightens hair; diaphoretic; golden red or yellow dye; (I) diaphoretic; antidepressant; regulates menstruation; used as catalyst with other herbs in Chinese medicine: F/H: ✦ may cause allergic reactions in those susceptible

sage: *sarubia. Salvia officinalis (Labiatae)*: leaf: (O) darkens hair; deodorizes; anti-cellulite; soothes sore muscles; cleanses; stimulates skin; (I) relaxes; antidepressant; reduces lactation; stimulates; tonic; darkens hair: H: ✦ may cause allergic reactions in those susceptible; avoid overdosage or prolonged use; epileptics and pregnant women abstain

sake see **rice, rice wine**

salt: *shio. sodium chloride.* powdered mineral: (O) cleanses; tones; heals; exfoliates; stimulates circulation: widely available

sandalwood: *byakudan. Santalum album L. (Santalaceae)*: wood, oil: (O) anti-cellulite; aromatic: disinfectant; antiseptic; rejuvenating: H

sassafras: *Sassafras albidum, S. officinale (Lauraceae)*: root bark: (O) diaphoretic; aromatic; soothes itching; soothes sore muscles; kills lice; antiseptic; eases poison ivy and poison oak rashes; (I) digestive; diaphoretic; diuretic; laxative; decreases lactation; reduces high blood pressure: H: ✦ may cause allergic reactions in those susceptible; a controversial 1960 study showed a possible link between cancer and safrole, an active constituent of sassafras, but many feel the study was severely flawed

savory: *Satureia hortensis, S. montana* (*Labiatae*): leaf: (O) soothes insect bites; stimulates; (I) stimulates; tonic; antibacterial; vermifuge; eliminates lung congestion: H

*seaweed: *kaisō*: whole plant: (O) revives; stimulates cell functions; tones; tightens; nourishes; refreshes; anticellulite; detoxifies; (I) beautifies hair, skin, nails; fights graying hair; aids in slimming; relaxes nerves; tonic; increases vitality; activates metabolism; diuretic; rich in iodine and other minerals; antibacterial; stimulates immune system; heals ulcers; reduces cholesterol; lowers blood pressure; prevents strokes; thins the blood: S/H/C/N

The following varieties of seaweed share similar properties:

> **arame:** *Eisenia bicyclis, E. arborea*
> **dulse:** *Palmaria palmata*
> **funori:** *Gloiopeltis furcata*
> **hijiki:** *Hizikia fusiformis*
> **Irish moss:** *Chondrus crispus*
> **kelp, kombu:** *Laminaria japonica Aresch* (*Laminariaceae*)
> **laver, nori:** *Porphyra tenera*
> **tengusa:** *Gelidium amansii*
> **wakame:** *Undaria pinnatifida*

sen-cha see **tea**

sesame: *goma* (**sesame oil:** *goma abura*): *zhima*: *Sesamum indicum* (*Pedaliaceae*): seed, oil: (O) nourishes; moisturizes; heals; useful for oily skin; nourishes hair; (I) beautifies hair; fights graying of hair: F/S/N

shiitake, black forest mushroom: *shiitake*: *Lentinus edodes, Cortinellis shiitake*: mushroom: (I) eliminates toxins; aids in weight control; lowers cholesterol; calms; activates metabolism; cleanses; beautifies skin: F/S/C/N

shōchū: distilled spirits containing 20–45% alcohol; tasteless; odorless; vodka may be substituted: S

shrimp: *ebi*: (I) beautifies skin and hair; aids in weight control: widely available: ✦ may cause allergic reactions in some

silk: *kinu*: (O) gives shine to hair: widely available

soybean: *daizu*: *Glycine max, G. soja Sieb. et Zucc.* (*Papilionaceae*): seed, curd, lees from curd, vinegar, fermented seed, sprout, fermented seed paste, oil, flour, sauce made from seed: (O) beautifies skin; soothes; nourishes; (I) weight control aid; high in calcium, B vitamins, estrogen, and protein; quickens metabolism; improves diges-

tion; cleanses; remineralizes; stimulates: S/C/N. The following soybean products share similar properties:

> **bean curd:** *tofu*
> **bean sprouts:** *moyashi*
> **fermented bean paste:** *miso*
> **fermented beans:** *nattō*
> **soy oil:** *daizu abura*
> **soy sauce:** *shōyu*
> **soybean flour (roasted):** *kinako*
> **soybean vinegar:** *sudaizu*
> **tofu lees:** *okara*

spearmint: *Mentha spicata* (*Labiatae*): leaf: (O) calming; sedative; (I) digestive; calming: H/G

spirits see **beer, rum,** *shōchū*, **rice wine** (*sake*), **champagne**

star anise: *hakkaku*: *bajiao*: *Illicium verum Hook. f.* (*Magnoliaceae*): fruit: (O) aromatic; (I) digestive; cough remedy; aids rheumatism; warming; affects spleen and kidneys: widely available

strawberry: *ichigo*: *Frageria vesca* (*Rosaceae*): fruit, leaf, rhizome: (O) (leaf) astringent; good for oily skin; (fruit) cleanses; heals; antifungal; calms acne; soothes sunburn; (I) (leaf) astringent; diuretic; refreshes; calms; (fruit) rich in vitamin C; anticancer; antioxidant; antiviral; reduces cholesterol and blood pressure; astringent; tonic; diuretic: widely available: ✦ may cause allergic reactions in those susceptible

sulfur: *io*: (O) beautifies skin; strengthens hair; lightens skin; detoxifies; softens; stimulates circulation: H

tabaschir see **bamboo**

tangerine, mandarin orange: *mikan*: (**rind of ripe fruit:** *chen pi*) (**rind of unripe fruit:** *qing pi*): *Citrus reticulata blanco* (*Rutaceae*): fruit, rind: (O) (unripe fruit rind) mobilizes *ki*; (ripe fruit rind) warms; cleanses; clears blemished skin; lightens skin; anti-aging; (I) (ripe fruit rind) mobilizes *ki*; digestive; stomachic; calms coughs; anti-aging; tonic; vitamins A, B, C: widely available

*tea: *cha/ocha*: *cha*: *Thea sinensis L.* (*Theaceae*): leaf: in general terms the various teas share the following similar effects: (O) soothes sunburn; dark varieties supply tint to skin and hair; soothes insect bites; reduces bleeding from superficial wounds; antioxidant; anticellulite; astringent; calms; prevents tooth decay; (I) cleanses; diuretic; eliminates fats; prevents tooth decay; aids in slimming; detoxifies; combats free radicals; anti-carcinogenic; calms: widely available: ✦ limit dosage during pregnancy and lactation; avoid if stomach ulcers or cardiac problems are present

green teas: *ocha*: (I) the green teas (varieties listed below) are noted particularly for their protective anticancer and cardiotonic properties:

ban-cha: the lowest grade of green tea

genmai-cha: *ban-cha* mixed with puffed brown rice kernels

gyokuro: high-grade green tea

hoji-cha: roasted ban-cha tea

kuki-cha: tea consisting of twigs and stems of the tea plant

matcha: powdered gyokuro green tea

sen-cha: medium-grade green tea

black teas: (l) activate fat-elimination process, reduce cholesterol, and lower hypertension:

oolong

puerh, polei

tengusa see **seaweed**

thyme: *Thymus vulgaris* (*Labiatae*): leaf: (O) deodorizes; aromatic; antiseptic; diaphoretic; stimulates; antidepressant; (l) soothes coughs; calms; stimulates; tonic; antiviral; antifungal: H: ✦ abstain during pregnancy

tofu, tofu lees see **soybean**

turmeric: *yu jin*: *Curcuma aromatica, Curcuma longa,* (*Zingiberaceae*): root: (O) brightens hair; antibacterial; (l) hemostatic; dissolves clots: F/S/H/C/N

ume, "plum": *ume*: *Prunus mume Sieb. et Zucc* (*Rosaceae*): unripe fruit, fruit kernel, blossom, pickled unripe fruit, cooked concentrate of unripe fruit, pickling vinegar brine, liquor: (Ol) antibacterial; detoxifies; blood purifier; heals; tonic; strengthener: S/N: ✦ pit is toxic

> **pickled plum, *umeboshi*:** (O) antibacterial; preservative; exfoliates; (l) cleanses; stomachic; tonic: S/N
>
> **plum extract:** *bainiku ekisu*: as for **pickled plum**
>
> **plum vinegar:** *umesu*: as for **pickled plum**
>
> **plum liquor:** *umeshu*: (l) digestive; refreshes: S

vanilla: *banira*: *Vanilla planifolia, V. aromatica* (*Orchidaceae*): dried seed pods: (O) aromatic; (l) aphrodisiac: widely available

vervain, verbena: *Verbena officinalis* (*Verbenaceae*): leaf: (O) antibacterial; heals; (l) relaxes; sedative; treats skin problems; liver and nerve tonic; promotes menstruation; increases lactation; digestive; anti-insomnia: H/N: ✦ avoid during pregnancy

vetivert, vetiver: *Vetiveria zizanioides* (*Gramineae*): root, oil: (O) aromatic; cools; tonic; (l) stimulates; tonic; digestive; encourages menstruation; kills parasites; diaphoretic: H/N

***vinegar:** *su*: (O) removes residues from hair; acid-balances skin and hair; purifies; stimulates circulation; strengthens skin; invigorates; soothes; smoothes; (l) tonic; strengthens; cleanses: widely available

violet: *Viola odorata* (*Violaceae*): leaf, flower, root, oil: (O) (leaf, flower) soothes; astringent; rich in vitamins A and C; contains salicylic acid; heals; good aftershave; beautifies skin; relieves swelling and inflammation; (l) (leaf, flower) relaxes; sedative; relieves respiratory congestion; cools; diaphoretic; eases headache: H/G: ✦ overdosage of leaf causes vomiting and diarrhea; do not ingest seeds

wakame see **seaweed**

walnut: *kurumi*: *Juglans nigra, J. Mandshurica* (*Jugliandiaceae*): hull, kernel, leaf: (O) (shell) darkens hair and skin; astringent; (l) weight control aid: widely available

wheat: *komugi*: *xiao mai*: *Triticum vulgare, T. aestivum* (*Graminae*): grain, bran, germ, oil from germ: (O) nourishes; soothes; heals; stimulates; (l) nourishes; sedative: widely available

witch hazel: *Hamamelis virginiana* (*Hamamelidaceae*): bark, leaf: (O) astringent; deodorizes; good for oily skin; cleanses; styptic; aromatic; good aftershave; soothes sunburn and insect bites; helps varicose veins; tones skin tissues; fights cellulite; (l) lowers blood pressure; benefits female reproductive system: H/G: ✦ do not use undiluted extract directly on skin; do not take commercial witch hazel internally

yarrow: *nokogirisō*: *Achillea millefolium* (*Compositae*): leaf: (O) stimulates hair growth; astringent; aromatic; diaphoretic; cleanses; good for oily skin; (l) astringent; diaphoretic; encourages circulation; lowers blood pressure; eases fevers and colds; reduces blood flow: H/G: ✦ may cause allergic reactions in those susceptible; avoid overdosage; abstain during pregnancy

yellow mullen, mullein: *Verbascum thapsus* (*Scrophulariaceae*): flower: (O) brightens hair; softens skin; soothes irritations; (l) relieves coughs: H: ✦ every part of this plant, except for the flower, is mildly toxic

yogurt: acidophilus-fermented milk: (O) soothes; antibacterial; softens; (l) nourishes; strengthens resistance: widely available

sources outside japan

mail-order sources for ingredients & supplies

In this era of multiculturalism, the entire world is now accessible in a multitude of ways. Shopping by mail from far-flung locations has become an international pastime, and one can locate just about anything imaginable by this wondrous method. You can have fresh *daikon* delivered in Boston, Chinese herbal tinctures flown to you in Peru, American megavitamins airmailed in to Katmandu. Wherever you reside, the following list will enlarge your East-West horizons in beauty and health.

Agraria
1051 Howard Street
San Francisco, CA
USA 94103
• Potpourri, bath products.

Alanese Ltd.
21 Bell Alley
Leighton Buzzard
Bedfordshire LU7 7DG
England
• Aromatherapy oils and a wide range of health and beauty products.

Aphrodisia
28 Carmine Street
New York, NY
USA 10014
• Herbs of every description.

Atlantis Rising
7915 SE Stark
Portland, OR
USA 97215
• Herbs, Oriental herbs, oils, seeds.

Bach Centre USA
P.O. Box 320
Woodmere, NY
USA 11598
• Bach Flower Remedies.

Basically Natural
109 East G Street
Brunswick, MD
USA 21716
• Natural, botanical products for hair.

Caswell-Massey Company
Catalog Order Department
320 West 13th Street
New York, NY
USA 10014
• Basic ingredients for cosmetics making, quality natural-bristle brushes, and sponges.

Chambers
P.O. Box 7841
San Francisco, CA
USA 94120
• Elegant items for the bath.

The Company of Women
102 Main Street
P.O. Box 742
Nyack, NY
USA 10960-0742
• Books of interest to women, electronic massagers, and gardening gloves are some of what this catalogue contains. Profits aid abused women and children.

Cosmetics to Go
Poole
Dorset BH15 1BR
England
• Beauty and bath.

Cosmos Herbs
329 Chiswick High Road
London W44HS
England
Tel: 081-995-7239
• Culinary and medicinal herbs, shop and mail order.

Culpeper Ltd.
Hadstock Road
Linton CB1 6NJ
England
• A wonderful source for oils, herbs, and potpourri of the highest quality.

The Daily Planet
P.O. Box 64411
St. Paul, MN
USA 55164-0411
Tel: 800-324-5950
• Ethnic/global things, including great books, bottles, mirrors, and a tabletop Tranquility Rock Garden, complete with gently trickling water.

Daniel Smith, Inc.
4130 1st Avenue South
Seattle, WA
USA 91834
• Fine art supplies, including a wide selection of Japanese brushes and rice paper, all at discount prices. High quality.

Derbe
Via O. Beccari 61/63
Firenze, Italia 50126
• Extraordinary skin and hair products, including a wonderful rosewater-based shampoo called "Blandissimo."

Diamond K Enterprises
RR 1, Box 30-A
St. Charles, MN
USA 55972
• Organic foods. Whole grains and flours (buckwheat, rice, soy, sesame, wheat), sea salt, honey.

Diamond Organics
P.O. Box 2159
Freedom, CA
USA 95019
Tel: 800-922-2396
• Full selection of fresh organic vegetables and fruits, including tangerines, Chinese cabbage, wheat grass, *kabocha*, burdock root, *daikon*, Asian greens, hearty greens and herbs. Same-day shipping available to any U.S. destination.

Earthen Joys
1412 Eleventh Street
Astoria, OR
USA 97103
• Beauty and the bath.

Ecco Bella
125 Pompton Plains Crossroad
Wayne, NJ
USA 07470
• Products not tested on animals, including skin care and fragrance.

Exotic Specialty Foods
20 Berkeley Street
Hull HU3 1PR
England
Tel/Fax: 0482-25236
• Mail-order service.

Felissimo
10 West 56th Street
New York, NY
USA 10019
Tel: 1-800-708-7690
Fax: 703-345-6546
• Extraordinary products for body and soul, including items for beauty and bath. Japanese implements of the highest quality.

Freshlands Natural Grocer
East-West Centre
196 Old Street
London EC1
England
• Mail order for the UK.

Frontier Direct
P.O. Box 127
Norway, IA
USA 52318-0127
Tel: 800-726-5404
• Herbs, including Japanese and Chinese herbs and ingredients, aromatic herbs and essential oils, and supplies. Among the selection, dried lotus pod, mugwort, apricot kernel oil, chrysanthemum blossoms, cassia, benzoin, sea plants, green and black teas, licorice root, plantain, safflower petals, sandalwood, cherry bark, *shiitake*, dried burdock, chickweed, ginseng, mortars and pestles, small cotton bags, wide-necked jars, spice mills. Many plant items are organic.

Garden Spot Distributors
Route 1, Box 729-A
New Holland, PA
USA 17557
• A wide selection of natural foods, including Japanese items.

George Ohsawa Macrobiotic Foundation
1511 Robinson Street
Oroville, CA
USA 95965
Tel: 916-533-7702
• Japanese ingredients, books, supplies.

Gold Mine Natural Food Company
1947 30th Street
San Diego, CA
USA 92102
Tel: 800-475-Food
• Macrobiotic and organic foods of high quality, with a wide selection of Japanese ingredients

and supplies. Carries the full line of top-notch Ohsawa America natural Japanese foods and ingredients. Eggplant toothpaste, burdock and *ume* concentrates, barley grass supplements, lotus root tea, green and black teas, *kuzu*, seaweeds, sea salt, black soybeans, *azuki* beans, all soybean products, dried *daikon*, mugwort, burdock, *shiitake*, brown rice vinegar, *wasabi* powder, pearl barley, rice bran, and much more. Also offers supplies like the Japanese mortar and pestle, Japanese cutlery and bamboo utensils, ginger and *daikon* graters, *tawashi* scrub brushes, and flour mills, including stone mills.

The Green Earth
2545 Prairie
Evanston, IL
USA 60201
Tel: 708-864-8949, 800-322-3662
- Fresh organic produce, delivery anywhere in the U.S. Carries Chinese cabbage, burdock root, *daikon*, ginger, lotus root, *kabocha*, taro root, many other vegetables and fruits, along with a range of natural foods, supplies, and supplements.

Green Farm Nutrition Centre
Burwash Common
East Sussex TN19 7LX
England
TEL: (0435) 882-482/ 883-457
- Extensive stock of natural products.

Health Innovations, Ltd.
Unit 10
Riverside Business Centre
Brighton Road
Shoreham, West Sussex
England BN43 6RE
Tel: 0273-440-177
Fax: 0273-465-325
- The source for "Imedeen," anti-aging tablets based on fish protein.

Herb Products Company
11012 Magnolia Boulevard
North Hollywood, CA
USA 81601
- Herbs, tinctures, essential oils, ginseng.

Hilltop Herb Farm
Box 886
Cleveland, TX
USA 77327
- Herbs, plants.

Humane Alternative Products
8 Hutchins Street
Concord, NH
USA 03301
Tel: 603-224-1361
- Colognes and perfumes guaranteed cruelty-free.

Indiana Botanic Gardens, Inc.
Hammond, IN
USA 46325
- Herbs, basic ingredients for cosmetics making.

Internatural
P.O. Box 580
Shaker St.
S. Sutton, NH
USA 03273
- Good selection of beauty and health products.

Jaffe Brothers, Inc.
P.O. Box 636
Valley Center, CA
USA 92082-0636
Tel: 619-749-1133
- Soybeans, *azuki* beans, sesame seeds, buckwheat, brown rice, sesame oil, safflower oil, dried persimmons, sea salt, honey, and more.

Macrobiotic Mall
18779-C
North Frederick Avenue
Gaithersburg, MD
USA 20879
- Macrobiotic items.

Maine Coast Sea Vegetables
Franklin, ME
USA 04634
Tel: 207-565-2907
- Harvests and processes sea plants from the Maine coast. High-quality, natural. Offers alaria, kelp, dulse, laver, seaweed seasonings, sea chips, seaweed candy.

Mendocino Sea Vegetable Company
P.O. Box 372
Navarro, CA
USA 95463
Tel: 707-895-3741
- Harvests and processes sea plants from the California coast. High-quality, natural. *Nori*, alaria, *kombu*, dulse, flaked *nori*, and even offer seaweed "feather boas" for the bath. A sea vegetable cookbook is available.

Mountain Ark Trading Company
120 South East Avenue
Fayetteville, AR
USA 72701
Tel: 800-643-8909
- High-quality organic and macrobiotic Japanese

foods, ingredients, and supplies. Carries Mitoku foods. Eggplant toothpaste, burdock concentrate, soybean products, sea plants, dried *shiitake*, bonito fish flakes, *ume* products, whole grains, beans, *kuzu*, pearl barley, green and black teas, sea salt, *wasabi* powder, *tawashi* scrub brushes, 100% cotton cheesecloth, grain, seed, and coffee mills, graters, bamboo and wooden utensils, Japanese mortars, pestles, and cutlery.

The Mystic Trader
1334 Pacific Avenue
Forest Grove, OR
USA 97116
• Books, meditation supplies, incense, Ayurvedic medicine, and more.

Natural Lifestyle Supplies
16 Lookout Drive
Ashville, NC
USA 28804
• Macrobiotic ingredients and supplies.

Nature's Herb Company
281 Ellis Street
San Francisco, CA
USA 94102
• Herbs and supplies.

Neal's Yard Remedies
15 Neal's Yard
Covent Garden
London WC2
England
Tel: 071-379-7222
• A wonderful source for products, herbs, and oils used in beauty and for healing. A good selection of books, too.

L'Officina Profumo-Farmaceutica di Santa Maria Novella
Via della Scala, 16n
Firenze, Italia 50123
Tel: 55-21-62-76
• Perfumes and potions originally formulated by alchemist-monks in the Middle Ages, with elegant and arcane remedies for everything from thinning hair to hysteria.

Ohsawa America
440 Valley Drive
Brisbance, CA
USA 94005
Tel: 800-475-3663
• Manufacturer of high-quality traditional, organic Japanese foods and macrobiotic items.

Organic Foods Express
11003 Emack Road
Beltsville, MD

USA 20705
Tel: 301-937-8608
• Fresh organic produce, reasonable prices. Carries *daikon*. Also offers oils, grains, seeds and nuts, flours, and other natural food items.

Paul's Grains
Rt. 1, Box 76
Laurel, IA
USA 50141
Tel: 515-476-3373
• High-quality, pesticide-free grains, flours, and bran.

Penn Herb Company
603 North 2nd Street
Philadelphia, PA
USA 19123
• Herbs.

Pyramid Books and the New Age Collection
P.O. Box 3333, Altid Park
Chelmsford, MA
USA 01824-0933
• Books, aromatherapy oils, New Age accoutrements.

San Francisco Herb and Natural Food Company
P.O. Box 40604
San Francisco, CA
USA 94103
—and—
113 Alder Street
West Babylon, NY
USA 11704
• Herbs.

Red Rose Collection
P.O. Box 280140
San Francisco, CA
USA 94128-0140
• Books, bath/body products, spirit-oriented items of every description.

Shojin Natural Foods
Bhagavan Buritz
P.O. Box 669
Captain Cook, HI
USA 96704
• Natural foods, organic items, herbs.

Star Herb Company
38 Miller Avenue
Mill Valley, CA
USA 94941
• Herbs and essential oils.

Starflower
885 McKinley Street
Eugene, OR
USA 97402
• Natural foods, organic items, herbs.

Steamboat Oriental Foods
P.O. Box 452
Bradford, West Yorkshire
England BD4 7TF
- Mail order in the UK for foods fresh and pre-served.

United Communications
Box 320
Woodmere, NY
USA 11598
- Detailed herb guide.

Walnut Acres
Walnut Acres Road
Penns Creek, PA
USA 17862
Tel: 800-433-3998 / 717-837-0601
- Organic and natural foods: whole grains, flours, high-quality oils, garlic capsules, kelp granules, molasses, honey, rice bran, and coffee, grain, and spice mills.

Whole Earth Access Company
Mail Order Department
2950 Seventh Street
Berkeley, CA
USA 94710
- A wide selection of food-preparation supplies and utensils.

Wide World of Herbs Ltd.
11 Saint Catherine Street East
Montreal 129
Quebec, Canada
- A wide selection of unusual herbs and essential oils.

Williams-Sonoma
Catalog for Cooks
Mail-Order Department
P.O. Box 7456
San Francisco, CA
USA 94120-7456
- A wide selection of food-preparation supplies and utensils. Imported and unusual items.

For bathtime background music, the following companies offer traditional Japanese *koto* and *shakuhachi* music on tape.

Folkways Records
632 Broadway
New York, NY
USA 10012

Music of the World
P.O. Box 258
Brooklyn, NY
USA 11209

mail-order sources for seeds and live plants

Many of the Asian vegetables and herbs may be successfully grown from seed in other areas of the world. The following Western seed suppliers offer catalogs.

Borchelt Herb Gardens
474 Carriage Shop Road
East Falmouth, MA
USA 02536
- Organic herb seeds.

Carl Odom
Pinola, MS
USA 39149
- Seeds.

Folklore Herb Company/Sanctuary Seeds
2388 West 4th Avenue
Vancouver, B.C.
CANADA V6K 1P1
- Medicinal herb seeds and vegetable seeds.

Harry E. Saier
Dimondale, MI
USA 48821
- Loofah seeds and many more.

Le Marché Seeds International
P.O. Box 566
Dixon, CA
USA 95620
- Baby-vegetable seeds and new/exotic food seeds.

Meadowbrook Herb Garden
Route 138
Wyoming, RI
USA 02898
- Herbs and herb seeds.

Nicols Garden Nursery
1190 N. Pacific Highway
Albany, OR
USA 97321
• Large selection of vegetable and herb seeds.

Richters
P.O. Box 26
Goodwood, Ontario
Canada L0C 1A0
• Herb seeds.

Taylor's Herb Gardens
1535 Lone Oak Road
Vista, CA
USA 92083
• Herbs and herb seeds.

Well-Sweep Herb Farm
317 Mt. Bethel Road
Port Murray, NJ
USA 07865
• Large selection of plants and seeds, rare herbs and flowers.

A World Seed Service
J.L. Hudson, Seedsman
P.O. Box 1058
Redwood City, CA
USA 94064
• Rare seeds from everywhere.

Further information on seed and live plant sources may be obtained by consulting the following directories:

Directory of Seed and Nursery Catalogs
National Gardening Association
180 Flynn Avenue
Burlington, VT
USA 05401

Seed, Bulb, and Nursery Supplies
Rodale's Organic Gardening Reader Service
33 East Minor Street
Emmaus, PA
USA 18049

retail sources for ingredients & supplies

The following list is a Western (America and England) potpourri of Japanese and Oriental food markets, natural foods stores, art supply stores, import stores, beauty goods stores, herb stores, and a Japanese department store or two.

UNITED STATES

ALABAMA

Oriental Super Market #1
3480 Springhills Avenue
Mobile 36608

ARIZONA

Crystal Castle
313 Highway 179
Sedona 86336
Tel: 602-282-5910
• Aromatherapy oils and other products.

Oriental Food Store
408 West Main
Jacksonville 72076

CALIFORNIA

Amsterdam Art
1013 University Avenue
Berkeley 94710
Tel: 415-548-9663

Bath & Body Works
Beverly Center
Beverly & La Cienega Blvds.
W. Hollywood 90048
• Natural beauty products, utensils, books.

Chinese Vegetable Center
709 N. Hill Street
Los Angeles 90012

Enbun
Japanese Village Plaza
1st St. & Central Ave.
Little Tokyo

Los Angeles 90012
Tel: 213-680-3280
• A wonderful Japanese market.

Erewhon Natural Foods
7660 Beverly Boulevard
Fairfax, District
Los Angeles 90036
Tel: 213-937-0777
• Top-quality natural foods.

Felton International Inc.
2242 Purdue Avenue
Los Angeles 90064
• Aromatics and essential oils.

Fillamento
2185 Fillmore Street
San Francisco 94115
• "Lifestyle" items and bath goods.

Fred Segal Essentials/ Fred Segal Scentiments
Fred Segal Santa Monica
500 Broadway
Santa Monica 90401
Tel: 310-458-3766
• Best of everything from all over the world for beauty.

Hathaway Allied Products
24002 Frampton Avenue
Harbor City 90710
• Herbs.

International Market
2019 Fillmore Street
San Francisco 94115
• Imported foods.

Kabuki Gifts and Imports
11355 Santa Monica Boulevard
West Los Angeles 90025
Tel: 213-477-2663

Kinokuniya
1581 Webster Street
San Francisco 94115
Tel: 415-567-7625
• Books and imports from Japan.

Macro Grocery
1050 40th Street
Oakland 94608
Tel: 415-653-6510

Mrs. Gooch's
239 N. Crescent Drive
Beverly Hills 90210
Tel: 310-274-3360
• High standards of purity in the products sold here.

Nowhere Natural Food Market
8001 Beverly Boulevard
Fairfax District
Los Angeles 90036
Tel: 213-658-6506

Oriental Grocery
418 Island Avenue
San Diego 92101

Pacific Supermarket
1620 W. Redondo Beach Boulevard
Gardena 90247
Tel: 310-323-7696
—and—
3030 W. Sepulveda Boulevard
Torrance 90505
Tel: 310-539-8899
• The largest Japanese market in the U.S., with products from all other Asian countries, too.

Sanwa Market
2122 Cabrillo Street
San Francisco 94121
• Oriental foods.

Shu Uemura Beauty Boutique
Century City Shopping Center
10250 Santa Monica Boulevard
Century City 90067
Tel: 310-284-8214
• Great skin-care and beauty tools, and make-up.

Sunflower Natural Foods
821 41st Avenue
Santa Cruz 90670

Superior Trading Company
867 Washington Street
San Francisco 94108
• Ginseng.

Thom's Natural Food
843 Clement Street
San Francisco 94118

COLORADO

Alfalfa's Market
1645 Broadway
Boulder 80302
Tel: 303-442-0909
• Comprehensive store with good Japanese selection, beauty and bath, fresh produce, books.

Essence
2080 Broadway (c/o The Upstairs)
Boulder 80302
Tel: 800-551-0701
• Custom fragrances, aromatherapy, and bath and body products.

Pacific Mercantile Grocery
1925 Lawrence Street
Denver 80202

Total Beauty Center
Upper Level, Village Inn Plaza
Vail 81657
Tel: 303-476-5933
• Beauty care and products of highest quality.

CONNECTICUT

East/West Trading Company
68 Howe Street
New Haven 00511
• Oriental foods.

Elysian Fields
5 Main Street
New Preston 06777
Tel: 203-868-7711
—and—
190 Main Street
Westport 06880
Tel: 203-226-2566
• A treasure trove of some of the best herbal skin-care and bath procuts.

En Avant
66 Railroad Street
New Milford 06776
Tel: 203-355-6907
• Beauty treatments.

Karel Art Materials
737 Canal Street
Stamford 06902
Tel: 203-348-8996

Kenko Natural
Kent-Cornwall Road
Kent, Litchfield County
Tel: 203-927-4079
• Natural foods.

KIRI Japanese Grocery, Inc.
35 Wilkes Road
Danbury 06811
Tel: 203-746-4591
Fax: 203-746-0826
• Everything Japanese, for home delivery only.

New Morning Country Store
15 Hollow Road
Woodbury 06798
Tel: 203-263-4868
• Wonderful Japanese and natural foods source.

DELAWARE

Newark Co-Op Natural Foods
280 East Main Street
Newark 19711
Tel: 302-368-5894

FLORIDA

Body Maintenance
1231 Washington Avenue
Miami
Tel: 800-428-0330
• Aromatherapy products.

Bread of Life Natural Food Market & Restaurant
2250 Wilton Drive
Fort Lauderdale 33305
Tel: 305-563-TOFU

Oriental Market
1202 S. Dale Mabry Highway
Tampa 33609

Shimmy
415 Española Way
Miami
Tel: 305-673-3523
• Fragrances and beauty products.

Sybara
762 Washington Avenue
Miami
Tel: 305-534-2346
• Scent in every form.

The Granary Whole Foods
1738 Kingsley Avenue
Orange Park 32073
Tel: 904-269-7222

GEORGIA

Makoto
1067 Oaktree Road
Decatur 30033
• Oriental foods.

Unity Natural Foods
2915 Peachtree Road
Atlanta 30305
Tel: 404-261-8776

IDAHO

Yuko's Gift
688 N. Holmes Avenue
Idaho Falls 83401
• Imports and Oriental foods.

ILLINOIS

Aiko's Art Materials Import
714 North Wabash Avenue
Chicago 60611
Tel: 312-943-0745

Ginza & Co.
315 E. University
Champaign 61820
• Oriental foods.

Herbarium, Inc.
2019 West Iowa Street
Chicago 60622
• Herbs.

Sherwyn's Health Food
645 W. Diversey
Chicago 60614
Tel: 312-477-1934

INDIANA

Asia Oriental Market
2400 Yeager Road
W. Lafayette 47906

IOWA

Tokyo Foods
1005 Pierce Street
Sioux City 51105

KANSAS

Sane Grains Natural Food Market
2900 E. Central
Wichita 67214
Tel: 316-684-3808

LOUISIANA

Belladonna
1720 St. Charles Avenue
New Orleans 70130
Tel: 504-581-6759
• Bath, beauty, and fragrance.

Oriental Merchandise Company
2636 Edenborn Avenue
Metairie 70002
• Oriental foods.

MARYLAND

Far East House
33 W. North Avenue
Baltimore 21201
• Oriental foods.

Organic Foods Express
12050 Parklawn Drive
Rockville 20852
Tel: 301-816-4944

MASSACHUSETTS

Always Natural
Dean's Plaza, Route 44
407 New State Highway
Raynham 02767
Tel: 617-823-9410

Aveline's Natural Food Store
42 Park Street (Route 20)
Lee 01238

Bread & Circus
15 Westland Avenue
Boston 02115
Tel: 617-375-1010
• Natural foods supermarket with well-stocked health and beauty section.

Colonial Drug
49 Brattle Street
Cambridge 02138
Tel: 617-864-2222
• Fragrances, with more than 500 essences in stock.

Fresh
121 Newbury Street
Boston 02116
Tel: 617-421-1212
• Fragrances, soaps, potpourri.

North Star Natural Foods
6 Monument Square
Leominster 01453
Tel: 617-537-4062

Organic Food Cellar
297a Newbury Street
Boston 02115

Yoshinoya
36 Prospect Street
Cambridge 02139

MICHIGAN

Harvest Health, Inc.
1944 Eastern Avenue
S.E., Grand Rapids 49507

Mt. Fuji Oriental Foods
22040 West 10 Mile
Southfield 48075

MINNESOTA

International House
75 W. Island Avenue
Minneapolis 55401
• Oriental foods.

Tao Natural Foods
2200 DuPont Avenue South
Minneapolis 55405
Tel: 612-377-4630

MISSOURI

Kim's Mart
6692 Enright
St. Louis 63130
• Oriental foods.

NEBRASKA

Oriental Market
611 N. 27th Street
Lincoln 68503

NEVADA

Tokyo-Plaza Shopping Center
3344 Kietzke Lane
Reno 89502

NEW JERSEY

The Health Shoppe
Midtown Shopping Center
66 Morris Street
Morristown 07960
Tel: 201-538-9131

Meer Corporation
North Bergen 07047
• Herbs and essential oils.

Miyako Oriental Foods
490 Main Street
Ft. Lee 07024

Yaohan Plaza
595 River Road
Edgewater 07020
Tel: 201-941-9113
• Everything Japanese under the sun! Almost like being there....

NEW MEXICO

Five Eggs–Everything Japanese
213 West San Francisco
Santa Fe 87501
Tel: 505-986-3403
• No food, but an exquisite selection of Japanese "lifestyle" items, like *tenugui*, teapots, and *tabi*. Owner Elaine McKay is happy to accept phone orders, to ship anywhere in the U.S.

Ten Thousand Waves
Hyde Park Road
Santa Fe 87504
Tel: 505-986-3403
• A wonderful Japanese-style spa with a full range of treatments, baths, and massage. A retail shop offers Japanese items and beauty products.

Wild Oats Market
1090 South St. Francis Drive
Santa Fe 87501
Tel: 505-983-5333
• Natural beauty and health products.

Yonemoto Bros.
8725 Fourth Street N.W.
Albuquerque 87114
• Oriental foods.

NEW YORK

Angelica's
147 First Avenue
New York 10003
Tel: 212-677-1549
• Herbs and spices.

Barneys New York
Barneys Apothecary
111 Seventh Avenue
New York 10011
—and—
61st & Madison Avenue
New York 10021
Tel: 212-929-9000
• The best in natural beauty from everywhere.

Boyd Chemists
655 Madison Avenue
New York 10021
• Wide selection of beauty supplies, brushes, sponges.

Carapan
5 West 16th Street
New York 10011
Tel: 212-633-6220
• A day spa with a shop: come here for any type of massage, Ayurvedic facials, aromatherapy,

shiatsu, and to buy books and beauty and health supplies.

Commodities (Biological Cultures)
117 Hudson Street
New York 10013
Tel: 212-334-8330
• Natural foods and supplies of every description

Devachan Salon & Spa
558 Broadway 2nd Floor
New York 10012
Tel: 212-274-8686
• No products, but an extraordinary East/West atmosphere in which to have hair cut or colored, aromatherapy, facials, and massage.

Erbe
196 Prince Street
New York 10012
Tel: 212-966-1445/ 800-432-ERBE
• Italian aromatherapy supplies, herbal beauty products and treatments.

Katagiri Company
224 East 59th Street
New York 10022
• Extensive selection of Japanese foods and supplies.

Kiehl Pharmacy
109 Third Avenue
New York 10003
• Herbs, essential oils, ingredients for making cosmetics.

New York Central Art Supply
62 3rd Avenue
New York 10003
• Rice paper, brushes.

New York Open Center Bookstore
83 Spring Street
New York 10012
Tel: 212-219-2527 ext.108
• A bookstore specializing in holistic learning and East-West topics.

Pearl River Mart
277 Canal Street
New York 10013
Tel: 212-431-4770
—and—
200 Grand Street
New York 10013
Tel: 212-966-1010
• A Chinese department store.

Rising Tide Natural Market
42 Forest Avenue
Glen Cove 11542
Tel: 516-676-7895

Takashimaya Department Store
693 Fifth Avenue
New York 10022
Tel: 212-350-0100
• Exquisite offerings from East and West, and a great bath/body department. High-quality teas.

Zen Oriental Bookstore
521 5th Avenue
New York 10175
Tel: 212-697-0840
—and—
115 W. 57th Street
New York 10019
Tel: 212-582-4622
• Imports and books.

NORTH CAROLINA

Asia Market
1325 Buck Jones Road
Raleigh 27606

OHIO

Brighter Day Natural Foods
Number 10, Tiber Way
Marietta 45750
Tel: 614-374-2429

Health Plus
4428 Milan Road
Sandusky 44870
Tel: 419-625-9149

Doc Heben's Heath Foods
11841 Detroit Avenue
Lakewood 44107
Tel: 216-529-9170

Soya Food Products, Inc.
2356 Wyoming Avenue
Cincinnati 45214
• Oriental foods.

OKLAHOMA

Japan Imported Foods
808 N.W. 6th Street
Oklahoma City 73106

OREGON

Ashland Community Food Store
37 3rd Street
Ashland 97520
Tel: 503-482-2237
• Organic, natural, macrobiotic foods.

Fred Meyers
7404 N. Interstate
Portland 97217
• Oriental foods.

Essene
719 South 4th Street
Philadelphia 19147
Tel: 215-922-1146
• Natural, organic, macrobiotic foods.

Haussman's Pharmacy
6th and Girard Avenue
Philadelphia 19127
• Herbs.

Imported Food Bazaar
2000 Market Street
Camp Hill 17011

RHODE ISLAND

East Sea Oriental Market
90-92 Warren Avenue
E. Providence 02914

SOUTH CAROLINA

Chieko Hardy
226 Jamaica Street
Columbia 29206
• Oriental foods.

SOUTH DAKOTA

Kitty's Oriental Food
P.O. Box 347
Box Elder 57719

TENNESSEE

Park & Shop Oriental
3664 Summer Avenue
Memphis 38122

TEXAS

Ault Bee Farms
Weslaco 78596
• Honey and aloe vera.

Good Food Store
1101 West 5th Street
Austin 78703
• Natural foods.

Japanese Grocery
14366-B Memorial Drive
Houston 77079

UTAH

Whole Earth Natural Foods
1026 2nd Avenue
Salt Lake City 84103

VIRGINIA

Tokyo Market
5312 Va. Beach Boulevard
Virginia Beach 23462

WASHINGTON

Umajimaya
519 6th Avenue South
Seattle 98104
• Oriental foods.

WASHINGTON, D. C.

Mikado
4709 Wisconsin Avenue NW
20016

WISCONSIN

Herbarium
Kenosha 53140

International House of Foods
440 West Gorham Street
Madison 53704

Outpost Natural Foods Co-Op
3500 North Holton Street
Milwaukee 53212
Tel: 414-961-2597

UNITED KINGDOM

Ajiro
27 Endell Street
London WC2
Tel: 071-240-6843
• Japanese foods.

Bushwacker Whole Foods
59 Goldhawk Road
Shepherds Bush
London W12 8EG
• Retailer of Japanese health foods.

City Herbs
Unit 28
Spitalfields Market
London E1
Tel: 071-247-4721
• Exotic fruits and vegetables, herbs and spices.

Clearspring Natural Grocer
196 Old Street
London EC1V 9BP
Tel: 071-250-1708
• Retailer and distributor of Japanese health foods in UK.

East West Herb Shop
3 Neal's Yard
London WC2
• Herbs.

Emporium Mercurius
291 Portobello Road
London W10
• Herbs and oils.

Green Farm Nutrition Centre
Burwash Common
East Sussex TN19 7LX
• Health foods.

JA Centre
348-356 Regents Park Road
London N3
Tel: 081-346-1042
• Huge selection of Japanese foods, including fresh produce.

Japan Centre
66-68 Brewer Street

London W1
Tel: 071-439-8035
• Japanese goods of all kinds.

Japan Foods
373-375 Uxbridge Road
London W3
Tel: 081-752-0212

Mysteries
9/11 Monmouth Street
London WC2
• Fragrances and oils, bath and beauty products.

New World Aurora
16a Neal's Yard
London WC2
• Oils and fragrances.

Ninjin Food Shop
244 Great Portland Street
London W1
Tel: 071-388-2511
• Japanese foods.

Wong Singh Jones
253 Portobello Road
London W11
• Incense.

Yoshino
15 Monkville Parade
Finchley Road
London NW11
Tel: 081-209-0966
• Delivers Japanese items anywhere in the UK.

suppliers, importers, manufacturers & distributors

The following companies may be contacted directly for information on the availability of their product lines.

UNITED STATES

high-quality natural japanese foods

Eden Foods
701 Tecumseh Road
Clinton, Michigan 49236
Tel: 517-456-7424
• Lima, Muso, and Eden brands.

Erewhon, Inc.
5 Waltham Street
Wilmington, Massachusetts 01887
Tel: 617-657-8120

Granum
2901 NE Blakely Street
Seattle, Washington 98105
Tel: 206-525-0051
• Mitoku products.

Great Eastern Sun
92 MacIntosh Road
Asheville, North Carolina 28806
Tel: 704-258-1821
• Mitoku products.

Edward & Sons
Box 3150
Union, New Jersey 07083
Tel: 201-964-8176

Imagine Foods, Inc.
299 California Avenue #305
Palo Alto, California 94306
Tel: 415-327-1444

Mount Ark
120 S. East Street
Fayetteville, Arkansas 72701
Tel: 800-643-8909

Nasoya Foods, Inc.
23 Jytek Drive
Leominster, Massachusetts 01453
Tel: 617-537-0713

Oak Feed Store
3030 Grand Avenue
Coconut Grove, Florida 33133
Tel: 305-448-7595

Ohsawa America
P.O. Box 12717
Northgate Station
San Rafael, California 94913
Tel: 800-647-2929

San-J International
384 Liberty
San Francisco, California 94114
Tel: 415-821-4040

Tree of Life, Inc.
P.O. Box 410, 315 Industrial Street
St. Augustine, Florida 32084
Tel: 904-824-8181

21st Century Foods, Inc.
30A Germania Street
Jamaica Plain, Massachusetts 02130

U.S. Mills, Inc.
395 Elliot Street
Newton Upper Falls, Massachusetts 02164
Tel: 617-969-5400

Usagiya Natural Foods
5711 37th Avenue, N.E.
Seattle, Washington 98105
Tel: 206-526-8173

Westbrae Natural Foods
4240 Hollis Street

Emeryville, California 94608
Tel: 415-658-7521

supplies

Nippon Kodo, Inc.
630 5th Avenue
New York, New York 10020
Tel: 212-581-2145
• Japanese incense.

Shoyeido Corporation
1700 38th Street, Suite 101
Boulder, CO 80301
Tel: 1-800-786-5476
• Japanese incense.

Shu Uemura USA Inc.
1901 Avenue of the Stars, Suite 582
Los Angeles, California 90067
Tel: 213-284-8854/8857
• Japanese Shu Uemura beauty products, cos-
  metics, utensils. Superb cosmetics brushes.

Truc International, Inc.
Box 167
Woodstock Hill, Connecticut 06281
• Bath accessories.

UNITED KINGDOM

high-quality natural japanese foods

Clearspring Unit 19A
Acton Park Estate
London W3 7QE
Tel: 081-749-1781
Fax: 081-746-2259

Felmore Limited
1 Lamberts Road
P.O. Box 1
Tunbridge Wells
Kent TN2 3EQ
Tel: 0892-34143
• Health publications, information on retail sources
  for health foods.

Kushi Institute
188 Old Street
London EC1V 9BP
• Macrobiotic center, information on sources for
  Japanese health foods.

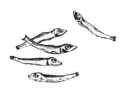

Sunwheel Foods Ltd.
Dukesway
Team Valley
Gateshead
Tyne and Wear NE11 0QP
Tel: 091-482-2611
• Distributor of Japanese health foods in the UK.

The Soil Association
86 Colston Street
Bristol BS21 5BB
Tel: 0272-290-661
• Publications listing organic food suppliers.

sources in japan

retail & mail-order sources for ingredients & supplies

Almost everything mentioned in this book may be easily obtained in Japan at the local food market, with a stop at the corner drugstore for specialty items. However, for those who wish to seek out the very best of everything, the following addresses may be useful.

foods, herbs, & supplies

Aroma Terrace
3-1-7 Ekoda
Hanmoku Azamino-ten 2F
Midori-ku, Yokohama
Kanagawa 225
Tel: 045-903-3134
• Along with a wide selection of herbs and related products, including Maurice Mességué's *tisanes* from France, this shop has a tearoom where herbal teas may be leisurely sipped. Open 10:30–7:00 daily except every third Wednesday.

Charis Seijo
Seijo 5-15-15
Setagaya-ku, Tokyo 157
Tel: 03-3483-1960
• Retailer-wholesaler of herbs, essential oils, and very special botanical products, with an herb garden, a restaurant, and aromatherapy classes among its offerings. Open 10:00–6:00 daily.

Culpeper House
3-6-20 Kita Aoyama
Minato-ku, Tokyo 107
Tel: 03-3486-8763
• Culpeper aromatherapy oils may be found here, along with a myriad other products. Open 11:00–7:30 daily. Also a branch in Ginza near Hotel Seiyo.

Dai-ichi Busan
Efuku 1-7-8
Suginami-ku, Tokyo 182
Tel: 03-3325-4861
• Organic foods retailer-wholesaler with shops all over Japan.

Herb Island
Odoro 255
Otaki-machi, Isumi-gun
Chiba-ken 298
Tel: 0470-82-2789
• Mail-order fresh and dried herbs, essential oils, herb seeds. There's a retail outlet and adjoining café in Shinjuku.

Mitoku Co., Ltd.
2-4-1 Marunouchi
Chiyoda-ku, Tokyo 100
Tel: 03-3201-6709
Fax: 03-3201-6709
• Mitoku offers to Japan residents a mail-order service of its high-quality traditional foods, all produced naturally. The company also carries such items as Katana knives and eggplant toothpaste.

Muso Co., Ltd.
Tanimachi 2-5-5
Chuo-ku, Osaka 540
Tel: 06-942-0343
Fax: 06-941-4760
• Produces traditional macrobiotic foods.

Natural House
3-6-18 Kita Aoyama
Minato-ku, Tokyo 107
Tel: 03-3498-2277
• Open from 10:00 to 10:00 daily, this retail store carries a wide selection of natural, traditional foods, supplies, and its own line of beauty products.

New Age Center
3-22-11 Jingumae
Shibuya-ku, Tokyo 150

Tel: 03-3470-5181
- Incense, oils, books, music, crystals, etc. Open 11:00–8:00 daily.

Nova
Kitamoto
Nakamaru 3-3-5
Saitama-ken 364
Tel: 0485-92-6491
- Organic foods.

San Francisco
17-5 Daikanyama
Shibuya-ku, Tokyo 150
Tel: 03-3463-0938
- The '60s reborn in '90s Tokyo, complete with potent Indian incense and love beads. Open 12:00–8:00, closed on Mondays.

Seikatsu no Ki
6-3-8 Jingumae
Shibuya-ku, Tokyo 150
Tel: 03-3409-1781
- A great selection of herbal products from Japan and elsewhere. Open 10:30–8:00 daily.

Shizenha Network
3570 Yatabe
Tsukuba-shi 305
Ibaraki-ken
Tel: 0298-37-0909
- Farming cooperative with synthetic-fertilizer-free produce.

Taneyama Ga Hara
Kotobuki 2-9-1
Taito-ku, Tokyo 111
Tel: 03-3842-2948
- Organic foods importer, natural fleece producer, wholesaler, distributor.

Yamamoto-Yama
2-52 Nihonbashi
Chuo-ku, Tokyo 103
Tel: 03-3271-3361
- A tea shop established in 1690, this shop is famous for its high-quality teas. Open 9:30–6:00 daily.

beauty items, cosmetics, & utensils

The Body & Bath Shop
Harajuku Kokun Bldg. 1F
5-7-5 Jingumae
Shibuya-ku, Tokyo 175
Tel: 03-3498-3618
- A wonderful selection of imported and Japanese products, all beautifully packaged. The Les Floralies products are available here. Open 11:00–8:00 daily.

Hyakusuke
2-2-14 Asakusa
Taito-ku, Tokyo 111
Tel: 03-3841-7058
- This is the only traditional make-up store left in Tokyo. Hyakusuke carries all the traditional products for skin care, beautiful traditional brushes, hair ornaments, Kabuki make-up. Open 11:00–5:00 approximately, this shop occasionally closes on Tuesdays.

Shu Uemura Beauty Boutique
5-1-3 Jingumae
Shibuya-ku, Tokyo 150
Tel: 03-3486-0048
- Open from 10:00 to 8:00 daily, this amazing shop is set up like a self-service cafeteria, with try-out counters for the hundreds of colors of make-up products, and elegant black trays upon which to pile one's choices. The brushes and beauty utensils are superb!

Yonoya
1-37-10 Asakusa
Taito-ku, Tokyo 111
Tel: 03-3844-1755
- The shop for traditional wooden combs and hair ornaments, open 10:00 to 7:00, closed Wednesdays.

incense

Kyukyodo
5-7-4 Ginza
Chuo-ku, Tokyo 104
Tel: 03-3571-4429
- Incense, brushes, rice paper. Open 10:00 to 8:00, except Sundays and holidays, when it's 11:00 to 7:00.

tenugui towels

Fujiya Tenuguiten
2-2-15 Asakusa
Taito-ku, Tokyo 111
Tel: 03-3841-2283
- A wide selection of cotton *tenugui* towels. Open 9:00 to 8:00, closed Thursdays.

tea ceremony utensils

Ryuzendo
5-8-6 Ginza
Chuo-ku, Tokyo 104
Tel: 03-3571-4321
- All tea ceremony items are carried here; this is the place to buy a bamboo tea whisk. Open 10:00 to 8:00, closed the third Sunday of each month.

stone, paper, scissors … & brushes

Gyokusendo
3-3 Jimbocho
Kanda
Chiyoda-ku, Tokyo 101
Tel: 03-3264-3741
- Beautiful brushes, inkstones. 9:00 to 7:00, closed on Sundays and holidays.

Haibara
2-7-6 Nihonbashi
Chuo-ku, Tokyo 103
Tel: 03-3272-3801
- Rice paper, handmade paper of all kinds. Open 9:30 to 5:30, 5:00 on Saturdays, closed Sundays and holidays.

Isetatsu
2-18-9 Yanaka
Taito-ku, Tokyo 110
Tel: 03-3823-1453
- Open 10:00–6:00 every day, this shop sells beautiful handmade paper.

Kiya
3-44-8 Yushima
Bunkyo-ku, Tokyo 113
Tel: 03-3831-8688
- A store for handmade paper and wonderful brushes, open 9:00–6:30, closed on Mondays.

Kiya
1-8 Muromachi
Nihonbashi
Chuo-ku, Tokyo 103
Tel: 03-3241-0111

- A store for stunning knives and scissors, open 10:00 to 5:30, 12:30 to 5:30 on Sundays and holidays.

Ubukeya
3-4 Ningyocho
Nihonbashi
Chuo-ku, Tokyo 103
Tel: 03-3661-4851
- Knives and scissors. Open 9:00 to 7:00, until 6:00 on Saturdays, closed Sundays and holidays.

Washikobo
1-8-10 Nishi Azabu
Minato-ku, Tokyo 106
Tel: 03-3405-1841
- A great handmade-paper store, open 10:00 to 6:00, closed Sundays and holidays.

wooden things

Hiratsuka
9-7-6 Ginza
Chuo-ku, Tokyo 104
Tel: 03-3571-1684
- Traditional chests made of paulownia wood. Open 10:00 to 7:00, closed on Sundays.

Ito-Oke-Ten
2-4-6 Tatekawa
Sumida-ku, Tokyo 130
Tel: 03-3633-7108
- Traditional cypress bath buckets, scoops, and basins. Open 8:00 to 5:00, closed on Sundays and holidays.

japanese natural/traditional cosmetics companies

There are many, many Japanese companies manufacturing products that contain traditional, natural ingredients. Following is a small sampling of some of these companies.

Clover Sekken Co., Ltd.
Kanro 2-1-4
Higashinari-ku, Osaka-shi
- Produces soaps and shampoos using seaweed, aloe, carrot extracts.

Hechima Colon Co., Inc.
Nakajima Isseido Co., Inc.

5-bancho 12
Chiyoda-ku, Tokyo
- Produces loofah-vine water, other loofah products, *azuki* bean powder scrub.

House of Rose Co., Inc.
Kita Aoyama 2-14-6
Minato-ku, Tokyo

- Produces many lines of skin care products, one of which is Kazusaya Kichibei, based on traditional recipes: loofah-vine water, cucumber water, pine water, horsetail water, black sugar and honey soaps, camellia oil shampoo, perfumed oil, hot-spring bath salts, rice bran soap, camellia oil. The company also markets pearl barley tea.

Meishoku Co.
Momoya-Juntenkan Co., Inc.
Cosmo Products Co., Inc.
Ichioka 2-4-30
Minato-ku, Osaka-shi
- A large company with many product lines, its Momotani Juntenkan line includes *azuki* bean powder and scrubbing bags. Products in other lines contain seaweed, apricot kernel, St. Johnswort, green tea, aloe, honey, shark's liver oil, safflower, chestnut.

Mimiran
Biyou-Bunka Co., Inc.
1-218, Takane-cho
Seto, Aichi
Tel: 0561-84-1433
- This is the best company for pure, natural, high-quality traditional treatments. They raise bush warblers for their prized droppings, and produce not only bush warbler droppings but powdered *kombu* and *funori* hair treatment, rice bran, rice bran bags, bean powder, cucumber water, loofah vine water, camellia oil, and creams and lotions containing pearl barley, rice germ oil, leaf chlorophyll. An old-fashioned treasure of a company.

Oshima Tsubaki Co.
Hamamatsucho 1-23-4
Minato-ku, Tokyo 105

Tel: 03-3438-3039
- Carries 100% pure camellia oil, camellia oil soap, camellia oil treatment shampoo. High quality.

Sunstar Co.
Asahimachi 3-1
Takatsuki-shi, Osaka 569
- A giant company, Sunstar produces many varieties of bath salts, some containing *yuzu* or *mikan* (tangerine).

Tsumurajuntendo Co.
Nihonbashi 3-4-10
Chuo-ku, Tokyo
- Produces hot-spring bath salts.

Yuen Cosmetics
Tokyo Branch
Casa Morii, 1F
3-2-11 Azabudai
Minato-ku, Tokyo 106
Tel: 03-3584-3468
- Produces high-quality products without mineral oil, alcohol, or added fragrance or color. Their natural, hypoallergenic products were developed by dermatologists for the treatment of post-cosmetic-surgery patients and patients with skin problems. Yuen products include such ingredients as algae extract, mulberry root, licorice root, and a variety of botanical extracts. The company produces an *azuki*-and-salt exfoliating scrub.

Yuzu Co., Inc.
Uwanakajima 27
Hanawa Aza
Kazuno-shi, Akita-ken
- This company produces a black sugar soap that also contains wheat germ oil and honey.

western natural cosmetics lines available in japan

Kiehl's
Sony Plaza
6-8-5 Ginza
Chuo-ku, Tokyo
TEl: 03-3575-2604

Neal's Yard
Living Motif
Axis Bldg. 1F
5-17-1 Roppongi

Minato-ku, Tokyo
Tel: 03-3587-2784
- This line is also available at Seibu's Loft outlets.

Sisley
5-4-2 Roppongi
Minato-ku, Tokyo
Tel: 03-3404-3959

japan beauty & health-care resources & services

Salon beauty-care is a fast-moving field; there's always something new to try. More and more, avant-garde beauty treatments combine luxuriousness with efficacy, sensual appeal with high-tech action. Tokyo offers the opportunity to experience cutting-edge technology applied to the art of feminine beauty. And for those who seek beauty treatments based on traditional or natural botanical substances, Chinese herbal medicine, or *tsubo* stimulation via massage or other means, there is no place like Tokyo.

Alexandra Nishiki, facial fitness specialist
Tel: 0422-46-0868 or Fax: 0422-48-0850
- Alexandra's imported beauty treatments always include the latest from New York and Paris. Acid peels (enzyme, glycolic, pumpkin, salycylic, Modified Jessnor's); body wraps; aromatherapy massage; oxygen treatments; electrocosmetologic treatments; Parisian Body Polish with crushed pearls; Liposomal facials; products by Catherine Atzen, Eva, Tissue Research, and Essensa. Alexandra is a specialist in skin rejuvenation, facial toning, and problem skin; she speaks English and Japanese.

Akahigedo Clinic
Nasu Bldg. 2F
1-38-8 Yoyogi
Shibuya-ku, Tokyo 151
Tel: 03-3370-5013
- A doctor of traditional medicine, Nobuyuki Takeuchi offers treatment based on *shiatsu* and acupuncture, herbal medicine, and a carefully monitored diet. As well, students are accepted for instruction in the traditional healing methods. Instruction is in Japanese and English. Although long-term students generally participate full-time in clinic work, there are also short-term seminars offered occasionally as well as regular classes in *kikō* standing meditation.

André Bernard
Houraiya Bldg. 4F
5-2-1 Roppongi
Minato-ku, Tokyo
Tel: 03-3404-0616
- A hair salon that also offers facials, manicures, pedicures, waxing. Open 9:00–6:00, closed Sundays. English spoken.

Asakusa Kannon Onsen
2-7-26 Asakusa
Taito-ku, Tokyo
Tel: 03-3844-4141
- A 45° C/112° F sodium bicarbonate hot-spring bath in old downtown Tokyo. Open 6:30 to 6:30 daily.

Azabu Juban Onsen
1-5-22 Azabu Juban
Minato-ku, Tokyo
Tel: 03-3405-4670
- A communal hot-spring bath, open from 3:00 to 11:00, closed on Tuesdays. Sauna too.

Bain Douche
Lions Mansion Hanzomon 1F
1-5-4 Kojimachi
Chiyoda-ku, Tokyo
Tel: 03-3263-4944
- A modern communal bathhouse, open 4:00 to 10:30, closed Sundays and holidays.

Do Sports Plaza
Sumitomo Bldg. B1
2-1-6 Nishi-Shinjuku
Shinjuku-ku, Tokyo
Tel: 03-3344-1971
- Sauna and massage, 10:00–10:30, until 9:00 on Sundays and holidays.

Gaien
4-23-6 Sendagaya
Shibuya-ku, Tokyo
Tel: 03-3403-3206
- Sauna and massage from 10:00 to 11:00 daily.

Green Plaza Shinjuku
1-29-3 Kabukicho
Shinjuku-ku, Tokyo
Tel: 03-3207-5411
- Sauna and massage 24 hours a day, until 11:00 on Sundays.

Hagiya Medical Beauty Research Institute

(Biyo Igaku Kenkyujo)
Ewan Bldg.
Tayuji-machi 8-2
Kita-ku, Osaka 530
Tel: 06-314-0818/06-311-0458

• Connected to the Hagiya Cosmetic Surgery Clinic, this is the place to go for the ultimate makeover—a restructuring of face or body. There is also an in-house dental clinic, an esthetic salon where the excellent Yuen products are used, and health and beauty counselors to advise on nutrition, lifestyle, exercise, and skin care. Takashi Morigaki, a kind of guru in the beauty field, oversees the Hagiya-Yuen total beauty concept program. Hagiya's research and development labs combine explorations of new technology with a natural, botanically oriented approach to skin care. Mr. Morigaki's daughter, Chieko Weiler, may be contacted in English for further information on Yuen or Hagiya, Tokyo Tel: 03-3584-3468.

Hotel Okura Steam Bath

Hotel Okura, 1F
2-10-4 Toranomon
Minato-ku, Tokyo
Tel: 03-3582-0111

• Massage and steam bath, 10:00 to 9:00 daily, reservations needed.

Isukura Yakkyoku

Suns Bldg. 2F
1-7-2 Jingumae
Shibuya-ku, Tokyo
Tel: 03-3478-4382

• Chinese herbal medicine custom-prepared from 10:00 to 8:00, closed the third Monday of each month. Only Japanese spoken.

Japan Health and Research Institute

Tel: 03-3274-2861

• Information on hot springs cures.

Japan Health Development Foundation

(Nihon Kenko Kaihatsu Zaidan)
Tokyo-Yaesu Bldg.
1-4-20 Yaesu
Chuo-ku, Tokyo 103
Tel: 03-3274-607

• Information on the *kurhaus* system, a network of European-inspired Japanese health spa establishments: Kurhaus for day use, Kurbad hot-spring centers, Kurhotel lodging facilities at hot springs, Aquahaus thermal centers, and Health Farms designed for extended stays. Facilities vary, but may include a wide variety of baths and pools, medical supervision for a hot-spring cure, basic health counseling, relaxation facilities, sports-training facilities, nature walks,

massage, nutritional counseling, acupressure and massage, and esthetic salon care.

Kazuno Balance Esute Roppongi

3-18-12 Roppongi
Gettsu Bldg. 6F
Minato-ku, Tokyo
Tel: 03-5570-9088

• Uses Chinese *kikō* technique to stimulate facial *tsubo* for total body balancing and healthy skin. From 10:00 to 9:00, closed Sundays and holidays. Reservation needed.

Kojimachi Rebirth

Kurhaus Bldg. 2F
4-2-12 Kojimachi
Chiyoda-ku, Tokyo
Tel: 03-3262-7561

• Acupuncture by appointment, some English spoken. Massage and sauna also available. 10:00–9:00, closed Sundays.

Ladies Sauna

Isetan-Kaikan Bldg. 4F
3-15-17 Shinjuku
Shinjuku-ku, Tokyo
Tel: 03-3356-2734

• Sauna, body treatments, massage. Open 10:00–8:30, closed Wednesdays.

Kuniko Maeda's Aroma Treatment Room

5-5-1 Seijo
SETAGAYA-KU, TOKYO 157
Tel: 03-3483-8920

• Essential oil massage, *shiatsu*, and acupuncture.

Mirror Mirror Esthetique Salon

Jingu Mansion 3F
3-5-33 Kita Aoyama
Minato-ku, Tokyo
Tel: 03-3404-5852

• Waxing and other services done by English-speaking staff.

Nagai Yakkyoku

1-8-10 Azabu Juban
Minato-ku, Tokyo
Tel: 03-3583-3889

• Traditional natural Chinese and Japanese medicine, consultations and prescriptions, with some English spoken. 9:00 to 8:00, closed Tuesdays.

Nagai Yakkyoku Hifu Koso Biganshitsu

1-8-10 Azabu Juban 2F
Minato-ku, Tokyo
Tel: 03-3583-1393

• Natural skin care, Asian herbs used. Open 10:00 to 5:00, closed Tuesdays.

Otomi-Yu

2-14-4 Akasaka

Minato-ku, Tokyo
Tel: 03-3583-7424
- A traditional communal bath in a beautiful old building. 4:00 to 11:30, closed Sundays.

Paru Onsen
Okazaki Bldg. 2F
2-14-13 Shibuya
Shibuya-ku, Tokyo
Tel: 03-3409-4882
- Jacuzzi bath, *shiatsu*, massage, plus seaweed tea or calcium water to drink. 10:00 to 11:00, closed the third Tuesday of each month.

Pharmacy
13 Togensha Bldg. 1F
4-12-1 Roppongi
Minato-ku, Tokyo
Tel: 03-3404-1518/1519
- A Shu Uemura establishment, this is a pharmacy dedicated to beauty. A beauty specialist trained in traditional herbal medicine offers consultations, diagnoses, and prescriptions. The holistic approach treats beauty problems both internally and externally. Japanese health insurance covers the cost of the prescribed herbal medicine! Quiet music and a gentle all-women staff contribute to the atmosphere of harmonious beauty. Open 11:00 to 8:00, closed Sundays.

Pink Pearl
Palace Hotel B1
1-1-1 Marunouchi
Chiyoda-ku, Tokyo
Tel: 03-3211-6975
- Massage, oil massage, steam bath. 1:00 to 7:00, closed Sundays.

Mona Roberts, aromatherapist
Tel: 03-3485-2567
- Aromatherapy treatments and workshops in English.

Salon de Linn
6-33-14 Jingumae
Shibuya-ku, Tokyo
Tel: 03-3498-9330
- This salon uses natural ingredients and emphasizes gentle and thorough skin cleansing. Skin care for sensitive skin. From 10:00 to 6:00, closed Tuesdays. Reservation needed.

Sanwa Massage
Imperial Hotel 4F
1-1-1 Uchisaiwaicho
Chiyoda-ku, Tokyo
Tel: 03-3580-5549
- Massage, pressure shower. Open 10:00 to 9:00 daily.

Shiawase Kenko Club
Noguchi Bldg. 5F
3-2 Sakuragaoka
Shibuya-ku, Tokyo
Tel: 03-3496-6422
- Traditional Asian medicine, from 8:30 am with no specified closing time; closed Tuesdays, Fridays, holidays.

Shizen Bikenko Biyo Center
1-9-2 Kajicho
Chiyoda-ku, Tokyo
Tel: 03-3254-7281
- Utilizes the traditional facial *tsubo* stimulation to heal skin imbalances. Counseling and sales of kampō medicine and natural foods on premises. From 10:00 to 7:00, closed Sundays and holidays. Reservation needed.

Shizenishobiyou Clinic
Sandai Bldg.
Misakamachi
Chiyoda-ku, Tokyo 101
Tel: 03-3230-4147
- Beauty consultations and treatment. Natural foods nutrition counseling, herbal treatments.

Shu Uemura Esthetic Salon
312 Bldg. 2F
3-12-12 Minami Aoyama
Minato-ku, Tokyo
Tel: 03-3401-4568
- 11:00 to 8:00, closed Tuesdays. This salon offers beauty counseling, relaxation facilities, facials, sauna, a make-up service, infrared rooms. Reservation needed.

Toyo Igaku Kenkyujo
(Oriental Medical Research Center)
Kitazato Daigaku Byooin
5-9-1 Shirogane
Minato-ku, Tokyo
Tel: 03-3444-6161
- Acupuncture, some English spoken. For the initial visit, the hours are 8:00 to 10:00, Monday through Saturday.

Uchi-Ike Shinkyu Seikotsu-in
Palaceo Aoyama Bldg. B2
2-7-13 Kita Aoyama
Minato-ku, Tokyo
Tel: 03-5411-0115
- A doctor of traditional medicine, Uchi-ike-*sensei*, with his staff, offers health and beauty treatments based on high-tech acupuncture and other methods of combined East/West research. A *ki*-measuring machine was recently acquired to facilitate the diagnosis of body imbalances. Dancers frequently come here for treatment. 9:00 to 7:00, closed Sundays and national holidays.

japan hair-care resources

What is a good hair stylist? Someone who possesses technical mastery, of course, but more than that, he or she must have the ability to understand your hair—and what's going on inside your head as well. A culture gap can get in the way of a good haircut.

The best way to find out who the good stylists are—and for our purposes, those who are experts in handling a broad range of hair types and cultural expectations—is via the grapevine. The following list of stylists and salons has been compiled from the recommendations of *Japan Times* readers. The technical focus, finesse, and sensitivity of the best stylists will make you want to stay in Tokyo forever! (That and the glorious pressure-point massage you receive from the shampooist.)

Stylist: Kenji
André Bernard
Horaiya Bldg. 4F
5-2-1 Roppongi
Minato-ku, Tokyo
Tel: 03-3404-0616
- Cuts and color for men and women. English is spoken and a complete range of aesthetic services is available. The Yokohama André Bernard is recommended as well. There, a stylist named Gary is the person to see.

Stylist: Kaoru-san & Hiroyoshi-san
K's Hair Salon
Ito Biru 4F
6-4-14 Roppongi
Minato-ku, Tokyo
Tel: 03-3479-0089
- Kaoru-san is the resident colorist; she has long experience with foreigners' hair. Her husband Hiroyoshi-san is highly regarded for his cuts. Henna and perms are handled well here.

Stylist: Aki Kubo
Lady Madonna
6-17-10 Nishibori
Urawa-shi, Saitama
Tel: 048-861-8576
- A specialist in fine hair, this stylist speaks English and is sensitive to foreign hair needs. The salon is 30 minutes outside Tokyo on the Keihin Tohoku line, and is open from 9:00–7:00 except Tuesdays.

Stylist: Kenji
MMK Hair International Salon
Roppongi TK Bldg. 4F
5-2-6 Roppongi (just behind McDonald's)
Minato-ku, Tokyo

Tel: 03-3423-1661
- Specialties: difficult, fine hair; cuts to give body; color; perms. Handles clients of all ages and hair types, both men and women. Described as brilliantly talented and kind, Kenji speaks English and is sensitive to his clients' needs.

Stylist: Isamu Ikeda
Nyozegamon
Shojibiru 4F
Meguro 1-6-16 (near Meguro Station)
Meguro-ku, Tokyo
Tel: 03-3493-8844
- The stylist Isamu Ikeda trained in London, speaks English, and is said to do both cuts and coloring of foreigners' hair very well. He is described as a true artist by his faithful clientele.

Panorama (any stylist)
6-5-2 Jingumae
Minami Aoyama
Shibuya-ku, Tokyo
Tel: 03-3400-3501
- Color and cuts for men and women, Japanese and non-Japanese. Highlighting is a specialty. English is spoken.

Salon de Junko (any stylist)
7-9-7 Roppongi
Minato-ku, Tokyo
Tel: 03-3479-8780
- Henna work.

Stylist: Kiyoji Sudo
Salon de Sudo
8-11-26 Akasaka
Minato-ku, Tokyo 107
Tel: 03-3479-0040/0050

- My favorite Tokyo stylist. Sudo-*sensei* is very gifted and enjoys a devoted professional clientele of models and performers along with people like you and me. Recommended highly, but some knowledge of Japanese would be useful. Open 10:00–7:00, closed on Sundays.

Stylist: Toshiyuki Iwazawa
Salon Québecois
3-21-12 Takamatsu
Tachikawa, Tokyo
Tel: 0425-27-4716
- Excellent color, cuts, and perms. Some English is spoken.

Stylist: Mr. Sen
Three's Company
179-1 Motomachi 4-chome

Naka-ku, Yokohama
Tel: 045-664-4765
- I've heard extravagant raves about this salon's hair-straightening technique—a process known as "Mr. Habit"—which evidently can make even the kinkiest curls turn into swingy shining silk! The cost as of this writing: $350!

Y.S. Park International Salon (any stylist)
Omotesando Bldg. B1
4-29-3 Jingumae
Shibuya-ku, Tokyo
Tel: 03-3746-2244
- Cuts and color for an international clientele.

learning resources

All Japan Judo Federation
Kodokan
1-16-30 Kasuga
Bunkyo-ku, Tokyo
Tel: 03-3811-7151
- Judo lessons.

Amateur Archery Federation of Japan
Kishi Memorial Hall 4F
1-1-1 Jinnan
Shibuya-ku, Tokyo
Tel: 03-3467-7949
- *Kyudō*, the Zen art of archery, is taught.

Hotaka Yojoen
7258-20 Ariake
Hotaka-cho
Minami Azumi-gun, Nagano-ken
Tel: 0263-83-5260
- This healing retreat offers stress-reducing programs, macrobiotic food, acupuncture, a natural hot springs, and workshops.

Iijuma Takuma
4-5-7 Roppongi
Minato-ku, Tokyo
Tel: 03-3401-7983
- Calligraphy lessons.

Ikebana International
Shufunotomo Bldg. 2F
1-6 Surugadai, Kanda

Chiyoda-ku, Tokyo
Tel: 03-3293-8188
- Ikebana (flower arrangement) lessons.

Ikenobo
2-3 Surugadai, Kanda
Chiyoda-ku, Tokyo
Tel: 03-3292-3071
- Ikebana lessons.

International Aikido Federation
102 Wakamatsucho
Shinjuku-ku, Tokyo
Tel: 03-3203-9236
- Lessons in aikido: "the way of the harmonious spirit".

Japan Kendo Federation
Nippon Budokan
2-3 Kitanomaru-koen
Chiyoda-ku, Tokyo
Tel: 03-3211-5804/5805
- *Kendō*—"the way of the sword"—is practiced with bamboo staves instead of samurai blades.

Ohara
Ohara Kaikan 2F
5-7-17 Minami Aoyama
Minato-ku, Tokyo
Tel: 03-3499-1200
- Ikebana lessons.

Sakura-kai
(Tea Ceremony Service Center)
3-2-25 Shimo-Ochiai
Shinjuku-ku, Tokyo
Tel: 03-3951-9043
• Ikebana and tea ceremony lessons.

Sho International
ICS Center Landic
Hirakawacho Bldg. 2F
2-6-2 Hirakawa-cho
Chiyoda-ku, Tokyo
Tel: 03-3234-8757; 03-3582-5679
• Calligraphy lessons.

Shu Uemura Facing Studio
5-7-17 Minami Aoyama
Minato-ku, Tokyo
Tel: 03-3407-4823
• Lessons in make-up and skin care, Japanese language only.

Sogetsu
Sogetsu Kaikan Bldg. 4F
7-2-21 Akasaka

Minato-ku, Tokyo
Tel: 03-3408-1126
• Ikebana classes in English

Terakoya Cultural House
2-34-3 Mejiro
Toshima-ku, Tokyo
Tel: 03-3989-9851
• Classes in tea, ikebana, calligraphy, *sumi-e* ink painting, Japanese cooking, and *shiatsu*.

Tochoji Zen Temple
4-34 Yotsuya
Sinjuku-ku, Tokyo 160
• Zazen meditation sessions open to the public one evening per week.

World Union of Karate-Do Organization
Sempaku Shinkokai Bldg. 4F
1-15-16 Toranomon
Minato-ku, Tokyo
Tel: 03-3503-6637
• Karate lessons.

tokyo restaurants of interest

A: High-priced
B: Medium-priced
C: Reasonable

Amanoya
2-18-15 Soto-Kanda
Chiyoda-ku, Tokyo
Tel: 03-3251-7911
• A famous old sweet-*sake* (*amazake*) drinking establishment established in 1579, open 9:00–6:00, closed on Sundays.

Bodaiju
4-3-14 Shiba
Minato-ku, Tokyo
Tel: 03-3456-3257
• Vegetarian Chinese. A·B. Open 11:30–2:30, 5:30–9:00.

Bon
1-2-11 Ryusen
Taito-ku, Tokyo

Tel: 03-3872-0375
• Zen Buddhist *shōjin ryōri*, traditional vegetarian temple cooking. Meals served at 12:00, 3:00, and 6:00. Closed on Tuesdays. A.

Buon Pesce
7-4-8 Roppongi
Minato-ku, Tokyo
Tel: 03-3403-9119
• A Shu Uemura establishment serving elegant seafoods said to be nourishing to beauty as well as health. Open 6:00 to midnight, closed Sundays and Flag Day. Reservations needed. A.

Goemon
1-1-26 Komagome
Bunkyo-ku, Tokyo
Tel: 03-3811-2015
• A menu based on a wide variety of tofu dishes. This restaurant with its traditional Japanese garden is open from 5:00 to 10:00 every day but Monday. B.

Gu
2-26-8 Kitazawa
Setagaya-ku, Tokyo
Tel: 03-3485-2187
• Natural foods restaurant. C.

Healthy-kan
4 Rokuban-cho
Chiyoda-ku, Tokyo
Tel: 03-3263-4023
• Health foods, herbal teas. C.

Mana
Kikusui Bldg. B1
1-16-5 Nishi-Shinjuku
Shinjuku-ku, Tokyo
Tel: 03-344-6606
• Natural Japanese and Western foods. B.

Mominoki House
2-18-5 Jingumae
Shibuya-ku, Tokyo
Tel: 03-3405-9144
• Health food in a hip ambiance, from 11:00 to 11:00 every day but Sunday. B.

Monk's Food
1-2-4 Gotenyama
Musashino-shi, Tokyo
Tel: 0422-48-3977
• Vegetarian/ macrobiotic food served with jazz. C.

Nataraj
3-19-1 Nishi Waseda
Shinjuku-ku, Tokyo
Tel: 03-3202-6987
• Vegetarian Indian cooking. C.

Natural House
6-14-15 Akasaka
Minato-ku, Tokyo
Tel: 03-3589-1077
• Natural foods. C.

Sankoin Temple
3-1-36 Honcho
Koganei-shi, Tokyo
Tel: 0423-81-1116
• Reservations a month in advance are advised for a meal at this convent restaurant for *shōjin ryōri*. 12:00 to 2:00 and 2:00 to 4:00, closed Thursdays, the month of August, and from Christmas Day to January 10th. Near Musashi Koganei station on the Chuo line. B.

Shizenkan
3-6 Maruyama-cho
Shibuya-ku, Tokyo
Tel: 03-3476-0591
• This small natural foods market has a wholefoods restaurant in the back, serving tasty vegetarian meals from 11:30 to 7:30. C.

Takaosan Yakuoin Temple
2177 Takaocho
Hachioji-shi
Tel: 0426-61-1115
• *Shōjin ryōri* lunches, reservations needed. From Takaosan station on the Keio line, take the cable car to Sanjo station and walk from there. B.

Tofu-ya
3-5-2 Akasaka
(Sanyo Akasaka Bldg. 1F)
Minato-ku, Tokyo
Tel: 03-3582-1028
• An enormous variety of tofu dishes. Open 11:30 to 1:30 and 5:00 to 11:00 Monday through Friday. B.

Tojinbo
New Shimbashi Bldg. B1
2-16-2 Shimbashi
Minato-ku, Tokyo
Tel: 03-3580-7307
• Health foods, traditional natural foods, *shōjin ryōri*, very fresh fish. Open 5:00 to 11:00, closed the 1st and 3rd Saturdays of each month, Sundays and holidays. C.

Tsubakiya
1-33-4 Senju
Adachi-ku, Tokyo
Tel: 03-3870-8761
• Good Japanese health food, weekday lunches only. C.

books of interest

the bath

Furo: The Japanese Bath
by Peter Grilli and Dana Levy, Kodansha International, Tokyo

The Book of the Bath
by C. Kanner, Fawcett, New York

beauty

Handbook of Natural Beauty
by Virginia Castleton Thomas, Rodale Press, Emmaus, Penn.

The Japanese Way of Beauty (hardback)
Inner Peace, Outer Beauty (paperback)
by Michelle Dominique Leigh, Birch Lane Press (Carol Publications), New York

The Joy of Beauty
by Leslie Kenton, Arrow, London

Vogue Complete Beauty
by Deborah Hutton, Harmony Books (Crown), New York

food

Chinese System of Food Cures
by Henry C. Lu, Pelanduk Publications (also by Sterling Publishing), Petaling Jaya, Malaysia

Diet for Natural Beauty
by Aveline Kushi with Wendy Esko and Maya Tiwari, Japan Publications, Tokyo

The Food Pharmacy
by Jean Carper, Bantam, New York

The Healing Foods
by Patricia Hausman and Judith Benn Hurley, Dell/Bantam (Doubleday), New York

The Heart of Zen Cuisine: A 600-year Tradition of Vegetarian Cooking
by Soei Yoneda, Kodansha International, Tokyo

Japanese Cooking: A Simple Art
by Shizuo Tsuji, Kodansha International, Tokyo

the garden

Oriental Vegetables: The Complete Guide for Garden and Kitchen
by Joy Larkcom, Kodansha International, Tokyo

Secret Teachings in the Art of Japanese Gardens: Design Principles Aesthetic Values
by David Slawson, Kodansha International, Tokyo

health and medicine

Chinese Folk Medicine
by Heinrich Wallnofer and Anna von Rottauscher, Signet Books, New York

Chinese Herbal Medicine
by Daniel P. Reid, Shambhala, Boston

Chinese Herbs: Their Botany, Chemistry, and Pharmacodynamics
by John D. Keys, Tuttle, Rutland, Vermont

Efective Tsubo Therapy
by Katsusuke Serizawa, Japan Publications, Tokyo

Massage: The Oriental Methods
by Katsusuke Serizawa, Japan Publications, Tokyo

Natural Healing for Women
by Susan Curtis and Romy Fraser, Pandora Press (HarperCollins), London

The Complete Book of Shiatsu Therapy
by Toru Namikoshi, Japan Publications, Tokyo

The Complete System of Chinese Self-Healing
by Dr. Stephen T. Chang, Aquarian/Thorsons (HarperCollins), London

The Shiatsu Way to Health
by Toru Namikoshi, Kodansha International, Tokyo

Tsubo: Vital Points for Oriental Therapy
by Katsusuke Serizawa, Japan Publications, Tokyo

Shiatzu: Japanese Finger Pressure for Energy, Sexual Vitality, and Relief from Tension and Pain
by Yukiko Irwin with James Wagenvoord, Arkana, London

herbs and botanicals

The Book of Tea & Herbs
by The Republic of Tea, The Cole Group, Santa Rosa, Cal.

The Illustrated Herbal
by Wilfred Blunt and Sandra Raphael, Thames & Hudson, London

The Illustrated Herb Encyclopedia
by Kathi Keville, Grange Books, London

japan

A Guide to Japanese Hot Springs
by Anne Hotta with Yoko Ishiguro, Kodansha International, Tokyo

Gateway to Japan, Revised and Updated
by June Kinoshita and Nicholas Palevsky, Kodansha International, Tokyo

Old Kyoto: A Guide to Traditional Shops, Restaurants, and Inns
by Diane Durston, Kodansha International, Tokyo

scent

Aromatherapy: The Art of Aromatherapy
by R.B. Tisserand, State Mutual, New York

The Book of Incense: Enjoying the Traditional Art of Japanese Scents
by Kiyoko Morita, Kodansha International, Tokyo

The Complete Book of Essential Oils & Aromatherapy
by Valerie Ann Worwood, New World Library, San Rafael, Cal.

the spirit

A Gathering of Spirit: Women Teaching in American Buddhism
edited by Ellen Sidor, Primary Point Press, Rhode Island

Even in Summer the Ice Doesn't Melt
by David K. Reynolds, Ph.D., William Morrow, New York

365 Tao: Daily Meditations
by Deng Ming-Dao, HarperCollins, San Francisco

Weavers of Wisdom: Women Mystics of the Twentieth Century
by Anne Bancroft, Arkana, London

Woman Awake: A Celebration of Women's Wisdom
by Christina Feldman, Arkana, London

Zen Seeds: Reflections of a Female Priest
by Shundo Aoyama, translated by Patricia Daien Bennage, Kosei, Tokyo

discipline and practice

Chado: The Japanese Way of Tea
by Soshitsu Sen, Weatherhill, Tokyo

Judo: The Gentle Way
by Alan Fromm and Nicholas Soames, Arkana, London

T'ai Chi Chuan and Meditation
by Da Liu, Arkana, London

The Book of Tea
by Kakuzo Okakura, Kodansha International, Tokyo

The Essence of Aikido: Spiritual Teachings of Morihei Ueshiba
translated by John Stephens, Kodansha International, Tokyo

The Spirit of Aikido
by Kisshomaru Ueshiba, Kodansha International, Tokyo

The Unfettered Mind: Writings of the Zen Master to the Sword Master
by Takuan Soho, Kodansha International, Tokyo

Zen and the Art of Calligraphy
by Omori Sogen and Terayama Katsujo, Arkana, London

retreats and sanctuaries

Fodor's Healthy Escapes
by Bernard Burt, Fodor's Travel Publications, New York

Sanctuaries: The Northeast
by Jack and Marcia Kelly, Bell Tower, New York

Sanctuaries: The West Coast and Southwest
by Marcia and Jack Kelly, Bell Tower, New York

Traveler's Guide to Healing Centers and Retreats in North America
by Martine Rudee and Jonathan Blease, John Muir Publications, Santa Fe, New Mexico

Bibliography

Belleme, Jan and John. *Cooking with Japanese Foods: A Guide to the Traditional Natural Foods of Japan.* Brookline, Mass.: East-West Health Books, 1986.

Blunt, Wilfrid and Raphael, Sandra. *The Illustrated Herbal.* London: Thames & Hudson, 1979.

Brelet-Rueff, Claudine. *Les Médecines Sacrées.* Paris: Albin Michel, 1991.

Bremness, Lesley. *Pocket Encyclopedia of Herbs.* London: Dorling Kindersley, 1990.

Carper, Jean. *The Food Pharmacy.* New York: Bantam, 1988.

Chang, Dr. Stephen T. *The Complete System of Chinese Self-Healing.* London: Aquarian/Thorsons; HarperCollins, 1989.

Chikamatsu, Monzaemon. *Koushoku Ichidai Onna.* Excerpted in *Keshoshi Bunken Shiryo Nenpyo.* Tokyo: Pola Bunka Kenkyujo, 1979.

Chikashige, Masumi. *Oriental Alchemy.* New York: Samuel Weiser, 1974.

Chotto Obaachan Oshiete. Ed. Mainichi Shimbun, Shakai-bu. Tokyo: Bunka Shuppan-kyoku, 1986.

Curtis, Susan and Fraser, Romy. *Natural Healing for Women.* London: Pandora Press; HarperCollins, 1991.

Dalby, Liza. *Geisha.* New York: Vintage Books, 1985.

Dyer, Sarah. *A Pocket Book on Herbs.* London: Octopus Books, 1982.

Ehon Edomurasaki. Excerpted in *Keshoshi Bunken Shiryo Nenpyo.* Tokyo: Pola Bunka Kenkyujo, 1979.

Ekiguchi, Kunio and McCreery, Ruth. *A Japanese Touch for the Seasons.* Tokyo: Kodansha International, 1989.

Fujiwara, Tokihira, Tadahira, et al. *Engishiki.* Excerpted in *Keshoshi Bunken Shiryo Nenpyo.* Tokyo: Pola Bunka Kenkyujo, 1979.

Haikara-Modan Keshoshi. Edited by Pola Bunka Kenkyujo. Tokyo: Pola Bunka Kenkyujo, 1986.

Hakim, Rashan Abdul. *Basic Herbs for Health and Healing.* New York: Sundial Product, 1989.

Harris, Ben Charles. *The Compleat Herbal.* New York: Larchmont Books, 1972.

Hausman, Patricia and Hurley, Judith Benn. *The Healing Foods.* New York: Dell/Bantam Doubleday, 1989.

Hiroidama Shin Chienoumi. Excerpted in *Keshoshi Bunken Shiryo Nenpyo.* Tokyo: Pola Bunka Kenkyujo, 1979.

Hotta, Anne and Ishiguro, Yoko. *A Guide to Japanese Hot Springs.* Tokyo: Kodansha International, 1986.

Hutton, Deborah. *Vogue Complete Beauty.* New York: Harmony Books; Crown, 1982.

Irwin, Yukiko and Wagenvoord, James. *Shiatzu.* London: Penguin Arkana, 1988.

Jingfeng, Cai. *La Diétothérapie Chinoise.* Beijing: Éditions en Langues Étrangères, 1989.

Kaptchuk, Ted and Croucher, Michael. *The Healing Arts.* New York: Summit Books, 1987.

Kenko. *Essays in Idleness: The Tsurezuregusa of Kenko.* Tokyo: Charles E. Tuttle, 1989.

Kenton, Leslie. *The Joy of Beauty.* London: Arrow Books, 1989.

Keville, Kathi. *The Illustrated Herb Encyclopedia.* London: Grange Books, Books & Toys Ltd., 1991.

Keys, John D. *Chinese Herbs.* Tokyo: Charles E. Tuttle, 1990.

Ko to Kodo. Edited by Kodo Bunka Kenkyukai. Tokyo: Yuzankaku Shuppan, 1989.

Kushi, Aveline with Esko, Wendy and Tiwari, Maya. *Diet for Natural Beauty*. Tokyo: Japan Publications, 1991.

Kushi, Michio. *Macrobiotic Home Remedies*. Tokyo: Japan Publications, 1985.

Loren, Sophia. *Women & Beauty*. London: Century Arrow; Arrow Books, 1986.

Lu, Henry C. *Chinese System of Food Cures*. Petaling Jaya, Malaysia: Pelanduk Publications, 1993.

Mizushima, Uraya. *Kewai Mayutsukuri Kuden*. Excerpted in *Keshoshi Bunken Shiryo Nenpyo*. Tokyo: Pola Bunka Kenkyujo, 1979.

Morishita, Keichi. *Yakukoshoku*. Tokyo: Hakujusha, 1986.

Mowrey, Daniel B., Ph.D. *The Scientific Validation of Herbal Medicine*. New Canaan, Conn.: Cormorant Books; Keats Publishing, 1986.

Murasawa, Hiroto and Tsuda, Norio, editors. *Keshoshi Bunken Shiryo Nenpyo*. Tokyo: Pola Bunka Kenkyujo, 1989.

Murata, Takako; Tsuda, Norio; Yamamura, Hiromi; and Tamaru, Eri, editors. Nihon no Kesho. Tokyo: Pola Bunka Kenkyujo, 1989.

Namikoshi, Toru. *The Complete Book of Shiatsu Therapy*. Tokyo: Japan Publications, 1981.

Ody, Penelope. *Les Plantes Médicinales: Encyclopédie Pratique*. Paris: Dorling Kindersley, 1993.

Okakura, Kakuzo. *The Book of Tea*. Tokyo: Charles E. Tuttle, 1960.

Polunin, Miriam and Robbins, Christopher. *La Pharmacie Naturelle*. Paris: Minerva, 1993.

Price, Shirley. *Practical Aromatherapy*. London: Thorsons, 1983.

Reid, Daniel P. *Chinese Herbal Medicine*. Boston: Shambhala, 1987.

Reynolds, David K. *Even in Summer the Ice Doesn't Melt*. New York: Quill, 1986.

Riva, Anna. *Golden Secrets of Mystic Oils*. Toluca Lake, California: International Imports, 1978.

Rose, Donna. *The Magic of Oils*. Hialeah, Florida: Mi-World Publishing Co., 1978.

Rose, Jeanne. *Jeanne Rose's Herbal Body Book*. New York: Perigree, 1982.

Secrets et Vertus des Plantes Médicinales. Edited by Reader's Digest. Paris: Sélection du Reader's Digest, 1985.

Serizawa, Katsusuke, M.D. *Effective Tsubo Therapy*. Tokyo: Japan Publications, 1984.

Serizawa, Katsusuke, M.D. *Massage: The Oriental Methods*. Tokyo: Japan Publications, 1972.

Serizawa, Katsusuke. *Tsubo: Vital Points for Oriental Therapy*. Tokyo: Japan Publications, 1976.

Takahashi, Yumiko. *Shimi, Shiwa o Totte, Kireini Wakagaeru*. Tokyo: Shufunotomo-sha, 1984.

Tanizaki, Junichiro. *In Praise of Shadows*. Translated by Thomas J. Harper and Edward G. Seidensticker. Tokyo: Charles E. Tuttle, 1990.

Thomas, Virginia Castleton. *Secrets of Natural Beauty*. London: Harrap, 1973.

Tsuda, Norio and Murata, Takako. *Mayu no Bunkashi* (*Mayu Kesho Kenkyu Hokokusho*). Tokyo: Pola Bunka Kenkyujo, 1984.

Tsuda, Norio and Murata, Takako. *Modan Keshoshi*. Tokyo: Pola Bunka Kenkyujo, 1986.

Tsuji, Shizuo. *Japanese Cooking: A Simple Art*. Tokyo: Kodansha International, 1984.

Tsutsui, Shoshi. *Mukashi kara Tsutae rarete iru: Shizen Butsu de Bihada Zukuri o*. Ushiyama: Biyo Bunka-sha.

Vogel, Dr. H.C.A. *The Nature Doctor*. Edinburgh: Mainstream Publishing, 1990.

Watashi no Kenko. (Issues published between 1985–1990.) Tokyo: Shufunotomo-sha.

Wyman, Donald. *Wyman's Gardening Encyclopedia*. New York: Macmillan, 1986.

Yamada, Ei. *Shizenkeshohin no Himitsu*. Tokyo: Nagoka Shoten, 1984.

Yamada, Kyoko. *Biyo to Shokuji no Daikenkyu*. Tokyo: Sanpo-sha, 1981.

Yu Koro: *Nihongami wa Kataru*. Tokyo: Pola Bunka Kenkyujo, 1985.

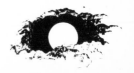

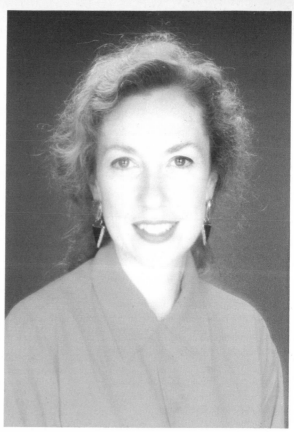

Author bio:

Michelle Leigh is a writer, poet, and illustrator, with an extensive anthropology background. She divides her time between northern Japan and a 270-year-old farm in Connecticut, and is at work on a line of beauty products of East-West inspiration.

notes

notes

notes

notes

notes

notes